# Diabetes Mellitus and Oral Health

T0176803

# Diabetes Mellitus and Oral Health

## An Interprofessional Approach

Edited by

Ira B. Lamster

WILEY Blackwell

*Library of Congress Cataloging-in-Publication Data*

Diabetes mellitus and oral health: an interprofessional approach / edited by Ira B. Lamster.
    p. ; cm.
  Includes bibliographical references and index.
  ISBN 978-1-118-37780-2 (pbk.)
  I. Lamster, Ira B., editor of compilation.
[DNLM: 1. Diabetes Complications–Case Reports.   2. Periodontal Diseases–etiology–Case Reports.
3. Diabetes Mellitus–Case Reports.   4. Periodontal Diseases–prevention & control–Case Reports.
WU 240]
  RK450.P4
  617.6′32–dc23

                            2013050122

A catalogue record for this book is available from the British Library.

*To my wife Gail, and our children and grandchildren, for the love and balance they provide.*

# Contents

# Contributors

**Nurit Bittner, DDS, MS**
Director of Postgraduate Prosthodontics
Assistant Professor of Clinical Dental
Medicine
Division of Prosthodontics
Section of Adult Dentistry
College of Dental Medicine
Columbia University
New York, New York

**Jeffrey M. Curtis, MD, MPH**
Medical Director, Diabetes Epidemiology
and Clinical Research Section
National Institute of Diabetes and
Digestive and Kidney Diseases
Phoenix, Arizona

**Dana T. Graves, DDS, DMSc**
Vice Dean for Scholarship and Research
Professor of Periodontics
School of Dental Medicine
University of Pennsylvania
Philadelphia, Pennsylvania

**Lewis W. Johnson, MD**
Professor of Medicine
Division of Endocrinology, Diabetes,
and Metabolism
SUNY Upstate Medical University
Syracuse, New York

**Harpreet Kaur, MD**
Staff Physician, Endocrinology, Diabetes,
and Metabolism
Mercy Diabetes Center
Mercy Medical Center-North Iowa
Mason City, Iowa

**William C. Knowler, MD, DrPH**
Chief, Diabetes Epidemiology and
Clinical Research Section
National Institute of Diabetes and
Digestive and Kidney Diseases
Phoenix, Arizona

**Evanthia Lalla, DDS, MS**
Professor of Dental Medicine
Division of Periodontics
Section of Oral and Diagnostic Sciences
College of Dental Medicine
Columbia University
New York, New York

**Ira B. Lamster, DDS, MMSc**
Dean Emeritus
College of Dental Medicine
Professor, Department of Health Policy
and Management
Mailman School of Public Health
Columbia University
New York, New York

**Daniel Lorber, MD**
Clinical Associate Professor
Weill Medical College
Cornell University
Director, Endocrinology
New York Hospital Queens
Flushing, New York

**Brian L. Mealey, DDS, MS**
Professor and Graduate Program Director
Department of Periodontics
University of Texas Health Science Center
San Antonio, Texas

**Ravichandran Ramasamy, PhD**
Associate Professor of Medicine
Diabetes Research Program
Division of Endocrinology
Department of Medicine
New York University School of Medicine
New York, New York

**Ann Marie Schmidt, MD**
The Iven Young Professor of
Endocrinology
Professor of Medicine, Pharmacology
and Pathology
Director, Diabetes Research Program
NYU School of Medicine
New York, New York

**George W. Taylor, DMD, DrPH**
Leland A. and Gladys K. Barber
Distinguished Professor in Dentistry
Chair, Department of Preventive and
Restorative Dental Sciences
School of Dentistry
University of California San Francisco
San Francisco, California

**Ruth S. Weinstock, MD, PhD**
SUNY Distinguished Service Professor
Chief, Division of Endocrinology,
Diabetes, and Metabolism
Medical Director, Clinical Research Unit
and Joslin Diabetes Center
Department of Medicine
SUNY Upstate Medical University
Syracuse, New York

**Dana Wolf, DMD, MS**
Associate Professor of Clinical Dental
Medicine
Division of Periodontics
Section of Oral and Diagnostic Sciences
College of Dental Medicine
Columbia University
New York, New York

# Acknowledgments

This book is the culmination of more than 20 years of work at the intersection of diabetes mellitus and oral health. There were many collaborators during that time, but Evanthia Lalla and Ann Marie Schmidt have been there throughout. Their insight and efforts were invaluable, and we continue to work together, as both are authors of chapters in this book.

My research focusing on the relationship of diabetes and oral disease has received generous funding from a number of sources. Thanks are due to Colgate Palmolive, Johnson & Johnson, as well as the National Institute of Dental and Craniofacial Research, the New York State Health Foundation, and the Juvenile Diabetes Research Foundation, and Enhanced Education.

Shelby Allen and Nancy Turner at Wiley Blackwell were very helpful and supportive during the preparation of this book, and early in the process they saw the importance of this project. My assistant Cynthia Rubiera helped make the task of translating thoughts to printed word far easier than it might have been. The Columbia University College of Dental Medicine (CDM) provided an environment that fostered interprofessional education and practice. The CDM culture emphasizes collaboration and a place for dental medicine in the larger health care environment. The faculty and students at CDM have always been a source of inspiration as we seek to define the future of the dental profession.

# Introduction

Diabetes mellitus is a group of endocrine disorders characterized by elevated levels of glucose in blood. The underlying cause is either an absence of insulin production, a lack of responsiveness to the actions of insulin, or some combination of both. The direct and indirect consequences of diabetes are enormous, resulting in significant morbidity and mortality. Diabetes is a chronic disease, and patients are required to manage their disease for decades. This reality can have a major impact on a person's lifestyle, and achieving the normal range of blood sugar in blood requires daily vigilance.

The financial cost of caring for patients with diabetes mellitus in the United States is estimated to be nearly a quarter of a trillion dollars per year [1]. Furthermore, the personal toll on patients and their families is enormous. Complications of the disease include vision problems leading to blindness, end-stage renal disease requiring kidney transplantation, increased incidence of myocardial infarction and strokes, and poor wound healing resulting in amputation.

Diabetes mellitus is of particular importance for dental professionals:

- The prevalence of diabetes is increasing. Based on data from 2011 [2], 25.8 million people in the United States have diabetes, representing 8.3% of the population. Furthermore, now there is interest in prediabetes, a condition in which the blood glucose level is above normal but not elevated enough to be classified as diabetes. Individuals with prediabetes are at risk for development of type 2 diabetes mellitus and its complications. It is estimated that more than 80 million adults in the United States have prediabetes [2]. Consequently, patients with dysglycemia are now, and will in the future, routinely be seen in dental offices.
- Older individuals in the United States and other developed countries are retaining their teeth, and in the future will require more dental services.
- There are a number of important oral manifestations of diabetes mellitus, including greater severity of periodontal disease, increased root caries, xerostomia, candidiasis, burning mouth syndrome, and benign parotid hypertrophy. Diabetes mellitus is the only systemic disease that is a recognized risk factor for periodontitis [3]. Because more than 25% of people with diabetes are unaware that they are affected [2], a person with undiagnosed diabetes may present to the dental office with an oral manifestation of the disease. Furthermore, because oral manifestations of diabetes are more common with poor metabolic control, an oral manifestation of diabetes may be an indication of a patient who requires medical attention to better manage his or her disease.

- There is mounting evidence that advanced periodontitis can adversely affect metabolic control in patients with diabetes [3]. Periodontal therapy provided to patients with periodontitis and diabetes has resulted in a significant decrease in the level of glycated hemoglobin.

As dental professionals consider the future of dental practice, and with the realization that an increasing number of patients with chronic diseases requiring multiple medications will be seen for dental care, an understanding of the etiology, prevalence, management, and clinical complications, including the oral complications of diabetes, is essential. This book will address this need, and is divided into three sections. There are four chapters in the medical considerations section, including (1) etiology, (2) epidemiology, classification, risk factors, and diagnosis, (3) medical complications, and (4) treatment. There are five chapters in the dental considerations section, including (5) management of the patients with diabetes in the dental office, (6) periodontal complications of diabetes, (7) the influence of periodontal disease on metabolic control, (8) non-periodontal oral complications of diabetes, and (9) assessment of diabetes mellitus in the dental office. The final section presents six case scenarios which describe patients with diabetes who are seen in the dental office, and illustrates how management of each requires dental professionals to have a thorough understanding of diabetes mellitus and work closely with other health care providers to deliver the most appropriate care. Furthermore, medical professionals must understand the importance of the oral cavity in the context of diabetes, identify oral problems when present, and refer patients for routine care.

Finally, this book is also notable because it makes a strong case for complete dental care being dependent upon an understanding of the entire patient. Dental care for medically complex patients demands that health care providers cooperate, and diabetes provides an excellent example of the importance of interprofessional practice. The result will be improved oral health, and health, outcomes. The results will benefit both patients and providers.

## References

1. American Diabetes Association. Economic costs of diabetes in the U.S. in 2012. *Diabetes Care.* 2012; 36:1033–46.
2. Centers for Disease Control and Prevention. National diabetes fact sheet: national estimate and general information on diabetes and prediabetes in the United States, 2011. Atlanta, GA: U.S. Department of Health and Human Services, Centers for Disease Control and Prevention, 2011.
3. Lalla E, Papapanou P. Diabetes mellitus and periodontitis: a tale of two common interrelated diseases. *Nat Rev Endocrinol.* 2011; 7(12):738–48.

# Section 1

# Medical considerations

# Chapter 1

# Etiology of diabetes mellitus

*Ravichandran Ramasamy, PhD*
*and Ann Marie Schmidt, MD*

## Introduction

The defining characteristics of diabetes, irrespective of the precise etiology, relate to the presence of hyperglycemia. The American Diabetes Association (ADA) has set forth specific criteria for the definition of diabetes. In the ADA guidelines, the following are necessary for the diagnosis of diabetes: (1) hemoglobin A1c (HbA1c) equal to or greater than 6.5% OR (2) fasting plasma glucose equal to or greater than 126 mg/dl OR (3) two-hour plasma glucose equal to or greater than 200 mg/dl during an oral glucose tolerance test (OGTT) (glucose load containing 75 grams anhydrous glucose dissolved in water) OR (4) in a patient with classic symptoms of diabetes or during a hyperglycemic crisis, a random glucose of equal to or greater than 200 mg/dl suffices to diagnose diabetes [1].

In this chapter, we will review the major types of diabetes and the etiologic factors that are known to or are speculated to contribute to these disorders. Furthermore, we will take the opportunity to present an overview of emerging theories underlying the pathogenesis of type 1 and type 2 diabetes. Types 1 and 2 diabetes constitute the vast majority of diabetes cases. Interestingly, both of these types of diabetes are on the rise worldwide [2, 3]. In addition to types 1 and 2 diabetes, we will also discuss gestational diabetes. Often a harbinger to the ultimate development of frank type 2 diabetes in the mother, this form of diabetes is potentially dangerous to both the mother and the developing fetus. Finally, we will discuss the syndromes known as MODY or maturity onset diabetes of the young. The disorders underlying MODY have very strong genetic components and are due to mutations in multiple distinct genes.

The greatest long-term danger of diabetes, irrespective of the etiology, lies in the potential for complications. The complications of the disease are insidious, deadly, and difficult to treat or reverse; hence, there is great urgency to identify specific means to prevent or mitigate these most common types of diabetes.

*Diabetes Mellitus and Oral Health: An Interprofessional Approach*, First Edition. Edited by Ira B. Lamster.
© 2014 John Wiley & Sons, Inc. Published 2014 by John Wiley & Sons, Inc.

# Type 1 diabetes

Type 1 diabetes accounts for approximately 5–10% of all cases of diabetes [1]. The countries with the highest incidence of type 1 diabetes include Finland and Sardinia [4]. Type 1 diabetes is usually diagnosed in childhood, hence the original classification "juvenile onset diabetes." Indeed, type 1 diabetes accounts for more than 90% of diabetes diagnosed in children and adolescents. Given that the disease is often diagnosed in adults, however, even into advanced age, the term "type 1 diabetes" has been adopted to more accurately reflect the diversity of affected ages. In type 1 diabetes, the primary etiology is due to a cellular-mediated autoimmune-mediated destruction of the β cells of the pancreas. Traditionally, in subjects with type 1 diabetes, autoantibodies may be detected that reflect the underlying attack against these cells [5]. These include autoantibodies to insulin, to GAD65, and to IA-2 and IA-2β (the latter two are tyrosine phosphatases). These antibodies are often detected up to years before the diagnosis of type 1 diabetes [6]. In most subjects with type 1 diabetes, one or more of these antibodies is evident. Indeed, in vulnerable subjects, such as first-degree relatives of affected individuals, the presence of these autoantibodies is often, but not always, a harbinger of the eventual diagnosis of diabetes. Hence, these antibody profiles may be used to predict the risk of diabetes in the siblings and relatives of affected subjects with type 1 diabetes [6].

## *Genetics of type 1 diabetes*

More than forty years ago, type 1 diabetes was found to have very strong links to the human leukocyte antigen (HLA)-encoding genes [7]. The largest study to address this issue was known as the Type 1 Diabetes Genetics Consortium (T1DGC). This group was composed of an international collaboration and amassed more than 14,000 samples [8]. By far, the greatest association to type 1 diabetes was found in the HLA, particularly in the HLA DR-DQ haplotypes. Furthermore, other genes found to have strong genetic association were in polymorphisms identified in the insulin gene [9]. The researchers of T1DGC earlier reported that beyond these two associations, two other loci were found to have odds ratios (ORs) greater than 1.5, and included *PTPN22* and *IL2RA* [9]. However, the ORs for these genes were relatively much lower than that of the HLA region, consistent therefore with the overall strong role of the HLA in the susceptibility to type 1 diabetes.

A number of groups have published the results of genome wide association studies (GWAS) in type 1 diabetes and identified more than 40 potential susceptibility loci in the disease [11]. Candidate genes identified in this approach included those encoding *IL10, IL19, IL20, GLIS3, CD69,* and *IL27*; these are all genes strongly linked to the immune/inflammatory response [10]. In their report, Bergholdt and colleagues integrated the data from these GWAS studies and translated them to a more functional level, that is protein-protein interactions and, finally, they tested their relevance in human islets and in a β cell line, INS-1 cells (rat insulimona-derived cells) [11]. First, they performed a meta-analysis of the type 1 diabetes genome wide Association studies that were available. From these, they identified 44 type 1 diabetes non-major histocompatibility complex (MHC) low density (LD) regions with significance; these regions contained more than 395 candidate genes. They then performed network analysis studies with the intention to more deeply

Table 1.1   Examples of non-HLA type 1 diabetes-associated loci.

| Locus | Description | Comments |
| --- | --- | --- |
| PTPN22 | Protein tyrosine phosphatase, non-receptor type 22 | Modulation of T and B cell function |
| INS | Insulin | Deficient in type 1 diabetes |
| IL2RA | Interleukin-2 receptor, α | T lymphocyte function |
| IL10 | Interleukin-10 | Immunoregulation Inflammation |
| IL19 | Interleukin 19 | Immunity/inflammation |
| GLIS3 | Gli-similar 3 protein | Pancreatic β cell generation Insulin gene expression Modulation of pancreatic β cell apoptosis |
| TRAF3IP2 | TRAF3 interacting protein 2 | Implicated in IL17 signaling Interacts with members of Rel/NF-κB transcription factor family |
| PLCG2 | Phospholipase C, γ 2 | Leukocyte signal transduction NK cell cytotoxicity |
| CCR5 | CC-chemokine receptor 5 | Major co-receptor for HIV entry into cells Immune cell recruitment |
| MYO1B | Myosin 1B | Cell membrane trafficking and dynamics |

probe network connections and protein-protein interactions. From this work, 17 protein networks were identified (which contained 235 nodes) containing at least two genes from different type 1 diabetes LD regions [11].

To follow up on these findings, human islets were exposed to pro-inflammatory cytokines and comparisons were made between the treated and untreated human islets (retrieved from eight donors). From this, the following genes were found to be significantly impacted by the cytokine stimulation in the human islets: *IL17RD, CD83, IFNGR1, TRAF3IP2, IL27RA, PLCG2, MYO1B*, and *CXCR7*. Interestingly, the study design suggested that perhaps these traditionally inflammation-associated factors were being produced by pancreatic β cells and not necessarily solely by immune cells. To test this specific point, rat INS-1 cells were treated with cytokines and the above eight genes were examined. Indeed, all but *IL27ra* were identified in the stimulated INS-1 cells [11]. In the case of cultured INS-1 cells, no immune cells are present, therefore suggesting the interesting possibility that these factors may be produced both by islet β cells themselves as well, likely, by infiltrating inflammatory cells. Examples of non-HLA genes linked to type 1 diabetes are illustrated in Table 1.1.

### Pathogenesis of type 1 diabetes

There is strong evidence that links the pathogenesis of type 1 diabetes to immune-mediated mechanisms of β cell destruction, including the detection of insulitis, the presence of islet cell autoantibodies, activated β cell-specific T lymphocytes and, as considered above, association of the disease with a restricted set of class II major histocompatibility alleles [12]. Importantly, the rate of the development of type 1 diabetes after the appearance of autoantibodies may be quite variable, reflecting perhaps the contribution of protective mechanisms (such as CD4+−T regulatory cells and other regulatory cells such as invariant natural killer T [NKT] cells). Such protective factors may differ among individuals, thereby possibly accounting for the variable progression of damaging autoimmunity and the appearance of diabetes. The diagnosis of type 1 diabetes, often made by the appearance of diabetic ketoacidosis [13], is linked to the absence or near absence of plasma C-peptide (N-terminus fragment of insulin that is used to monitor the ability to produce insulin) [14]. It has been suggested that particularly in adults, residual β cell function may be retained for years after the appearance of autoantibodies without manifestation of ketoacidosis. In the sections to follow, we consider some of the specific factors that have been linked to the pathogenesis of type 1 diabetes.

## Type 1 diabetes and the environment: infectious agents

As discussed above, the incidence of type 1 diabetes is on the rise at a rate of 3–5% per year that is doubling every 20 years. This is occurring particularly in very young children and is present more often in subjects bearing the low risk alleles [15, 16]. What accounts for these findings? Certainly, genetic risk cannot explain the overall rise in this disorder over relatively short time periods, thereby placing a spotlight on so-called "environmental" factors. For example, it has been suggested that acute infections such as those that are bacterial or viral in nature may precipitate the disease. After such an acute onset, subjects may often enter so-called "honeymoon" periods during which time hyperglycemia abates and the subjects do not require insulin for survival. Examples of viruses linked to type 1 diabetes include cytomegalovirus, coxsackie B, mumps, rubella, Epstein-Barr virus, rotavirus, and varicella zoster virus [17]. An intriguing example of an association between an environmental trigger and type 1 diabetes was speculated to have occurred in Philadelphia in 1993. During the first six months of that year, a substantial rise in the incidence of type 1 diabetes among children was observed. It had been noted that in the two years prior to this event, an outbreak of measles had occurred in the same location, thereby raising the hypothesis that the viral infection stimulated factors that caused type 1 diabetes to emerge in vulnerable children [18].

## Type 1 diabetes: the microbiome

In the human intestine, it is estimated that more than 100 trillion bacteria reside and colonize the organ [19]. Far from being a passive factor in the host, these bacteria critically interface with the immune and metabolic systems. Studies have suggested that specific classes of bacteria may exert effects on the immune system. For example, Bacteroidetes were shown to reduce intestinal inflammation [20]. Segmented filamentous bacteria were suggested to induce Th17 immune responses [21]. Th17 immune responses are usually linked to the clearance of extracellular pathogens during periods of infection; Th17 T cells produce major cytokines that induce inflammation such as IL6 and IL8 [22].

In animal models, interference with the normal gut microbiota has impacted the incidence of type 1 diabetes. For example, raising two major mouse and rat models of type 1 diabetes in germ-free or altered flora environments resulted in the animals developing insulitis and type 1 diabetes at accelerated rates [23, 24]. In contrast, feeding type 1 diabetic-vulnerable animals antibiotics significantly delayed or prevented type 1 diabetes [25]. Based on these considerations, the hunt is on to identify the specific phyla of bacteria that display adaptive/anti-type 1 diabetes impact. So called "probiotics" might one day be identified as treatments to alter the course of type 1 diabetes development, such as the protective effects shown by treatment of type-1-diabetes-vulnerable rats with *Lactobacillus johnsonii* [26].

In the context of the microbiome, it is interesting that type 1 diabetes may appear more frequently in individuals born by Cesarean section vs. natural deliveries [27]. It was shown that in the earliest time of life, the gut microbiome constituents differ in these two states with skin vs. vaginal microbes, respectively, reflecting the major microbiota in subjects born by these two methods. Hence, via Cesarean birth, there is a delay in the colonization of the gut with organisms such as *Bacteroides, Bifidobacterium, and Lactobacillus*; the extent to which this might account for increased type 1 diabetes is not clear [28]. The possibility that the distinct phyla of bacteria may influence the types of immune/inflammatory cells in the gut is under consideration as a contributing factor in type 1 diabetes. In this context, type 1 diabetes manifests with an increased number of intestinal inflammatory cells in parallel with reduced numbers of FoxP3+CD4+CD25+ T lymphocytes [28]. Hence, it is possible that alteration of the gut microbiota might lead to alterations in immune cell patterns in the gut.

In studies in Finnish subjects with type 1 diabetes, experimental analyses have shown that within the gut microbiome, there is a change in the ratio of two key phyla of bacteria—an increased percentage of Bacteroidetes in parallel with a lower percentage of Firmicutes [29]. Whether this association is linked mechanistically to type 1 diabetes has yet to be clarified. 16S sequencing and metagenomics are current strategies under way to determine if there are actual mechanistic links between alterations in the gut microbiome and the susceptibility to type 1 diabetes.

## Type 1 diabetes: vitamin D

Vitamin D, or 1,25-dihydroxyvitamin D3 ($1,25(OH)_2D_3$), has been linked at multiple levels to the pathogenesis of type 1 diabetes. Most importantly, vitamin D plays immunomodulatory roles in cells that express the vitamin D receptor (VDR). Included among such cells are antigen presenting cells, activated T cells, and pancreatic islet β cells [30]. Studies have shown that administration of vitamin D or analogues may exert protection against type 1 diabetes in non-obese diabetic (NOD) mice [31]. Experimental studies to discern the underlying mechanisms showed that administration of $1,25(OH)_2D_3$ reduced inflammatory cytokine (such as IL6) production in parallel with increased regulatory T cells. On the contrary, mice deficient in $1,25(OH)_2D_3$ were shown to be at higher risk of developing type 1 diabetes [32].

What is the evidence in human subjects linking vitamin D to type 1 diabetes? Insights into this question became evident in the study of vitamin D receptor (VDR) polymorphisms. The gene encoding the VDR is located on chromosome 12q12-q14 in the human and single nucleotide polymorphisms (SNPs) have been shown to alter the function of the receptor. The results of studies examining these SNPs have yielded contrary data but the largest meta-analysis to date showed that one of the VDR polymorphisms, *BsmI*, was associated with significantly increased risk of T1D but other SNPs, including *FokI, ApaI, and TaqI*, did not display a significant association with T1D [33]. It remains possible that the

*VDR* locus is not itself the disease affecting locus; rather, the *VDR* may in fact be a marker locus in linkage equilibrium with the true disease locus. Certainly greater functional studies on the SNPs and vitamin D actions are essential to mechanistically link the SNPs to pathological function of the receptor and associations with the pathogenesis of T1D.

What about the levels of vitamin D? Multiple studies in different countries have addressed this question and suggest that lower levels of vitamin D might be related to type 1 diabetes. For example, studies in Switzerland, Qatar, North India, the northeastern United States, and Sweden suggested that levels of vitamin D were lower in type 1 diabetic subjects vs. control subjects. In contrast, in the sun-enriched state of Florida no differences in vitamin D levels were noted between type 1 diabetic subjects and their unaffected first degree relatives and control subjects [30].

Interestingly, support for the North to South incidence of type 1 diabetes emanates from the fact that sun exposure, which is strongly linked to latitude, has possible relationships with type 1 diabetes. Specifically, a number of observational studies have suggested increased type 1 diabetes prevalence in the northern, less sun-exposed latitudes vs. more sun exposed regions. In the EURODIAB study, the incidence of diabetes was found to be higher in the northern region study centers vs. the southern centers, with the exception of Sardinia. Sardinia is considered to be in the southern region but it reported higher rates than those observed in neighboring southern region sites [34, 35]. Not taken into account in these studies are the genetic variations and other vulnerabilities and associations with type 1 diabetes, such as affluence (the latter associated with type 1 diabetes) [36].

The above considerations suggest that supplementation with vitamin D might be protective in type 1 diabetes. When a meta-analysis of multiple observational studies was performed, the results suggested that the incidence of type 1 diabetes was reduced by up to 29% in subjects given supplementation with vitamin D [37]. It is notable, however, that in these studies, concerns regarding many factors, such as reporting of vitamin D levels, doses of vitamin given, and the absence of documentation of vitamin consumption, as examples, limited the overall interpretability of these studies. Hence, a prospective randomized clinical trial is definitely needed to rigorously address these questions and establish possible causality between vitamin D and type 1 diabetes. At this time, no specific answer is available to unequivocally address this issue. Despite these caveats, however, it is essential to address this issue as supplementation with vitamin D should be feasible.

### Type 1 diabetes and insulin resistance

In the sections above, we discussed some of the major factors impacting the etiology of type 1 diabetes. Of late, the issue of "double diabetes" has emerged; this term, first employed to describe this concept in 1991, suggests that there is an emergence of insulin resistance in subjects with type 1 diabetes [38, 39]. For example, in type 1 diabetic subjects with obesity or in whom even very high levels of exogenous insulin did not achieve euglycemia, insulin resistance was speculated to be present [38, 39]. The Diabetes Control and Complications Trial/Epidemiology of Diabetes Interventions and Complications (DCCT/EDIC) study suggested that a family history of type 2 diabetes significantly predicted excess weight gain in type 1 diabetic subjects [40]. Thus, the degree of peripheral insulin resistance might result from genetic and/or environmental factors (such as energy intake and physical activity).

In fact, in the Pittsburgh cohort of the Epidemiology of Diabetes Complications (EDC) study, there is evidence that the prevalence of obesity has risen significantly in type 1 diabetic subjects, similar to the findings reported in the general population. From 1987 to 2007, this study showed that the prevalence of obesity rose seven-fold and that the prevalence of overweight rose 47% [41]. Although some of these changes might be attributable to insufficient glycemic control in the past decades, the overall premise is that the general increase in obesity/overweight has also impacted the type 1 diabetic subject population.

Finally, it is plausible that the development of insulin resistance might be accounted for, in part, by the route of administration of therapeutic exogenous insulin. When insulin is administered by the subcutaneous route, this has been associated with relative peripheral hyperinsulinemia together with hepatic hypoinsulinemia. Such a regimen might ultimately lead to reductions in peripheral insulin-mediated glucose uptake and increased hepatic glucose production [42]. It remains to be seen which factors may underlie the observed insulin resistance in type 1 diabetes and how these might best be managed in type 1 diabetes.

### Type 1 diabetes: summary

In summary, the incidence of type 1 diabetes is on the rise. As Figure 1.1 illustrates, there are multiple contributing factors. Although genetic factors are a major underlying cause, emerging evidence suggests that subjects with traditionally lower genetic risk alleles are being diagnosed with type 1 diabetes. These considerations strongly implicate so-called "environmental" factors in the multiple steps beyond genetic risk that are required before frank type 1 diabetes results. Insights into the interactions between the host and microbiome with respect to modification of genetic risk highlight the complexity of the factors that may significantly modify type 1 diabetes risk.

## Type 2 diabetes

Type 2 diabetes is the most prevalent form of diabetes, accounting for up to 90–95% of diagnosed cases of diabetes, and is on the rise [1]. The International Diabetes Foundation (IDF) reported that in the age range of 20–79 years, approximately 285 million adults suffer from diabetes, a number which is expected to rise to approximately 438 million in the year 2030 [2]. In fact, about 90–95% of these cases will be in the type 2 diabetes classification. Older nomenclature referred to this form of diabetes as "non-insulin dependent" or "adult-onset diabetes." In this form of diabetes, at least early in the course of the disease, subjects display insulin resistance with a "relative" deficiency of insulin. However, in the later stages of disease, some subjects are not able to produce sufficient amounts of insulin to compensate for the hyperglycemic stress [1]. This reflects underlying dysfunction of the pancreatic β cell. In type 2 diabetes, ketoacidosis seldom occurs; where it does occur, it may be precipitated by events such as infections. In cases in which very high levels of glucose are present, subjects may present with coma [43].

In general, the risk of developing type 2 diabetes rises with age and is associated with obesity and diminishing physical activity. Type 2 diabetes occurs more frequently in women who displayed gestational diabetes (GDM) during their pregnancies. Further,

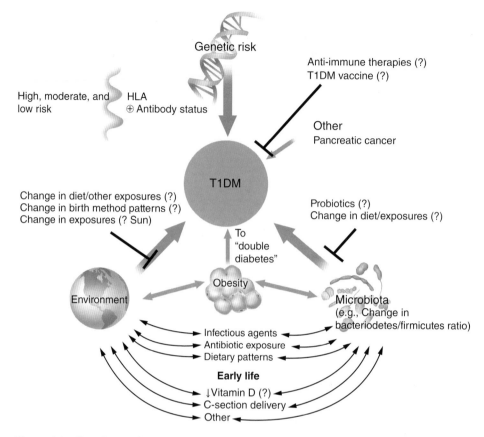

**Figure 1.1**  Contributory factors to the development of type 1 diabetes. Multiple factors, from genetic risk to environmental influences and perhaps the interface with the gut microbiome, contribute to the pathogenesis of type 1 diabetes. Given that in the vast majority of subjects, genetic risk/antibody status may be discerned and tracked, novel interventions hold promise, ultimately, for the prevention of type 1 diabetes. Dangers in type 1 diabetes, however, include the possible influence of obesity on the rise in "double diabetes." Efforts to minimize possible contributory risks for type 1 diabetes are essential.

epidemiological evidence suggests that the incidence of type 2 diabetes is rising in childhood and adolescence, presumably due to increased obesity and reduced physical activity [44]. In type 2 diabetes, there is a very strong association with genetic factors. Many studies have addressed this issue and will be considered in the sections that follow.

### Genetics of type 2 diabetes

The genetics of type 2 diabetes must take into account two key underlying etiologies of the disease, that is, β cell function (insulin secretion) and insulin resistance [1]. In the pre-GWAS era, the strong genetic contribution to type 2 diabetes was determined via family and twin studies [45]. From these efforts, a major gene found to be linked to type 2 diabetes included *CAPN10* (first described in a Mexican-American population) [46].

Others found that regions within chromosomes 5 and 10 were linked to type 2 diabetes, including within the latter, the *TCF7L2* gene [47, 48]. Multiple independent studies confirmed that SNPs in *TCF7L2* were linked to type 2 diabetes. The association of this gene with type 2 diabetes was confirmed in multiple distinct populations [49, 50]. Candidate gene approaches also identified *PPARG* and *KCNJ11* (the latter a potassium inwardly rectifying channel subfamily J member 11) as susceptibility genes for type 2 diabetes [51, 52]. It was not until the GWAS era that more modern and effective approaches were used to identify susceptibility genes in type 2 diabetes.

The first reported GWAS in type 2 diabetes was performed in a French cohort and was composed of 661 cases and 614 control subjects. The number of SNP loci covered in this study was 392,935. From this study, the following genes were identified as association signals in type 2 diabetes: *SLC30A8*, *HHEX*, *LOC387761*, and *EXT2*, and the study validated the association of the disease with *TCF7L2* [53]. Following this study, the Icelandic company deCODE Genetics and its colleagues confirmed the association of type 2 diabetes with *SLC30A8* and *HHEX* and added *CDKAL1* [54]. Following this, three collaborating groups (Wellcome Trust Case Control Consortium/United Kingdom type 2 Diabetes Genetic consortium, the Finland-United States Investigation of NIDDM [FUSION] and the Diabetes Genetics Initiative [DGI]) published the findings confirming the association of type 2 diabetes with *SCL30A8* and *HHEX* and added newly discovered associations with *CDKAL1*, *IGF2BP2*, and *CDKN2A/B* [55–57].

Following these discoveries, the need to increase sample size led to the above groups combining efforts to form the Diabetes Genetics Replication and meta-analysis, or DIAGRAM, consortium. Upon testing of an additional 4,549 cases and 5,579 controls, an additional five loci were discovered including *JAZF1*, *CDC123/CAMK1D*, *TSPAN/LGR5*, *THADA*, and *ADAMTS9* [58]. By the continued addition of new subjects into these studies, an additional 12 new loci were reported in 2010 [59].

What has emerged from these studies is that many of the type 2 diabetes susceptibility loci are linked to insulin secretion based on human studies examining these loci with functional indices [45]. Hence, it is plausible that pancreatic $\beta$ cell dysfunction may be a major factor linked to the susceptibility to type 2 diabetes. Examples of genes linked to type 1 diabetes are illustrated in Table 1.2.

The limitations of GWAS have been uncovered by results in a European twin study in which it was found that only approximately 10% of the known type 2 diabetes heritability might be explained by the loci identified in the GWAS [45]. To the extent that SNPs that might be important clues for type 2 diabetes but not be included in the screening modalities will influence missing heritability. In addition, it is quite possible that low-frequency risk variants may indeed possess large effects. Therefore, the next steps include next-generation sequencing strategies such as genome-wide (exome) sequencing [60]. It is hoped that such strategies, as well as utilization of other genetic tools (such as analysis of small RNAs and epigenetics analyses), will fill in the gaps of the missing heritability.

## Pathogenesis of type 2 diabetes

In the sections to follow, we will consider the major factors speculated to contribute to the pathogenesis of type 2 diabetes.

Table 1.2   Examples of type 2 diabetes-associated loci.

| Locus | Description | Comments |
|-------|-------------|----------|
| TCF7L2 | Transcription factor 7-like 2 | Wnt signaling and regulation of glucose metabolism |
| PPARG | Peroxisome proliferator activated receptor γ | Regulation of lipid and glucose homeostasis, anti-inflammation, and fatty acid oxidation |
| KCNJ11 | Potassium inwardly rectifying Channel J, member 11 | Roles in insulin secretion |
| IGF2BP2 | Insulin-like growth factor-2 mRNA binding protein | Binds mRNA encoding IGF2 |
| WFS1 | Wolfram syndrome 1 | Rare recessive neurodegenerative disorder, one component of which is diabetes |
| CDKAL1 | CDK5 regulatory subunit associated protein1-like 1 | Glucose homeostasis; likely roles in insulin secretion and sensitivity |
| SLC30A8 | Soluble carrier family 30 (zinc transporter), member 8 | Putative roles in insulin secretion |
| HHEX | Hematopoietically expressed homeobox | Putative roles in insulin secretion |
| FTO | Fat mass and obesity associated gene | Roles in methylation, associated with obesity and energy metabolism |
| HNF1B | Hepatocyte nuclear factor-1beta | Roles in pancreatic exocrine function; related to MODY (maturity onset diabetes of the young) |

## Type 2 diabetes and obesity

Obesity is considered a major risk factor for the development of type 2 diabetes. How does obesity mediate insulin resistance and diabetes? This is a intensely active area of investigation stimulated by the pioneering studies of Hotamisligil and Spiegelman. They set the stage for linking adipose tissue "inflammation" to insulin resistance in obesity. In 1993, they showed that tumor necrosis factor (TNF)-α mRNA was highly expressed in the adipose tissue of at least four different rodent models of obesity with consequent diabetes and that when TNF-α was neutralized in obese fa/fa rats, insulin sensitivity was improved, as evidenced by increased peripheral uptake of glucose [61]. In 2003, Weisberg and Ferrante showed that obesity in human subjects and in animal models was associated with increased infiltration and/or retention of macrophages in the perigonadal, perirenal, mesenteric, and subcutaneous adipose tissue [62]. Ferrante's later work linked CCR2 and its chemoattractant functions to the increased infiltration of macrophages to adipose tissue in high fat feeding in mice [63]. Further work on the macrophage populations by Olefsky and colleagues suggested that expression of CD11c was a key contributor to obesity-associated insulin resistance [64]. Other studies have suggested that macrophage populations cause increased activation of NF-κB and JNK MAP kinase signaling pathways, both linked to insulin resistance [65, 66]. Various genetic modification studies in mice suggest that these pathways are required for the link between high fat feeding/obesity and the development of insulin resistance. Taken together, these seminal findings suggest that in obesity, inflammatory cells and their inflammatory mediators contribute to metabolic dysfunction, insulin resistance, and the ultimate development of type 2 diabetes, and that targeting these pathways may be beneficial in suppression of the adverse effects of obesity [67, 68].

## Type 2 diabetes and the microbiome

As in type 1 diabetes, emerging evidence suggests links of the gut microbiome to type 2 diabetes [69]. Jumpertz and colleagues studied the effects of altering energy balance in human subjects on gut microbiota profiles; these studies were performed in 12 lean and 9 obese subjects who consumed two calorically different diets. Simultaneous monitoring of the gut microbiota was performed, together with pyrosequencing of 16S rRNA in feces and monitoring of stool calories by bomb calorimetry. These findings revealed that changes in the diet (nutrient load) altered the bacterial composition of the microbiome rapidly [70]. Specifically, increased proportions of Firmicutes and reductions in Bacteroidetes taxa were linked to increased energy harvest [70]. Such data directly link gut microbiota and nutrient absorption in the human subject. Interestingly, the ratio of Bacteroidetes and Firmicutes is also altered in animal models when the animals are subjected to dietary modulation [71]. Importantly, the specific mechanisms by which these distinct taxa exert these effects have yet to be identified.

It has been shown that the gut microbiome interfaces with the host to a exert specific impact on catabolism of dietary toxins, micronutrient synthesis, absorption of minerals and electrolytes, and short chain fatty acid (SCFA) production which affects the growth and differentiation of gut enterocytes and colonocytes, as examples [69]. In germ-free raised mice, studies have revealed that the gut microbiome plays major roles in whole body metabolism including regulation of phosphocholine and glycine levels in the liver [72]. Further, germ-free rats displayed increased concentrations of conjugated bile acids which accumulate in tissues such as the liver and heart [73].

Work by Cho and Blaser revealed that the administration of subtherapeutic doses of antibiotics to young mice resulted in increased adiposity. In parallel, multiple effects on metabolism were noted, including changes in gene expression patterns linked to metabolism of carbohydrates to short chain fatty acids, increased levels of colonic short chain fatty acid levels, and altered hepatic metabolism of lipids and cholesterol. Examination of the taxa revealed that although there was no change in overall bacterial census, an increase in the relative concentrations of Firmicutes vs. Bacteroidetes was noted in the antibiotic-fed mice vs. the controls. These effects were found to parallel the changes in adiposity in the mice [74].

These and other studies reflect and underscore the dynamic nature of the composition of the gut microbiome. Indeed, in human subjects who underwent bariatric surgery, it was shown that the fecal material displayed significant changes in the composition of the microbiome. Specifically, Graessler and colleagues performed metagenomic sequencing and showed that overall the surgery resulted in a reduction in Firmicutes and Bacteriodetes and an increase in Proteobacteria [75]. Overall, establishing causality between the gut microbiome constituents and obesity has not yet been accomplished; much work is under-way to discern the specific means by which these varied taxa of bacteria may impact energy utilization and metabolism in processes linked to obesity.

## Type 2 diabetes and vitamin D

As in the case of type 1 diabetes, vitamin D levels have been speculated to contribute to the pathogenesis of type 2 diabetes. Mezza and colleagues reviewed the available litera-ture from human studies linking vitamin D deficiency to type 2 diabetes; their conclusion was that the results are "mixed"; whereas some studies suggested that deficiency of vita-min D was associated with increased type 2 diabetes, others identified no such association [76]. Similar caveats to the reported studies in type 1 diabetes prevailed in this setting as well. Specifically, many of the studies were cross-sectional, they did not take into account dietary factors, the subjects often displayed varied diabetes risk profiles as well as differ-ent patterns of serum vitamin D levels, and only single measurements of vitamin D were reported in many of the studies.

Others performed meta-analyses to identify potential relationships between levels of vitamin D and type 2 diabetes as follows: First, Forouhi and colleagues only considered prospective studies and reported a significant inverse association between the incidence of type 2 diabetes and the levels of vitamin D. Causality was not identified by the work of this report [77]. Second, in therapeutic interventions, George and colleagues reviewed the impact of supplementation with vitamin D and suggested that there was no evidence that such treatment was beneficial in terms of prevention of type 2 diabetes or improvement in glycemic control [78].

In addition to potential links to type 2 diabetes, vitamin D levels have also been explored with respect to insulin resistance. *In vitro* studies suggested a potential role of Vitamin D in preventing free fatty acid mediated insulin resistance in C2C12 (skeletal muscle) cells [79]. Several potential molecular mechanisms by which vitamin D may be associated with insulin include the following: (1) vitamin D may influence insulin action by stimulation of the expression of insulin receptors and amplifying glucose transport, and (2) the effects of vitamin D on the intracellular calcium pool may contribute to regu-lation of peripheral insulin resistance. Further links between vitamin D and type 2 diabe-tes have been suggested by relationships between vitamin D and insulin secretion [76]. In animal models, vitamin D-deficient diets have been associated with reduced insulin secretion [80].

Interventional studies on administration of vitamin D to insulin resistant/glucose intol-erant subjects have yielded conflicting results that have not resolved the issue. At this time, several interventional clinical trials are under way to rigorously test the effects of vitamin D supplements on pancreatic $\beta$ cell function and insulin resistance in human subjects highly vulnerable to the development of type 2 diabetes, and in other studies, in subjects newly diagnosed with type 2 diabetes or prediabetes syndromes [76].

Hence, although studies to date have not yielded clear results, the underlying concept that vitamin D supplementation may be of utility in type 2 diabetes and prediabetes syn-dromes remains an unanswered question and one that may be addressed when the results of ongoing trials are finalized and released. Clearly, however, this is an area that requires further and standardized investigation; it is intriguing to link vitamin D metabolism to the composition and function of the gut microbiome. Indeed, Bargenolts reviewed the links between vitamin D metabolism and the gut microbiome and suggested a two hit model: First, an obesity-provoking diet shifts the microbiome from symbiosis to dysbiosis and the double hit of steatosis (fat accumulation in the various target organs) and inflammation together with the second hit (such as vitamin D deficiency) are necessary to activate signaling pathways that suppress adaptive insulin receptor signaling. Barengolts hypothesized that alterations in dietary patterns, such as vitamin D supplementation and prebiotics, might improve prediabetes and type 2 diabetes management if initiated early in the process of obesity [81].

## Type 2 diabetes and environmental pollution

Multiple epidemiologic studies, performed in such locations as Ontario, Canada; Ruh, Germany; the United States (multiple cohorts); Denmark; Iran; and Taiwan have shown associations between exposure to particulate matter (PM), such as in air pollution, and type 2 diabetes as well as insulin sensitivity. In those studies, varied measures of type 2 diabetes, glycosylated hemoglobin levels, or HOMA-IR were reported—all reflective of significant metabolic dysfunction [82].

Intriguingly, these studies suggest that primary inhalation of these PMs is linked mechanistically to inflammatory signals that are related to metabolism. How is this possible? Rajagoplan and Brooks summarized the work of various authors whose work implicated specific mechanisms by which this might occur [82]. For example, first, it is possible that alveolar macrophages subjected to PM exposure might release pro-inflammatory cytokines that secondarily cause a systemic inflammation, which might contribute to metabolic dysfunction. Second, it is possible that oxidative stress triggered by PM might activate local inflammatory signaling pathways whose products may impact the organism via systemic release. Third, it is plausible that the update of the PM by macrophages may cause presentation via dendritic cells to T lymphocytes within the secondary lymphoid organs, thereby triggering an immune/inflammatory-mediated response. Fourth, it is possible that the PM and their components may be able to gain direct access to the circulation and thereby cause inflammation and, potentially, contribute to insulin resistance. Finally, pathways linking the lung to the brain might be directly responsible for inflammation which might contribute to insulin resistance and metabolic dysfunction [82].

Based on these epidemiological and basic research studies, it is possible that strict efforts to combat air pollution and PM may ultimately lead to reduction in type 2 diabetes, prediabetes, and the metabolic dysfunction syndromes in human subjects.

## Type 2 diabetes: summary

As Figure 1.2 illustrates, type 2 diabetes is associated with a very strong genetic predisposition based on the results of GWAS that were performed/confirmed in multiple populations. To date, although a number of the linked genes have been identified through earlier candidate and GWAS efforts, it is believed that the great majority have yet to be discovered. Interestingly, many of the genes uncovered by these approaches are linked to

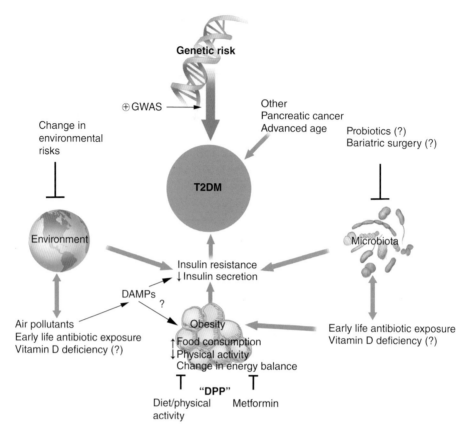

**Genetic risk**

⊕GWAS

Other
Pancreatic cancer
Advanced age

Probiotics (?)
Bariatric surgery (?)

Change in
environmental
risks

**T2DM**

Environment

Microbiota

Insulin resistance
↓ Insulin secretion

DAMPs
?

Air pollutants
Early life antibiotic exposure
Vitamin D deficiency (?)

Obesity
↑Food consumption
↓Physical activity
Change in energy balance

Early life antibiotic exposure
Vitamin D deficiency (?)

**"DPP"**

Diet/physical
activity

Metformin

**Figure 1.2**   Contributory factors to the development of type 2 diabetes. A major cause of type 2 diabetes is accounted for by obesity and the reductions in physical activity. Strong genetic risk along with multiple influences in the environment and in the microbiome may substantially modify the risk of type 2 diabetes. The DPP study showed that in highly vulnerable subjects, metformin or change in diet/physical activity were able to prevent type 2 diabetes vs. placebo control. Efforts to augment protective therapies for type 2 diabetes are essential.

a greater extent to insulin secretion rather than resistance. Obesity, physical activity, and changes in lifestyle are believed to be the cause of the striking increases in type 2 diabetes world-wide. The rapid success of certain forms of bariatric surgery in reversing type 2 diabetes even before significant weight loss suggests that host interfaces with the gastro-intestinal tract and other neuro/immune/metabolic systems contribute integrally to type 2 diabetes. Perhaps future studies will uncover roles for the gut microbiome directly in these findings; this remains to be determined.

Taken together, evidence suggests roles for the gut microbiome, vitamin D metabolism, and PM in air pollution in the exacerbation of type 2 diabetes and prediabetes syndromes. The extent to which type 2 diabetes may be reversed by adaptive modulation of body mass, gut bacteria, vitamin D levels, and air pollution remains an open question. However, the identification of putative aggravating factors to this disease hold promise for the ultimate prevention/reversal of type 2 diabetes, at least in certain subjects.

# Gestational diabetes

## Epidemiology and diagnosis

Oliveira and colleagues reiterated the definition of gestational diabetes (GDM) as follows: "glucose intolerance with onset or first recognition during pregnancy or as carbohydrate intolerance of variable severity diagnosed during pregnancy, which may or may not resolve afterward" [83]. GDM is important to diagnose and treat because it is linked to increased complications for both the mother and the developing child throughout the pregnancy and delivery. It is estimated that one-third of women with GDM remain affected with either type 2 diabetes or altered glucose metabolism post-delivery [1].

The consensus from epidemiological studies is that GDM is on the rise, at least in part due to increased obesity that is observed in women of child-bearing age. Barbour and colleagues reported in 2007 that the incidence of GDM had doubled over the prior six to eight years and that this paralleled the obesity epidemic [84]. Importantly, about 40–60% of pregnant women have no apparent risk factors for GDM, thereby stressing the urgent need to carry out screening on all pregnant women [85]. It is estimated that 15–50% of women afflicted with GDM will ultimately develop diabetes in the decades after pregnancy [86].

The diagnosis of GDM is generally based on the following algorithm: first, a fasting plasma glucose level is determined at the first surveillance visit for pregnancy. A normal value is considered less than 92 mg/dl. This is followed up by a 75-gram oral glucose tolerance test (OGTT) between weeks 24 and 28 of pregnancy. If the first visit fasting plasma glucose exceeds 92 mg/dl, then this suffices for the diagnosis of GDM and follow-up OGTT is not performed. If the initial fasting plasma glucose exceeds 126 mg/dl, this likely indicates that diabetes existed prior to the pregnancy [1, 83, 85]. By World Health Organization criteria, a level of glycosylated hemoglobin equal to or greater than 6.5% suffices for the diagnosis of probably diabetes. Based on the above findings, the 75-gram OGTT may be indicated. This consists of a fast between 8 and 14 hours; following the consumption of 75 grams glucose, plasma glucose is assessed at 1 and 2 hours. GDM is diagnosed when one or more of the values exceeds or is equal to 180 mg/dl or 153 mg/dl at 1 or 2 hours, respectively [1, 83, 85].

## Metabolic factors and etiology of GDM

As in other forms of diabetes, the key to hyperglycemia in GDM rests on the forces that modulate insulin sensitivity and the ability of the pancreatic β cell to produce and release insulin. Human pregnancy is naturally characterized by an increase in insulin resistance; in normal pregnancy, both skeletal muscle and adipose tissue develop insulin resistance [87, 88]. In the normal setting, an approximately 50% reduction in insulin-mediated glucose disposal occurs in parallel with a 200–250% increase in insulin secretion, the latter required to maintain normal levels of blood glucose in the mother [88, 89]. Placental-derived hormones are critical in the mechanisms by which euglycemia is maintained [85]. For example, human placental lactogen (hPL) has been shown to increase up to 30 times during pregnancy; its role is to induce release of insulin from the pancreas during the pregnancy [90]. A second placenta-derived hormone, human placental growth hormone (hPGH), also increases in pregnancy. This hormone, similar in its sequence and effects to human growth hormone, causes a severe decline in peripheral insulin sensitivity during pregnancy [91].

How are these changes manifested at the molecular level? Barbour and colleagues obtained access to skeletal muscle fibers from non-pregnant women, pregnant women without GDM, and pregnant women with GDM and examined the various key components of the insulin signaling pathway. They reported that skeletal muscle IRS-1 was reduced in normal pregnancy and even further reduced in GDM pregnancy vs. non-pregnant controls. Skeletal muscle levels of p85α of PI3K (which normally blocks the association of PI3-kinase with IRS-1, overall leading to reduced GLUT4 translocation to the plasma membrane and, hence, less insulin-stimulated glucose uptake to the skeletal muscle) is higher in normal and GDM pregnancy vs. non-pregnant controls. However, small but significantly lower levels of p85α in skeletal muscle were observed in GDM pregnancy vs. normal pregnancy. In adipose tissue, levels of IRS-1 were lower than those observed in the absence of pregnancy or in pregnancy without GDM and the levels of p85α were higher in the adipose tissue of non-pregnant and normal pregnant subject tissue [85]. Furthermore, in GDM pregnancy, alterations in serine and tyrosine phosphorylation of IR and IRS-1 further suppress insulin signaling. Overall, the effect is to reduce GLUT-4 translocation to the membrane and thereby reduce glucose uptake even further in GDM pregnancy than in normal pregnancy [85].

In addition, inflammatory markers are altered in GDM pregnancy. For example, pregnant women with GDM display higher levels of tumor necrosis factor (TNF)-α in skeletal muscle than in non-GDM pregnancy, which persists even in the post-partum period [92]. Furthermore, levels of adiponectin, a hormone that serves to enhance insulin sensitivity, is reduced in GDM adipose tissue, thereby suggesting it may be linked to the syndrome of insulin resistance in pregnancy and especially in GDM pregnancy [93]. In addition, levels of PPAR-gamma decline to greater degrees in GDM adipose tissue [94]. Such a change favors and increases lipolysis, thereby increasing the release of free fatty acids, molecular mediators that may serve to mediate insulin resistance and hepatic glucose production.

Taken together, these underlying factors serve to significantly increase insulin resistance, particularly in GDM pregnancy. Furthermore, together with impaired β cell function and reduced adaptation of the β cell during pregnancy, multiple factors converge to increase risk and severity of GDM in pregnant women.

### Gestational diabetes and potential roles for vitamin D

Alzaim and Wood have reviewed the existing literature for potential roles of vitamin D deficiency in GDM. They summarize the results of five cross-sectional studies which suggested that women with GDM had poorer vitamin D status vs. pregnant women without GDM [95]. However, these authors provided a number of caveats to these five studies, as follows: First, all of the studies were cross-sectional in design. Second, there was inconsistent accounting for such factors as ethnicity, season during pregnancy, physical activity of the subjects, the number of pregnancies (particularly the order of the current pregnancy under study), and body mass index pre-pregnancy. Third, in most of the studies the levels of vitamin D were measured late in the pregnancy and after GDM had already developed. There were no reports of the vitamin D levels pre-pregnancy; hence, the potential predictive value of the pre- to pregnancy state were not available for consideration [95].

In fact, in only one study by Zhang and colleagues was a prospective cohort study performed among mostly non-Hispanic Caucasian pregnant women in the United States (Tacoma, Washington). In the study, the levels of vitamin D were measured at approximately the 16th week of pregnancy. Overall, the authors concluded that (1) vitamin D deficiency was found in 33% of women who developed GDM vs. 15% in the women who did not develop GDM; (2) at 24–28 weeks gestation, the risk of developing GDM was 2.66-fold higher in vitamin D-deficient women vs. the non-vitamin D-deficient pregnant women; and (3) when the results were limited to non-Hispanic Caucasian women only, the risk of developing GDM was 3.77-fold higher with vitamin D deficiency vs. without vitamin D deficiency [96]. The researchers pointed out that a caveat to this study is that the levels of vitamin D were only measured once during the course of the study; therefore, it remains possible that those levels as reported were not consistent during the entire course of the pregnancy.

At this time, interventional studies on the use of vitamin D in pregnancy are quite limited. In one study by Rudnicki and Pedersen, vitamin D was administered by intravenous route followed by oral supplementation to pregnant women with established GDM. The study showed that after the intravenous dose of vitamin D, fasting serum glucose declined significantly. However, these benefits were not sustained after the patients began to take the oral supplementation [97]. It was speculated that perhaps the oral doses might have been too low or that pharmacologic factors based on the precise form of vitamin D administered to the subjects accounted for the reduced efficacy.

Taken together, the available data strongly suggest that definitive conclusions will be essential to determine if and when to administer vitamin D to pregnant subjects and whether or not specific subsets of pregnant women are most likely to benefit.

### GDM: Summary

In summary, epidemiologic evidence indicates a rise in GDM that, perhaps not surprisingly, parallels the increase in obesity and its consequences. Given that GDM exerts potentially damaging effects to both mother and the developing fetus, prevention and therapeutic efforts are essential to ensure safer pregnancies and improved outcome for the fetuses. In this context, the potential benefits of vitamin D supplementation have yet to be conclusively addressed. However, preliminary evidence from cross-sectional studies might suggest a link between deficiency in vitamin D and GDM. Further studies are required to address this question.

## Maturity onset diabetes of the young

Maturity onset diabetes of the young (MODY) is a group of monogenic disorders, inherited in an autosomal dominant manner, in which specific genetic mutations causing defects in insulin secretion but not generally with insulin action result in hyperglycemia, usually before the age of 25 years. MODY is believed to be responsible for approximately 2–5% of all cases of diabetes [1, 98]. To date, mutations in at least six distinct genes have been identified to account for MODY [99].

The most common form of MODY is a mutation in chromosome 12 in the gene *HNF1α*. This gene encodes for hepatic nuclear factor 1 α [100]. A second form of MODY is associated with mutations in the gene encoding glucokinase; this mutation is located on chromosome 7p [101, 102]. Glucokinase serves to convert glucose to glucose-6-phosphate; the metabolism within this pathway is then responsible for stimulation of insulin secretion. In this setting, higher levels of glucose are thus required for stimulation of insulin secretion. Other forms of MODY result from mutations in the following genes: *HNF4α* [103], *HNF1β* [104], *IPF1* (insulin promoter factor) [105], and *NEUROD1* [106]. Beyond these mutations, numerous others have been reported that account for the MODY syndrome; however, they are much rarer.

Because of the age of onset, MODY disorders are often misdiagnosed as type 1 or type 2 diabetes. Key components for diagnosis therefore include diagnosis before age 45 years, the absence of β cell autoimmunity (auto-antibodies), absence of obesity or any features of the metabolic syndrome, sustained production of insulin despite hyperglycemia, and because of the genetic nature of the disease, a strong family history [107]. It is important to note that the presence of MODY does not, of course, exclude obesity. These criteria are meant to inform possible clues to direct the practitioner to a diagnosis of MODY vs. a more typical form of diabetes (type 1 or type 2).

## Summary

### *Other notable causes of diabetes*

In addition to the most common causes of diabetes detailed above, it is important to note that there are many other less common causes that require mention, such as those forms of diabetes induced by drugs (e.g., corticosteroids) or as components of distinct autoimmune syndromes. Refer to the review [11] which details the myriad etiologies underlying the most common and the very rare causes of this disease [1]. One seminal link to note is the association between pancreatic cancer and diabetes. Pancreatic cancer is the fourth leading cause of death due to cancer in the United States and the sixth leading cause of cancer death in Europe and Japan [108]. Cigarette smoking remains an extremely strong risk factor; given the decline of smoking in the last decades, the incidence in this form of cancer has declined, but only in countries in which smoking has generally declined as well [108]. Pancreatic cancer remains highly intractable to curative efforts; the five-year survival rate is less than 5%. Diabetes has important "bidirectional links" to pancreatic cancer. Type 2 diabetes has been shown to increase the risk of pancreatic cancer [109]. On the other hand, it has also been noted that new-onset diabetes may be a spotlight that uncovers the presence of undiagnosed pancreatic cancer, especially in patients with weight loss or in those with a strong family history of the disease [109].

### Prevention of diabetes: on the horizon?

Given the sobering epidemiological data on the rise in types 1 and 2 diabetes, it is essential to query, Are the current trends in increases in the most common forms of diabetes, types 1 and 2 diabetes, a foregone conclusion? Is all hope lost? The answer is a firm "no." In the case of type 1 diabetes, clinical trials aimed at new-onset and at-risk type 1 diabetes (the latter antibody-positive subjects), using various forms of immunotherapy and other strategies, are well under way. A key challenge and benchmark in this regard will be the identification and validation of prognostic and predictive biomarkers for the eventual diagnosis of type 1 diabetes. Such immune interventions are now viewed as best when used in "combination" strategies [110].

What about type 2 diabetes? As discussed above, obesity and reduced physical activity clearly are major risk factors. In the Diabetes Prevention Program (DPP) trial, subjects at high risk for type 2 diabetes (elevated fasting and post-load plasma glucose concentrations) were randomized to placebo, metformin, or lifestyle modification (weight loss and physical activity). Over a 2.8-year follow-up, the incidence of diabetes development was 11%, 7.8%, and 4.8% in the placebo, metformin, and lifestyle groups, respectively. Lifestyle intervention reduced the incidence of type 2 diabetes by 58% and metformin reduced the incidence of type 2 diabetes by 31% compared to that observed in placebo treatment. Interestingly, the lifestyle modification strategy arm was significantly more beneficial than the metformin arm [111].

These data strongly suggest that there is likely no "point of no return" in types 1 and 2 diabetes. Intense efforts aimed at reducing the development of type 1 and type 2 diabetes hold great promise to mitigate the devastation of these diseases.

Additional discussion about prevention of diabetes mellitus can be found in chapters 2 and 4.

## References

1. American Diabetes Association. Diagnosis and classification of diabetes mellitus. *Diabetes Care* 2010; 33 (Suppl 1): S62–S69.
2. International Diabetes Federation. *IDF Diabetes Atlas*, 5th ed. International Diabetes Federation: Belgium, 2012.
3. Lipman TH et al. Increasing incidence of type 1 diabetes in youth: Twenty years of the Philadelphia Pediatric Diabetes Registry. *Diabetes Care* 2013; 36: 1597–1603.
4. Lammi N et al. A high incidence of type 1 diabetes and an alarming increase in the incidence of type 2 diabetes among young adults in Finland between 1992 and 1996. *Diabetologia* 2007; 50: 1393–1400.
5. Lernmark A et al. Islet cell-surface antibodies in juvenile diabetes mellitus. *New Engl J Med* 1978; 299: 375–380.
6. Gorus FK et al. IA-2 autoantibodies complement GAD65-autoantibodies in new-onset IDDM patients and help predict impending diabetes in their siblings. The Belgian Diabetes Registry. *Diabetologia* 1997; 40: 95–99.
7. Singal DP, Blajchman MA. Histocompatibility (HL-A) antigens, lymphocytoxic antibodies and tissue antibodies in patients with diabetes mellitus. *Diabetes* 1973; 22: 429–432.

8. Noble JA, Erlich HA. Genetics of type 1 diabetes. *Cold Spring Harb Perspect Med* 2012; 2: 007732.
9. Pociot F et al. Genetics of type 1 diabetes: what's next? *Diabetes* 2010; 59: 1561–1571.
10. Barrett JC et al. Genome-wide assocation study and meta-analysis find that over 40 loci affect risk of type 1 diabetes. *Nat Genet* 2009; 41: 703–707.
11. Bergholdt R et al. Identification of novel type 1 diabetes candidate genes by integrating genome-wide association data, protein-protein interactions, and human pancreatic islet gene expression. *Diabetes* 2012; 61: 954–962.
12. Boitard C. Pancreatic cell autoimmunity. *Presse Med* 2012; 41: e636–650.
13. Richie RH Jr, Talbot NB. The management of diabetic ketoacidosis and coma. *Pediatr Clin North Am* 1962; 9: 263–276.
14. Cahill GF Jr. C-peptide: a new method of assessing pancreatic beta cell function. *New Engl J Med* 1973; 288: 1181–1182.
15. Kontiainen S et al. Differences in HLA types in children with insulin-dependent diabetes diagnosed in the 1960s, 1970s, and 1980s. *Lancet* 1988; 332: 219.
16. Vehik K et al. Islet autoantibody seroconversion in the DPT-1 study. *Diabetes Care* 2011; 34: 358–362.
17. Hara N et al. The role of the intestinal microbiota in type 1 diabetes. *Clin Immunol* 2013; 146: 112–119.
18. Lipman TH et al. the epidemiology of type 1 diabetes in children in Philadelphia 1990–1994: evidence of an epidemic. *Diabetes Care* 2002; 25: 1969–1975.
19. Qin J et al. A human gut microbiome catalogue established by metagenomic sequencing. *Nature* 2010; 464: 59–65.
20. Mazmanian SK et al. A microbial symbiosis factor prevents intestingal inflammatory disease. *Nature* 2008; 453: 620–625.
21. Ivanov II et al. Induction of intestingal Th17 cells by segmened filamentous bacteria. *Cell* 2009; 139: 485–498.
22. McGeachy MJ, McSorley SJ. Microbial-induced Th17: superhero or supervillain? *J Immunol* 2012; 189: 3285–3291.
23. Patrick C et al. Promotion of autoimmune diabetes by cereal diet in the presence or absence of microbes associated with gut immune activation, regulatory imbalance, and altered cathelicidin antimicrobial Peptide. *Diabetes* 2013; 62: 2036–2047.
24. King C, Sarvetnick N. The incidence of type 1 diabetes in NOD mice is modulated by restricted flora not germ-free conditions. *PLoS One* 2011; 6: e17049.
25. Brugman S et al. Antibiotic treatment partially protects against type 1 diabetes in the Bio-Breeding diabetes prone rat. Is the gut flora involved in the development of type 1 diabetes? *Diabetologia* 2006; 49: 2105–2108.
26. Valladares R et al. *Lactobacillus johnsonii* N6.2 mitigates the development of type 1 diabetes in BB-DP rats. *PLoS One* 6:e10507.
27. Cardwell CR et al. Caesarean section is associated with an increased risk of childhood-onset type 1 diabetes mellitus: a meta-analysis of observational studies. *Diabetologia* 2008; 51: 726–735.
28. Atkinson MA, Chervonsky A. Does the gut microbiota have a role in type 1 diabetes? Early evidence from humans and animal models of the disease. *Diabetologia* 2012; 55: 2868–2877.
29. Giongo A et al. Toward defining the autoimmune microbiome for type 1 diabetes. *ISME J* 2010; 5: 82–91.
30. Chakhtoura M, Azar ST. The role of vitamin D deficiency in the incidence, progression, and complications of type 1 diabetes mellitus. *Intl J Endocrinol* 2013; 2013: 148673.

31. Zella JB et al. Oral administration of 1,25-dihydroxyvitamin D3 completely protects NOD mice from insulin-dependent diabetes mellitus. *Arch Biochem Biophys* 2003; 417: 77–80.
32. Giulietti A et al. Vitamin D deficiency in early life accelerates type 1 diabetes in non-obese daibetic mice. *Diabetologia* 2004; 47: 451–462.
33. Zhang J et al. Polymorphisms in the vitamin D receptor gene and type 1 diabetes mellitus risk: an update by meta-analysis. *Mol Cell Endocrinol* 2012; 355: 135–142.
34. Casu A et al. Bayesian appraoch to study the temporal trend and the geographical variation in the risk of type 1 diabetes: the Sardinian Conscript type 1 diabetes registry. *Pediatric Diabetes* 2004; 5: 32–38.
35. Mohr SB et al. The association between ultraviolet irradiance, vitamin D status and incidence rates of type 1 diabetes in 51 regions worldwide. *Diabetologia* 2008; 51: 1391–1398.
36. Liese AD et al. Neighborhood level risk factors for type 1 diabetes in youth: the SEARCH case-control study. *Int J Health Geogr* 2012; 11: 1.
37. Zipitis CS, Akobeng AK. Vitamin D supplementation in early childhood and risk of type 1 diabetes: a systematic review and meta-analysis. *Arch Disease Childhood* 2008; 93: 512–517.
38. Cleland SJ et al. Insulin resistance in type 1 diabetes: what is "double diabetes" and what are the risks? *Diabetologia* 2013; 56: 1462–1470.
39. Teupe B, Bergis K. Epidemiological evidence for "double diabetes." *Lancet* 1991; 337: 361–362.
40. Purnell JQ et al. Relationship of family history of type 2 diabetes, hypoglycemia, and autoantibodies to weight gain and lipids with intensive and conventional therapy in the Diabetes Control and Complications Trial. *Diabetes* 2003; 52: 2623–2629.
41. Conway B et al. Adiposity and mortality in type 1 diabetes. *Int J Obes* 2009; 33: 796–805.
42. Taylor AM et al. Somatomedin-C/IGF-1 measured by radioimmunoassay and somatomedin bioactivity in adolescents with insulin-dependent diabetes compared with puberty matched controls. *Diabetes Res* 1988; 9: 177–181.
43. Fadini GP et al. Characteristics and outcomes of the hyperglycemic hyperosmolar non-ketotic syndrom in a cohort of 51 consecutive cases at a single center. *Diabetes Res Clin Pract* 2011; 94: 172–179.
44. Sinha R et al. Prevalence of impaired glucose tolerance among children and adolescents with marked obesity. *New Engl J Med* 2002; 346: 802–810.
45. Imamura M, Maeda S. Genetics of type 2 diabetes: the GWAS era and future perspectives. *Endocrine J* 2011; 58: 723–739.
46. Horikawa Y et al. Genetic variation in the gene encoding calpain-10 is associated with type 2 diabetes mellitus. *Nat Genet* 2000; 26: 163–175.
47. Reynisdottir I et al. Localization of a susceptibility gene for type 2 diabetes to chromosome 5q34-q35.2. *Am J Hum Genet* 2003; 73: 323–335.
48. Grant SF et al. Variant of transcription factor 7-like2 (*TCF7L2*) gene confers risk of type 2 diabetes. *Nat Genet* 2006; 38: 320–323.
49. Zhang C et al. Variant of transcription factor 7-like 2 (*TCF7L2*) gene and the risk of type 2 diabetes in large cohorts of US women and men. *Diabetes* 2006; 55: 2645–2648.
50. Hayashi T et al. Replication study for the assocation of *TCF7L2* with susceptibility to type 2 diabetes in a Japanese population. *Diabetologia* 2007; 50: 980–984.
51. Altshuler D et al. The common PPAR gamma Pro12Ala polymorphism is associated with decreased risk of type 2 diabetes. *Nat Genet* 2000; 26: 76–80.
52. Gloyn AL et al. Large scale association studies of variants in genes encoding the pancreatic beta cell KATP channel subunits Kir6.2 (*KCNJ11* and SUR1 (*ABCC8*) confirm that the *KCNJ22* E23K variant is associated with type 2 diabetes. *Diabetes* 2003; 52: 568–572.

53. Sladek R et al. A genome-wide association study identifies novel risk loci for type 2 diabetes. *Nature* 2007; 445: 881–885.
54. Steinthorsdottir V et al. A variant in *CDKAL1* influences insulin response and risk of type 2 diabetes. *Nat Genet* 2007; 39: 770–775.
55. Saxena R et al. Genome-wide association analysis identifies loci for type 2 diabetes and triglyceride levels. *Science* 2007; 316: 1331–1336.
56. Zeggini E et al. Replication of genome-wide association signals in UK samples reveals risk loci for type 2 diabetes. *Science* 2007; 316: 1336–1341.
57. Scott LJ et al. A genome-wide associaton study of type 2 diabetes in Finns detects multiple susceptibility variants. *Science* 2007; 316: 1341–1345.
58. Zeggini E et al. Metaanalysis of genome wide association data and large-scale replication identifies additional susceptibility loci for type 2 diabetes. *Nat Genet* 2008; 40: 638–645.
59. Voight BF et al. Twelve type 2 diabetes susceptibility loci identified through large-scale association analysis. *Nat Genet* 2010; 42: 579–589.
60. Roukos DH et al. Novel next-generation sequencing and networks-based therapeutic targets: realistic more effective drug design and discovery. *Curr Pharm Des* 2013; In press.
61. Hotamisligil GS et al. Adipose expression of tumor necrosis factor alpha: direct role in obesity linked insulin resistance. *Science* 1993; 259: 87–91.
62. Weisberg SP et al. Obesity is associated with macrophage accumulation in adipose tissue. *J Clin Invest* 2003; 112: 1796–1808.
63. Weisberg SP et al. CCR2 modulates inflammatory and metabolic effects of high fat feeding. *J Clin Invest* 2006; 116: 115–124.
64. Patsouris D et al. Ablation of CD11c positive cells normalizes insulin sensitivity in obese insulin resistant animals. *Cell Metab* 2008; 8: 301–309.
65. Arkan MC et al. IKK-beta links inflammation to obesity-induced insulin resistance. *Nat Med* 2005; 11: 191–198.
66. Hirosumi J et al. A central role for JNK in obesity and insulin resistance. *Nature* 2002; 420: 333–336.
67. Goran MI, Alderete TL. Targeting adipose tissue inflammation to treat the underlying basis of the metabolic consequences of obesity. *Nestel Nutr Inst Workshop Ser* 2012; 73: 49–60.
68. Wang X et al. Inflammatory markers and risk of type 2 diabetes: a systematic review and meta-analysis. *Diabetes Care* 2013; 36: 166–175.
69. Devaraj S et al. The human gut microbiome and body metabolism: implications for obesity and diabetes. *Clin Chem* 2013; 59: 617–628.
70. Jumpertz R et al. Energy-balance studies reveal associations between gut microbes, caloric load, and nutrient absorption in humans. *Am J Clin Nutr* 2011; 94: 58–65.
71. Hooper LV, Gordon JI. Commensal host-bacterial relationships in the gut. *Science* 2001; 292: 1115–1118.
72. Claus SP et al. Systemic multicompartmental effects of the gut microbiome on mouse metabolic phenotypes. *Mol Syst Biol* 2008; 4: 219.
73. Swann JR, et al. Systemic gut microbial modulation of bile acid metabolism in host tissue compartments. *Proc Natl Acad Sci USA* 2010; 108 (Suppl): 4523–4530.
74. Cho I et al. Antibiotics in early life alter the murine colonic microbiome and adiposity. *Nature* 2012; 488: 621–626.
75. Graessler J et al. Metagenomic sequencing of the human gut microbiome before and after bariatric surgery in obese patients with type 2 diabetes: correlation with inflammatory and metabolic parameters. *Pharmacogenomics J* 2012; In press.
76. Mezza T et al. Vitamin D deficiency: a new risk factor for type 2 diabetes? *Ann Nutr Metab* 2012; 61: 337–348.

77. Forouhi NG et al. Circulating 25-hydroxyvitamin D concentration and the risk of type 2 diabetes: results from the European Prospective Investigation into Cancer (EPIC)- Norfolk cohort and updated meta analysis of prospective studies. *Diabetologia* 2012; 55: 2173–2182.

78. George PS et al. Effect of vitamin D supplementation on glycaemic control and insulin resistance: a systematic review and meta-analysis. *Diabet Med* 2012; 29: e142–e150.

79. Zhou QG et al. 1,25-dihydroxyvitamin D improved the free fatty acid induced insulin resistance in cultured C2C12 cells. *Diabetes Metab Res Rev* 2008; 24: 459–464.

80. Ayesha I et al. Vitamin D deficiency reduces insulin secretion and turnover in rats. *Diabetes Nutr Metab* 2001; 14: 78–84.

81. Barengolts E. Vitamin D and prebiotics may benefit the intestinal microbacteria and improve glucose homeostasis in prediabetes and type 2 diabetes. *Endocr Pract* 2013; May-Jun; 19(3): 497–510.

82. Rajagopalan S, Brook RD. Air pollution and type 2 diabetes: mechanistic insights. *Diabetes* 2012; 61: 3037–3045.

83. Oliveira D et al. Metabolic alterations in pregnant women: gestational diabetes. *J Pediatr Endocr Met* 2012; 25: 835–842.

84. Barbour LA et al. Cellular mechanisms for insulin resistance in normal pregnancy and gestational diabetes. *Diabetes Care* 2007; 30 (Suppl 2): S112–S119.

85. Ramos-Levi AM et al. Risk factors for gestational diabetes mellitus in a large population of women living in Spain: implications for preventative strategies. *Int J Endocrinol* 2012; 2012: 312529.

86. England LJ et al. Preventing type 2 diabetes: public health implications for women with a history of gestational diabetes mellitus. *Am J Obstet Gynecol* 2009; 200: 365.e1-8.

87. Catalano PM et al. Carbohydrate metabolism during pregnancy in control subjects and women with gestational diabetes. *Am J Physiol* 1993; 264: E60–E67.

88. Catalano PM et al. Longitudinal changes in glucose metabolism during pregnancy in obese women with normal glucose tolerance and gestational diabetes mellitus. *Am J Obstet Gynecol* 1999; 180: 903–916.

89. Kuhl C. Etiology and pathogenesis of gestational diabetes. *Diabetes Care* 1998; 21 (Suppl 2); B19–B26.

90. Brelje TC et al. Effect of homologous placental lactogens, prolactins, and growth hormones on islet B-cell division and insulin secretion in rat, mouse and human islets: implications for placental lactogen regulation of islet function during pregnancy. *Endocrinology* 1993; 132: 879–887.

91. Handwerger S, Freemark M. The roles of placental growth hormone and placental lactogen in the regulation of human fetal growth and development. *J Pediatr Endocrinol Metab* 2000; 13: 343–356.

92. Friedman JE et al. Increased skeletal muscle tumor necrosis factor alpha and impaired insulin signaling persist in obese women with diabetes mellitus 1 yr. postpartum. *Diabetes* 2008; 57: 606–613.

93. Ranheim T et al. Adiponectin is reduced in gestational diabetes in normal weight women. *Acta Obstet Gynecol Scand* 2004; 83: 341–347.

94. Catalano PM et al. Downregulated IRS1 and PPAR gamma in obese women with gestational diabetes: relationship to FFA during pregnancy. *Am J Physiol Endocrinol Metab* 2002; 282: E522–E533.

95. Alzaim M, Wood RJ. Vitamin D and gestational diabetes. *Nutr Rev* 2013; 71: 158–167.

96. Zhang C et al. Maternal plasma 25-hydroxyvitamin D concentrations and the risk of gestational diabetes mellitus. *PLoS One* 2008; 3:e3753.

97. Rudnicki PM, Molsted-Pederson L. Effect of 1,25-dihyroxycholecalciferol on glucose metabolism in gestational diabetes mellitus. *Diabetologia* 1997; 40: 40–44.

98. Giuffrida FM, Reis AF. Genetic and clinical characteristics of maturity-onset diabetes of the young. *Diabetes Obes Metab* 2005; 318: 326.
99. Fujiwara M et al. Detection and characterization of two novel mutations in the *HNF4A* gene in maturity-onset diabetes of the young type 1 in two Japanese families. *Horm Res Paediatr* 2013; 79: 220–226.
100. Yamagata K et al. Mutations in the hepatocyte nuclear factor 1 alpha gene in maturity onset diabetes of the young (MODY3. *Nature* 1996; 384: 455–458.
101. Froguel P et al. Close linkage of glucokinase locus on chromosome 7p to early onset non insulin dependent diabetes mellitus. *Nature* 1992; 356: 162–164.
102. Vionnet N et al. Nonsense mutation in the glucokinase gene causes early onset non-insulin dependent diabetes mellitus. *Nature* 1992; 356: 721–722.
103. Yamagata K et al. Mutations in the hepatocyte nuclear factor 4a gene in maturity onset diabetes of the young (MODY1). *Nature* 1996; 384: 458–460.
104. Horikawa Y et al. Mutation in hepatocyte nuclear factor-1beta gene (TCF2) associated with MODY. *Nat Genet* 1997; 17: 384–385.
105. Stoffers DA et al. Early onset type II diabetes mellitus (MODY4). *Nat Genet* 1997; 17: 138–139.
106. Malecki MT et al. Mutations in NEUROD1 are associated with the development of type 2 diabetes mellitus. *Nat Genet* 1999; 23: 323–328.
107. Kavvoura FK, Owen KR. Maturity onset diabetes of the young: clinical characteristics, diagnosis and management. *Pediatr Endocrinol Rev* 2012; 10: 234–242.
108. Partensky C. Toward a better understanding of pancreatic ductal adenocarcinoma: glimmers of hope? *Pancreas* 2012; 42: 729–739.
109. Yadav D, Lowenfels AB. The epidemiology of pancreatitis and pancreatic cancer. *Gastroenterology* 2013; 144: 1252–1261.
110. Staeva TP et al. Recent lessons learned from prevention and recent-onset type 1 diabetes immunotherapy trials. *Diabetes* 2013; 62: 1–17.
111. Knowler WC et al. Reduction in the incidence of type 2 diabetes with lifestyle intervention or metformin. *New Engl J Med* 2002; 346: 393–403.

# Chapter 2

# Classification, epidemiology, diagnosis, and risk factors of diabetes

*Jeffrey M. Curtis, MD, MPH*
*and William C. Knowler, MD, DrPH*

## Introduction

Diabetes mellitus is a heterogeneous group of metabolic disorders grouped together due to their common feature of hyperglycemia. The incidence and prevalence of diabetes have increased markedly in recent decades, mostly due to increases in type 2 diabetes rates, which have paralleled the increasing rates of obesity in the developed world during the same time. The increasing prevalence of diabetes is important because of the associated morbidity and mortality and the associated costs, in terms of both the personal cost of decreased quality of life and the economic impact of providing health care to a growing population with a chronic disease and the accompanying loss of productivity.

The fact that diabetes mellitus is more than one disease has important implications. The age and setting of onset, the mechanism responsible for elevated blood glucose, and the expected complications of one type of diabetes mellitus may be different from those in another type. Therefore, the approaches to treatment for different types of diabetes differ. Thus, accurately classifying a particular patient's diabetes facilitates choice of the most effective glucose-lowering treatment and interventions to prevent complications.

## Classification

The current nomenclature for diabetes mellitus was formalized by the American Diabetes Association in 1997 [1]. At that time the older terms insulin-dependent diabetes mellitus (IDDM) and non-insulin-dependent diabetes mellitus (NIDDM) were eliminated due to the confusion they caused over misclassifying patients on the basis of their treatment rather than on the pathophysiology of their particular disease. Rather, the terms type 1 and type 2 diabetes mellitus were adopted for the most common types of diabetes mellitus.

The overwhelming majority of cases of diabetes mellitus can be placed in one of three categories: type 1, type 2, or gestational. A fourth category includes diabetes caused by other factors, including medicines (some medicines used to treat HIV infection and agents used to prevent rejection after organ transplant, for example), genetic defects affecting

*Diabetes Mellitus and Oral Health: An Interprofessional Approach*, First Edition. Edited by Ira B. Lamster.
© 2014 John Wiley & Sons, Inc. Published 2014 by John Wiley & Sons, Inc.

insulin production or action, and other insults to the pancreas that cause a secondary inability to secrete insulin appropriately.

Type 1 diabetes, which constitutes less than 10% of all diabetes mellitus cases, is characterized by marked or absolute deficiency of insulin production by the β cells of the pancreatic islets of Langerhans. Because insulin is required for most cells in the body to take up glucose, which they use to fuel metabolic processes, this insulin deficiency results in glucose remaining extracellular, including in the blood. The hyperglycemia of diabetes mellitus occurs while the cells are starved for fuel due to their inability to internalize the glucose that is just outside their cell membranes. Type 1 diabetes requires treatment with insulin for the patient to survive.

The insulin deficiency of type 1 diabetes is usually caused by T-cell—mediated autoimmune destruction of β cells, as discussed in Chapter 1. Due to the technical and ethical limitations of obtaining pancreatic biopsy specimens from humans with type 1 diabetes, much of what is known about the pathophysiology of the disease has been learned from mouse models, most often the nonobese diabetic (NOD) mouse [2]. In NOD mice, activation of autoreactive T lymphocytes is the main pathway to β cell destruction and the resulting insulin deficiency.

Type 1 diabetes can occur at any time in a person's life. In fact, at least one study [3] has shown that the incidence of type 1 diabetes may be stable or possibly even increase with age (Figure 2.1). However, it characteristically is associated with rapid onset in childhood, when it is often first recognized when the afflicted child develops diabetic ketoacidosis, a life-threatening complication associated with dramatically high blood glucose levels. For unknown reasons, when type 1 diabetes occurs later in life, its onset is usually slower, sometimes making it difficult to distinguish from type 2 diabetes.

Type 2 diabetes, which accounts for approximately 90% of diabetes mellitus in the developed world, is characterized by a combination of insulin resistance and β cell failure, both of which are required for the disease to develop. Normally insulin sensitive cells throughout the body, most notably adipose, skeletal muscle, and liver, become less sensitive to insulin, which results in the β cells secreting larger quantities of insulin to overcome the resistance and prevent hyperglycemia. Eventually the β cells are no longer able to overcome the insulin resistance, and hyperglycemia results. Insulin resistance is an early pathophysiologic derangement in the development of type 2 diabetes. Whether β cell failure begins simultaneously or develops after insulin resistance has not been definitively shown; however, some predisposition to β cell failure may predate even the development of insulin resistance [4].

The insulin resistance characteristic of type 2 diabetes tends to occur more frequently in more obese people, which is why rates of both obesity and type 2 diabetes have risen in parallel over recent decades. However, even lean people can develop insulin resistance and type 2 diabetes, and some obese people remain insulin sensitive and do not develop diabetes. This incomplete association of obesity with insulin resistance and diabetes suggests that other factors are at play, which has been interpreted as indirect evidence for a genetic component to the cause of type 2 diabetes. However, the strength of the association between obesity and type 2 diabetes, even if it is incomplete, suggests that the primary causes are environmental, as will be discussed under risk factors.

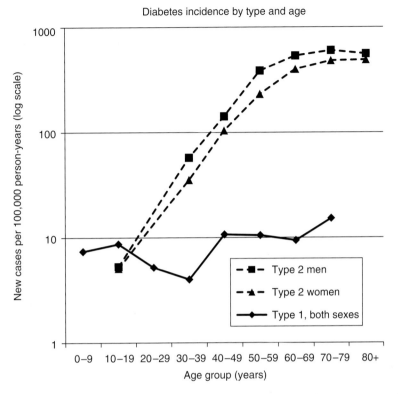

**Figure 2.1**   Incidence of diabetes by type and age. The definitions of diabetes type used for the data represented here are not those used currently for diagnosing or classifying diabetes; however, they provide an estimate of the incidence of diabetes by type in the Rochester, Minnesota, area from 1945 to 1969. Glucose criteria were the same regardless of type of diabetes diagnosed. Type 1 diabetes (IDDM in the original publication) was defined as requiring insulin therapy, evidence of ketosis-proneness, and relative weight less than 1.2; type 2 (NIDDM in the original publication) was defined as relative weight of 1.2 or more and/or no evidence of ketosis, regardless of type of therapy. Relative weight was calculated from recommended height-weight tables. Due to small numbers, the rates shown for the youngest three age groups (0–9, 10–19, and 20–29 years) were collapsed into a single average value at the middle age range, consistent with the original publication. Data from Melton LJ, Palumbo PJ, Chu CP. Incidence of diabetes mellitus by clinical type. *Diabetes Care* 1983; 6: 75–86.

In most cases, distinguishing between type 1 and type 2 diabetes is not difficult. People with type 1 diabetes tend to be leaner at the onset of the disease, and this form of diabetes is more common than type 2 diabetes in younger people. Those with type 2 diabetes tend to be older and heavier. However, the obesity epidemic has begun to affect children, and with childhood obesity has come a trend toward younger people developing type 2 diabetes. Also, as mentioned above, sometimes lean people develop insulin resistance and type 2 diabetes. Thus, in some cases, making the distinction between type 1 and type 2 diabetes can be difficult. Patients with type 2 diabetes sometimes require insulin to control their blood glucose; however, the use of insulin does not change the type of diabetes they have. The classification scheme is based on the pathophysiologic defect causing hyperglycemia, not on the type of treatment used.

In contrast with the absolute insulin deficiency characteristic of type 1 diabetes, people with type 2 diabetes continue to make insulin, albeit at a rate that does not overcome their insulin resistance sufficiently to normalize blood glucose levels [4]. Therefore, measuring circulating insulin levels would seem to be an easy way to distinguish type 1 from type 2 diabetes. However, insulin administered as a medicine, necessary for the survival of a patient with type 1 diabetes, would be measured and result in a false negative test for insulin deficiency. In addition, insulin has historically been difficult to measure routinely as a clinical test. Therefore, simply measuring insulin levels in a newly diabetic person has not been an effective method to distinguish between type 1 and type 2 diabetes in cases in which the diagnosis is not obvious. However, another protein, the C peptide, can be measured as a surrogate for endogenous insulin and can aid in making the correct diagnosis. The C peptide is part of the initial polypeptide chain that eventually is processed into insulin. It is cleaved from the rest of the chain and remains in the secretory granules within the β cells until it is secreted, in equimolar amounts, with insulin. The C peptide is relatively easy to measure in a clinical laboratory. If the level of C peptide in the patient's blood is undetectable or very low, a diagnosis of type 1 diabetes is suggested. If the level of C peptide is normal or high, despite hyperglycemia, then type 2 diabetes is more likely.

Gestational diabetes is defined as impaired glucose regulation (elevated fasting glucose or abnormal glucose tolerance) that develops or is first recognized during pregnancy [5, 6]. This definition leaves open the possibility that some women diagnosed with gestational diabetes may have had preexisting diabetes (of any type) that was not recognized prior to pregnancy. Because pregnancy is a time of more frequent contact with health care providers, and because screening for diabetes in pregnancy is common, it is likely that some women with diabetes that predated their pregnancy are first diagnosed during pregnancy and categorized as having gestational diabetes despite having diabetes that could have been diagnosed prior to pregnancy had the women been tested.

As is discussed later, gestational diabetes is diagnosed with lower blood glucose thresholds than diabetes mellitus outside pregnancy. Therefore, a nonpregnant woman with nondiabetic glucose test results who becomes pregnant could be diagnosed with gestational diabetes even with no change in her glucose concentrations. However, pregnancy is believed to be a time of increased insulin resistance [7], so it may be a time when women with a predisposition to hyperglycemia, as a result of either insulin resistance or β cell defects, even if subclinical outside pregnancy, may develop sufficient hyperglycemia to be diagnosed with gestational diabetes. Indeed, the first criteria for diagnosing gestational diabetes [8] were designed to predict those women who would develop type 2 diabetes after pregnancy. After the pregnancy, women who had gestational diabetes should be reclassified as having type 1 diabetes, type 2 diabetes, another type of diabetes, or not having diabetes. Therefore, gestational diabetes is not a "type" of diabetes in the same sense as the other types, but a designation of the condition under which diabetes or impaired glucose regulation is first diagnosed.

Other, rarer types of diabetes mellitus include those caused by single gene mutations affecting β cell function. These genetic defects are inherited in an autosomal dominant fashion and cause maturity onset diabetes of the young (MODY), with onset usually in adolescence or early adulthood. MODY generally is not associated with insulin resistance or autoimmunity against insulin or islet cells. Other conditions that damage the pancreas, including trauma, pancreatitis, cystic fibrosis, and pancreatic carcinoma, can destroy β cells and lead to diabetes from insulin deficiency. While technically not type 1 diabetes, these rare types of diabetes are treated with exogenous insulin just as type 1 diabetes would be.

## Epidemiology

A report [9] published in 2013, including data from the 2005–2010 National Health and Nutrition Examination Survey (NHANES), stated that the prevalence of diabetes during this period in the U.S. population aged at least 20 years was 12.1%, with 8.2% previously diagnosed and 3.9% undiagnosed. This overall prevalence represents a 45% increase from 1988. The figure for previously diagnosed diabetes was based on self-reports to questionnaires. The undiagnosed figure was based on a combination of fasting plasma glucose and HbA1c. This report did not distinguish between the types of diabetes; however, presumably, the large majority was type 2. Using HbA1c alone to detect diabetes in the NHANES population resulted in a lower prevalence.

The Centers for Disease Control and Prevention (CDC) reported [10] in 2011 that approximately 25.9 million Americans, or 8.3% of the U.S. population, had diabetes, of whom 7 million had not been diagnosed. The difference between this figure and the 12.1% cited in the previous paragraph is due to methodological differences in the calculation and, importantly, because this latter figure includes those under 20 years of age, in whom diabetes is less prevalent. Approximately 215,000 of those under 20 years of age had diabetes, whereas 10.9 million of those over 65 (26.9%) did. Among non-Hispanic blacks over 20 years of age, 18.7% had diabetes, whereas the figure was 10.2% for non-Hispanic whites. American Indians and Alaska Natives also had a disproportionately high prevalence of diabetes, at 14.2%. However, regional differences were striking: Alaska Native adults had a prevalence of only 5.5%, whereas American Indian adults in southern Arizona had a prevalence of 33.5%.

The CDC tracks diabetes and obesity prevalence by county throughout the United States. The most recently available maps (Figure 2.2) provide a visual indicator of the strong association of geographic areas with high prevalence rates of diabetes and obesity.

As is discussed in more detail later, "prediabetes" is defined by abnormalities of fasting glucose, two-hour post-load glucose, or HbA1c that do not meet diagnostic levels for diabetes. The CDC estimates that 35% of the U.S. population over 20 years of age (79 million Americans) has prediabetes, based on fasting glucose or HbA1c levels obtained in the National Health and Nutrition Examination Survey, the National Health Interview Survey, data from the Indian Health Service, and 2010 U.S. resident population estimates [10]. The estimated prevalence of prediabetes in those over 65 years of age is 50%. Prediabetes does not have the dramatic racial/ethnic differences in prevalence that diabetes has, with estimated prevalence among adults being 35% for non-Hispanic whites, 35% for non-Hispanic blacks, 36% for Mexican Americans, and 20% for American Indians. It should be noted, however, that the data source and method used to estimate the prevalence for American Indians was different from those used for the other racial/ethnic groups.

(A)

Age-adjusted county-level estimates of diagnosed diabetes among adults aged ≥ 20 years:
United States 2010

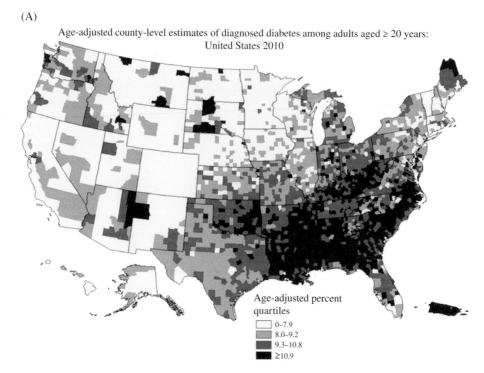

Age-adjusted percent
quartiles

- 0–7.9
- 8.0–9.2
- 9.3–10.8
- ≥10.9

Figure 2.2A   Age-adjusted prevalence of diagnosed diabetes among U.S. adults.

(B)

Age-adjusted county-level estimates of obesity among adults aged ≥ 20 years:
United States 2010

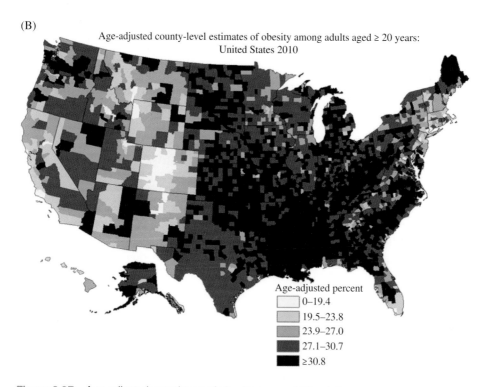

Age-adjusted percent

- 0–19.4
- 19.5–23.8
- 23.9–27.0
- 27.1–30.7
- ≥30.8

Figure 2.2B   Age-adjusted prevalence of obesity among U.S. adults.

The CDC figures cited above include both type 1 and type 2 diabetes; however, the large majority is type 2 [10]. Among people younger than 20 years, type 1 diabetes remains more common. In children under 10 years of age, 19.7 new cases of type 1 diabetes occur per 100,000 children per year, compared with 0.4 new cases of type 2 diabetes per 100,000 children per year. Among those between 10 and 20 years of age, 18.6 new cases of type 1 diabetes are diagnosed per 100,000 youth per year, compared with 8.5 cases per year of type 2 diabetes.

According to the CDC [10], gestational diabetes occurs in 2–10% of pregnancies in the U.S., which is consistent with the estimates of 1.7–11.6% from Schneider [11], whose figures were for the world's advanced economies, not just the United States. Based on data from the Hyperglycemia and Adverse Pregnancy Outcomes (HAPO) study [12], and using International Association of Diabetes in Pregnancy Study Groups (IAPDSG) criteria [13] that diagnose more women than do many previous criteria, the prevalence of gestational diabetes in the United States is estimated to be 18%. Of women diagnosed with gestational diabetes, 5–10% are believed to have type 2 diabetes that was present but not diagnosed before pregnancy [10].

## Diagnosis

The diagnostic criteria for diabetes mellitus for nonpregnant patients [6] (Table 2.1) include HbA1c at least 6.5% (48 mmol/mol), fasting plasma glucose at least 126 mg/dl (7.0 mmol/l), or 2-hour plasma glucose at least 200 mg/dl (11.1 mmol/l) after drinking the equivalent of 75 gm of anhydrous glucose dissolved in water. HbA1c is a test that estimates the average plasma glucose over the previous two to three months, although the result is a percentage of the circulating adult hemoglobin (HbA) that is glycated, rather than an estimate of average glucose in mg/dl or mmol/l. Any of these test results, if positive, should be confirmed by repeat testing to make the diagnosis. However, if a patient has symptoms of hyperglycemia or is in a hyperglycemic crisis, a random plasma

Table 2.1   Diagnostic criteria[1] for diabetes and prediabetes in nonpregnant people.[2]

| | Normal if all values are as shown below | Prediabetes if any one value is as shown below, but diabetes criteria not met | Diabetes if any one value is as shown below |
|---|---|---|---|
| FPG (mg/dl)[3] | <100 | 100–125 | ≥126 |
| Two-hour PG (mg/dl)[4] | <140 | 140–199 | ≥200 |
| HbA1c (%) | <5.7 | 5.7–6.4 | ≥6.5 |

[1]Diagnosing diabetes (but not prediabetes) requires repeating the abnormal test on another day unless the patient has HbA1c ≥6.5% and either FPG or two-hour PG exceeds the diabetes threshold or if random plasma glucose ≥200 mg/dl with symptoms of hyperglycemia.
[2]Adapted from American Diabetes Association. Diagnosis and classification of diabetes mellitus. *Diabetes Care* 2013; 36 (suppl 1): S67–S74.
[3]Fasting plasma glucose.
[4]Plasma glucose obtained two hours after ingestion of 75 gm of anhydrous glucose dissolved in water, or an equivalent glucose load.

glucose, without regard to the timing of the last meal, of at least 200 mg/dl (11.1 mmol/l) is diagnostic, without the need for confirmation testing.

These fasting and two-hour plasma glucose criteria were established on the basis of increased risk of diabetic retinopathy, which is, using currently available diagnostic methods, the complication most specific to diabetes. Figure 2.3 shows prevalence of retinopathy by glucose value, with the glucose values shown on the X axis divided into deciles of the population to allow superimposition of the curves for fasting and 2-hour glucose and HbA1c. The prevalence of retinopathy remains low through most of the glucose distribution, by any of the three tests, until it begins to increase in the second highest decile and increases exponentially thereafter. There is no discrete inflection point; however, the diagnostic cutpoints were established to approximate an inflection point on these curves. The association of 2-hour plasma glucose and retinopathy was first shown [14] among the Pima Indians of central Arizona, a population with a very high prevalence of type 2 diabetes. In the same population the similar association with the other glycemic measures (fasting plasma glucose and HbA1c) by deciles was then shown [15] and subsequently confirmed in an Egyptian population [16] and in a broader cross-section of U.S. adults [1], using data from NHANES III. The HbA1c diagnostic

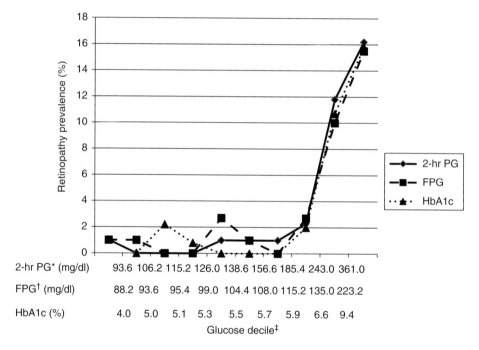

**Figure 2.3**   Retinopathy prevalence by deciles of fasting plasma glucose, two-hour plasma glucose, and HbA1c.
*Plasma glucose two hours after a 75-gm oral glucose load.
†Fasting plasma glucose.
‡The numbers shown are the boundaries between deciles.
Adapted from McCance DR, Hanson RL, Charles MA, *et al.* Comparison of tests for glycated hemoglobin and fasting and two hour plasma glucose concentrations as diagnostic methods for diabetes. *BMJ* 1994; 308: 1323–1328.

threshold was added by the American Diabetes Association in 2010 [17] after having been recommended the previous year by the International Expert Committee [18]. The delay in acceptance of the HbA1c as a diagnostic test for diabetes was largely due to slow standardization of this test across laboratories and to its being influenced by non-glycemic factors including conditions that may alter the stability or type of hemoglobin, such as anemia and hemoglobinopathies.

Despite its somewhat higher laboratory cost, HbA1c as a diagnostic test has the advantage of offering a more stable view of glucose values over a longer period than is possible with any single plasma glucose result. It is also more convenient for patients and possibly less costly overall because it does not require fasting, ingestion of a glucose load, or properly timed phlebotomy. However, HbA1c results are affected by non-glycemic factors, mentioned above.

The American Diabetes Association [6] has also defined glucose and HbA1c ranges that are less than those diagnostic of diabetes but indicative of increased risk of developing diabetes (Table 2.1). The high-risk conditions defined by these values have been termed impaired fasting glucose (IFG) if based on the fasting value, impaired glucose tolerance (IGT) if based on the two-hour value from a 75-gm OGTT, or prediabetes if based on either of these or HbA1c. The term prediabetes may be misleading if it is erroneously understood to mean that progressing to diabetes is inevitable. In fact, the term merely defines a condition of heightened risk of developing diabetes. To be classified with prediabetes, a person must not meet diagnostic criteria for diabetes or have been previously diagnosed with diabetes but must have at least one glucose or HbA1c value within the high-risk range. The range that defines prediabetes is 100–125 mg/dl (5.6–6.9 mmol/l) for the fasting plasma glucose, 140–199 mg/dl (7.8–11 mmol/l) for the two-hour plasma glucose, and 5.7–6.4% for the HbA1c [6]. Each of these ranges is associated with an increased risk of developing diabetes; however, the lower limits do not indicate a threshold above which diabetes risk suddenly increases. The risk of diabetes increases progressively across the entire range of glucose values. Therefore, the specific lower limits of these prediabetes ranges are somewhat arbitrary. The fasting glucose lower bound (100 mg/dl) was lowered from 110 mg/dl in 2003 to make the prevalence of IFG similar to that of IGT. As with diabetes diagnostic criteria, the HbA1c range indicating prediabetes was first recommended by the American Diabetes Association in 2010 [17]. It is important to note that in each case, despite the lack of a clear lower limit at which risk begins to increase, a higher glucose or HbA1c value is associated with an increased risk of developing diabetes.

Different criteria are used to diagnose gestational diabetes. Further complicating the screening and diagnosis process during pregnancy, several organizations have recommended different screening procedures and diagnostic tests and cutpoints for gestational diabetes. Some of the various criteria used in the United States are shown in Table 2.2. Still more criteria, not shown here, are used in other countries. The American College of Obstetricians and Gynecologists (ACOG) [19] recommends that all women be screened for gestational diabetes, using either patient history and clinical risk factors or a non-fasting 50-gm oral glucose challenge with a single plasma glucose drawn one hour after the glucose drink. ACOG does not specify a screening cutpoint; however, in common practice, the 50-gm test is considered positive if the subsequent glucose value is at least 130 or 140 mg/dl, with either threshold being considered acceptable. After a positive

Table 2.2  Diagnostic criteria for gestational diabetes by different organizations.

| | ACOG[1] | | | IADPSG/ADA[2] | WHO[3] |
|---|---|---|---|---|---|
| | 50-gm screen | 100-gm OGTT[4] | | 75-gm OGTT[4] | 75-gm OGTT[4] |
| | | Carpenter and Coustan | NDDG[5] | | |
| FPG (mg/dl)[6] | | 95 | 105 | 92 | 126 |
| One-hour PG (mg/dl)[7] | 130 or 140 | 180 | 190 | 180 | |
| Two-hour PG (mg/dl)[8] | | 155 | 165 | 153 | 140 |
| Three-hour PG (mg/dl)[9] | | 140 | 145 | | |

[1] American College of Obstetricians and Gynecologists. To be diagnosed with gestational diabetes by ACOG criteria, a woman must meet at least two of the 100-gm OGTT glucose values, by either Carpenter and Coustan or NDDG criteria.
[2] International Association of Diabetes in Pregnancy Study Groups/American Diabetes Association. To be diagnosed with gestational diabetes by IADPSG/ADA criteria, a woman must meet at least one of the glucose values listed.
[3] World Health Organization. To be diagnosed with gestational diabetes by WHO criteria, a woman must meet at least one of the glucose values listed.
[4] Oral glucose tolerance test.
[5] National Diabetes Data Group.
[6] Fasting plasma glucose. All tests shown are performed with a fasting glucose except for the 50-gm screen, which is performed without regard to the timing of prior food intake. The 50-gm screen is not a diagnostic test, but a screening test that leads, if abnormal, to a3-hour OGTT, according to ACOG guidelines.
[7] Plasma glucose obtained one hour after ingestion of a glucose load.
[8] Plasma glucose obtained two hours after ingestion of a glucose load.
[9] Plasma glucose obtained three hours after ingestion of a glucose load.

screen, ACOG recommends that the woman undergo a 100-gm, three-hour oral glucose tolerance test (OGTT). ACOG allows the diagnosis to be made when a woman's plasma glucose meets either Carpenter and Coustan or National Diabetes Data Group (NDDG) thresholds. Of the four glucose values drawn in a three-hour OGTT, the woman must meet at least two to be diagnosed. The Carpenter and Coustan plasma glucose criteria are 95 mg/dl (5.3 mmol/l) fasting, 180 mg/dl (10.0 mmol/l) at one hour, 155 mg/dl (8.6 mmol/l) at two hours, and 140 mg/dl (7.8 mmol/l) at three hours. The NDDG criteria are 105 mg/dl (5.8 mmol/l) fasting, 190 mg/dl (10.6 mmol/l) at one hour, 165 mg/dl (9.2 mmol/l) at two hours, and 145 mg/dl (8 mmol/l) at three hours.

By contrast with the ACOG procedure, the International Association of the Diabetes and Pregnancy Study Groups (IADPSG) [13] in 2010 recommended a one-step screening/diagnostic test, using a two-hour, 75-gm OGTT, at 24–28 weeks of gestation in all women not previously diagnosed with diabetes, and that earlier screening with the same test be performed in women from high risk groups. The thresholds proposed by the IADPSG, diagnostic of gestational diabetes if any one is met, are 92 mg/dl (5.1 mmol/l) fasting, 180 mg/dl (10 mmol/l) at one hour, and 153 mg/dl (8.5 mmol/l) at two hours. These cutpoints are primarily based on results of the HAPO study [20], an observational study (without an intervention) that examined levels of maternal glycemia, measured by a 75-gm OGTT, in approximately 25,000 ethnically diverse pregnant women, and found that above these approximate cutpoints, the risk of exceeding the 90th percentile in birth weight, neonatal C-peptide level (a marker for insulin resistance), or neonatal percent body fat was nearly doubled, compared with the baseline population risk. These results agree with earlier findings [21–24] among Pima Indians who underwent similar 75-gm OGTTs and had long-term follow-up of both mothers and offspring.

The World Health Organization (WHO) recommends [25] that the same procedure used outside pregnancy (75-gm OGTT) be used during pregnancy, with gestational diabetes diagnosed when a woman's results meet or exceed the thresholds used for impaired glucose tolerance (two-hour plasma glucose at least 140 mg/dl [7.8 mmol/l]) or diabetes by fasting criteria (fasting plasma glucose at least 126 mg/dl [7 mmol/l]).

The ACOG criteria, initially proposed by O'Sullivan and Mahan [8], were developed for their ability to predict subsequent type 2 diabetes in pregnant women. They were not developed to prevent potential negative effects of diabetes during pregnancy. ACOG specifically does not endorse using the one-step screening and diagnostic test recommended by the IADPSG, in part because the recommendations are based on observational data rather than clinical trials demonstrating a clinical outcome benefit from revising the diagnostic criteria [19]. However, as mentioned above, the IADPSG criteria were developed to provide thresholds above which some of the complications of diabetic pregnancies are more likely. Whether interventions in women exceeding these thresholds will prevent adverse pregnancy outcomes or longer term metabolic outcomes in the mother or offspring has yet to be shown. The American Diabetes Association has adopted the IADPSG recommendations [26].

## Risk factors

The primary risk factor for diabetes mellitus is elevated blood glucose. While this statement seems circular, having elevated blood glucose, not high enough to be diagnostic of diabetes, indicates high short-term risk of developing diabetes. As described in the previous section, this high-risk condition is termed prediabetes [6]. The ranges of various glucose tests that define prediabetes are shown in Table 2.1.

Type 1 diabetes risk is increased by genetic factors, including certain HLA types. People at risk for type 1 diabetes can also often be identified by autoantibodies long in advance of hyperglycemia developing. However, routinely testing for such autoantibodies is not recommended because of the lack of effective preventive measures for those with autoantibodies.

Risk factors for type 2 diabetes and gestational diabetes are similar, although the prerequisite for the latter, pregnancy, is not required for the former. Important risk factors [26] for both include sedentary lifestyle, history of gestational diabetes in a previous pregnancy or of delivering a baby weighing over 9 pounds, cardiovascular disease, being a member of a high-risk racial or ethnic group, older age, hypertension, polycystic ovary syndrome, obesity, or a history of elevated blood glucose. Some racial and ethnic groups, especially indigenous populations of economically developed nations and some Pacific Islanders, are at particularly high risk of developing type 2 diabetes. Some of this racial/ethnic risk may be mediated by increased obesity, whether due to genetic or environmental factors. The risk conferred by a history of gestational diabetes merits some particular mention. Among women without type 2 diabetes predating pregnancy, an estimated 35–60% will develop diabetes over the 10–20 years following a pregnancy complicated by gestational diabetes [10].

Because type 2 diabetes rates have increased along with increasing rates of obesity, and because sedentary lifestyle is a risk factor for both type 2 diabetes and obesity, the availability of relatively inexpensive, calorie-dense food and the lack of need to exert strenuous effort on a regular basis (both recent phenomena in human history) are certainly factors in the development of type 2 diabetes. These risk factors, overconsumption and inadequate physical activity, are considered environmental, as opposed to genetic, factors. Western society has created an environment in which foods that predispose to obesity are available in large quantities and physical exertion, even for movement, is largely unnecessary.

A family history of type 2 diabetes could potentially impart risk through either genetic or shared environmental factors [27]. In fact, both appear to be important. The results [28] of a detailed search of the National Human Genome Research Institute's database conducted in July 2011 included more than 60 genetic regions robustly associated with type 2 diabetes. That number has certainly increased since the search was conducted, and it will likely continue to increase. However, the effect sizes from any individual genetic association discovered to date are small; therefore, genetic risk factors discovered to date explain only slightly more than 10% of the heritability of developing diabetes [29].

## Screening

Screening for a disease in asymptomatic people is only recommended if detecting the disease at an earlier stage or detecting a high-risk condition would allow an opportunity to favorably alter the eventual course of the disease. The American Diabetes Association currently recommends that relatives of people with type 1 diabetes be screened with antibody testing only in the context of a clinical research study [26]. More widespread screening for type 1 diabetes has not been shown to offer a clinical advantage to those screened. Therefore, screening for HLA types, serologic markers, or other potential risk factors for type 1 diabetes is not yet recommended [30].

In the case of type 2 diabetes, tests used for screening are also used for diagnosis, so screening could also be termed detection or simply testing. The American Diabetes Association recommends testing for type 2 diabetes in asymptomatic adults if they are overweight or obese (BMI equal to or greater than $25 \, kg/m^2$) and have one or more additional risk factors for diabetes [26] (listed in the previous section). Without additional risk factors, the association recommends that screening begin at age 45. If results are normal, the person should be retested every three years, or more frequently if his or her risk status is particularly high (e.g., the person has prediabetes). Any of the tests used for diagnosing diabetes (FPG, an OGTT with two-hour glucose, or HbA1c) could be used for testing asymptomatic people. However, providers should be aware that each of these tests may detect diabetes or prediabetes in different individuals. Detecting prediabetes provides an opportunity to intervene to prevent progression to diabetes. Diagnosing type 2 diabetes earlier in the course of the disease, through screening, allows the patient

and the diabetes treatment team to take specific, proven steps to prevent diabetes complications, as will be discussed in Chapter 3. Screening should take place in the health care
setting, where correct laboratory test interpretation, patient education, and follow-up
of results can occur. Screening in community settings is not recommended. Laboratory
instruments used for screening should be approved for such use. Glucometers used by
patients to self-monitor their blood glucose are not sufficiently accurate [31] and should
not be used for screening.

Screening for GDM is performed in association with diagnostic testing. Both are
covered under Diagnosis, above.

## Prevention

Effective methods for preventing type 1 diabetes have not yet been found. However, clinical
trials of immunosuppressive therapy before the onset of diabetes in those showing evidence
of autoimmunity toward the β cells may show promise [32].

Several clinical trials have shown that type 2 diabetes can be prevented, either through
a lifestyle intervention [33, 34] or with medicines [34–41]. The lifestyle interventions
that have proven effective in preventing diabetes have focused on weight loss through a
combination of caloric restriction (with emphasis on fat restriction) and physical activity.
Specifically, the intervention used by the Diabetes Prevention Program (DPP) [34]
attempted to induce a weight loss of at least 7% from the baseline. Participants in this
study were encouraged, through a 16-lesson curriculum with frequent follow-up with an
interventionist, to follow a low-fat, reduced calorie diet and to exercise at the intensity
of brisk walking for at least 150 minutes per week. Similarly, the Finnish Diabetes
Prevention Study (DPS) [33] had a goal of at least 5% weight loss, which participants
were encouraged to achieve through a reduction in fat intake to less than 30% of total
energy, a reduction in saturated fat intake to less than 10% of total energy, an increase
in fiber intake to at least 15 g/1,000 kcal consumed, and moderate exercise for at least
30 minutes daily. Coincidentally, the interventions in each of these two studies, which
were conducted in people with prediabetes, showed a 58% reduction in the incidence of
type 2 diabetes in the intervention group, compared with the control group.

The DPP also tested whether metformin, a medicine used to treat diabetes, would reduce
the incidence of diabetes, compared with the control group. Metformin's action is incom-
pletely understood; however, it is known to decrease hepatic glucose production and to
decrease insulin resistance. Participants in the metformin arm were treated with 850 mg of
metformin twice daily. They were not given the lifestyle intervention. This group experienced a 31% reduction in the incidence of diabetes. The youngest and heaviest participants
responded best to metformin. However, all subgroups of participants responded well to the
lifestyle intervention.

Several medications from the thiazolidinedione family (trogligazone [35, 36], pioglitazone [37, 38], and rosiglitazone [39]) have demonstrated the ability to prevent diabetes
in different populations. Unfortunately, each is associated with adverse effects that may
limit its usefulness. Thiazolidinediones work by improving insulin sensitivity, especially
in the muscles and liver. Troglitazone was removed from the U.S. market due to rare but

potentially fatal liver damage. Pioglitazone remains on the market but is associated with an increased risk of bladder cancer and worsening congestive heart failure [42]. Rosiglitazone also remains on the market but is used only rarely due to an association with cardiovascular events [43]. All of the thiazolidinediones cause weight gain. There may be a role for thiazolidinediones in preventing diabetes, but due to their associated risks, they are not commonly used for this purpose.

Orlistat, a gastrointestinal lipase inhibitor used for weight loss, was reported to decrease the incidence of diabetes by 37% in obese people with prediabetes, although the conclusion is uncertain because of the high drop-out rate in this study [40]. By blocking gastrointestinal lipase, orlistat works by decreasing the amount of fat absorbed in the intestines. Unfortunately, orlistat carries a high risk of gastrointestinal side effects that limit its use for either weight loss or diabetes prevention.

Another gastrointestinal enzyme blocker, acarbose, which inhibits $\alpha$-glucosidase and thereby decreases carbohydrate absorption in the gut, has also decreased the incidence of type 2 diabetes by 25% [41]. Possibly due to the gastrointestinal side effects of acarbose, the study showing its effectiveness in preventing diabetes was also limited by a high drop-out rate: 31% in the acarbose group and 19% in the placebo group.

Bariatric (weight loss) surgery is the most effective intervention to prevent diabetes currently available. The largest examination of bariatric surgery is the Swedish Obese Subjects (SOS) study, which has been conducted since 1987. For practical reasons, SOS is a non-randomized study comparing those undergoing gastric banding, vertical banded gastroplasty, or gastric bypass (together termed bariatric surgery or sometimes metabolic surgery), with a matched control group with similar levels of obesity and similar other characteristics, for various outcomes. A recent publication [44] from this cohort examined the effect of bariatric surgery in obese subjects without diabetes at the baseline on the development of diabetes over a follow-up period of up to 15 years. Bariatric surgery was associated with an 82% reduction in the incidence of diabetes (28.4 vs. 6.8 cases/1,000 person-years in the standard care and surgery groups, respectively). Eligibility for bariatric surgery in the United States is currently restricted by most payers to those who meet criteria [45] established in 1992 by the National Institutes of Health. These criteria require that people with a BMI between 35 and 40 kg/m$^2$ have at least one comorbid condition that would be expected to improve as a result of the surgery, for example, a cardiovascular disease risk factor. The SOS study group examined [46] the effect of bariatric surgery on those who met or did not meet the NIH criteria (NIH criteria are not inclusion criteria for the SOS study). They found that even in those who did not meet NIH criteria for bariatric surgery eligibility, diabetes incidence decreased by 67%, compared with those who did not undergo surgery.

Another important strategy that is beginning to be explored for preventing type 2 diabetes is intervention during pregnancy. Diabetes during pregnancy increases the risk of obesity and type 2 diabetes in the offspring of that pregnancy [47, 48]. If the offspring is a girl, then she is at increased risk of having diabetes during her pregnancy and increasing the risk of early-onset type 2 diabetes in her offspring (Figure 2.4). Intervening with the mother to prevent gestational diabetes or at least improve blood glucose levels during pregnancy to break this vicious cycle is being explored as one way to prevent a feared further increase in type 2 diabetes that may otherwise occur.

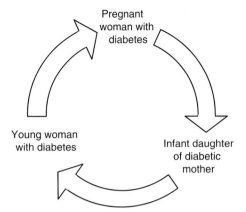

**Figure 2.4**   Vicious cycle of type 2 diabetes in mothers and daughters.
Adapted from Knowler WC, Pettitt DJ, Saad MF, *et al*. Diabetes mellitus in the Pima Indians:
incidence, risk factors, and pathogenesis. *Diabetes/Metabolism Rev* 1990; 6: 1–27.

Currently the type of diabetes for which prevention has proven most feasible is type 2 diabetes. To prevent this most common type of diabetes, lifestyle interventions focused on weight loss, medicines, and bariatric surgery all have compelling evidence of effectiveness, even among people at the highest risk for the disease. Choosing the best intervention for a particular patient is important. Both lifestyle intervention and bariatric surgery have the advantage of additionally improving cardiovascular disease risk factors. The lifestyle intervention used in the DPP and DPS is labor intensive. Participants in the DPP met individually with a case manager for a 16-session curriculum over the first 24 weeks of the study and then met monthly for the remainder of the study, with additional group sessions periodically [34]. The case managers helped them to identify and overcome barriers to healthy nutrition and regular exercise.

As described above, the medicines shown to prevent diabetes all have potential side effects. Thiazolidinediones induce weight gain. Rosiglitazone is suspected to increase the risk of cardiovascular events. Pioglitazone is associated with worsening congestive heart failure and bladder cancer [42], albeit at a low rate. Metformin, orlistat, and acarbose each can cause troubling gastrointestinal side effects that often limit their use. Bariatric surgery is costly and not universally available, although its proponents suggest that as a weight loss treatment overall, it is cost effective in the long term [49]. Many patients believe it to be an effort-free approach to weight loss. However, it requires a drastic lifestyle change that some patients find difficult over time, and it carries its own risk of complications.

## Conclusion

Diabetes mellitus is currently recognized as several different diseases, each with its own pathophysiologic basis, but all with the common abnormality of elevated blood glucose. By far the most common form of diabetes mellitus is type 2, which is associated with obesity, and which develops only in those with both insulin resistance and a defect in insulin secretion. Type 2 diabetes has become a common condition among U.S. adults, and it will likely become more common as the population ages. However, type 2 diabetes has been shown to be preventable by several interventions, including lifestyle changes focused on weight loss; certain medicines that improve insulin sensitivity, decrease hepatic glucose production, or decrease macronutrient absorption in the gut; and weight loss surgery. Much research is still needed to identify methods to prevent type 1 and gestational diabetes.

Additional discussion about prevention of diabetes mellitus can be found in chapters 1 and 4.

## Acknowledgment

This research was supported by the Intramural Research Program of the NIH, The National Institute of Diabetes and Digestive and Kidney Disease (NIDDK).

## References

1. The Expert Committee on the Diagnosis and Classification of Diabetes Mellitus. Report of the Expert Committee on the Diagnosis and Classification of Diabetes Mellitus. *Diabetes Care* 1997; 20: 1183–1197.
2. Anderson MS, Bluestone JA. The NOD mouse: a model of immune dysregulation. *Annu Rev Immunol* 2005; 23: 447–485.
3. Melton LJ, Palumbo PJ, Chu CP. Incidence of diabetes mellitus by clinical type. *Diabetes Care* 1983; 6: 75–86.
4. Weyer C, Bogardus C, Mott DM, et al. The natural history of insulin secretory dysfunction and insulin resistance in the paghogenesis of type 2 diabetes mellitus. *J Clin Invest* 1999; 104: 787–794.
5. ACOG Practice Bulletin. Clinical management guidelines for obstetrician-gynecologists. Number 30, September 2001. Gestational Diabetes. *Obstet Gynecol* 2001; 98: 525–38.
6. American Diabetes Association. Diagnosis and classification of diabetes mellitus. *Diabetes Care* 2013; 36 (suppl 1): S67–S74.
7. Barbour LA, McCurdy CE, Hernandez TL, et al. Cellular mechanisms for insulin resistance in normal pregnancy and gestational diabetes. *Diabetes Care* 2007; 30: S112–S119.
8. O'Sullivan JB, Mahan CM. Criteria for the oral glucose tolerance test in pregnancy. *Diabetes* 1964; 13: 278–285.
9. Cheng YJ, Imperatore G, Geiss LS, et al. Secular changes in the age-specific prevalence of diabetes among U.S. adults. *Diabetes Care* 2013 (Published ahead of print online May 1, 2013).
10. Centers for Diseases Control and Prevention. *National diabetes fact sheet: national estimates and general information on diabetes and prediabetes in the United States, 2011*. Atlanta, GA: U.S. Department of Health and Human Services, Centers for Disease Control and Prevention, 2011.
11. Schneider S, Bock C, Wetzel M, et al. The prevalence of gestational diabetes in advanced economies. *J Perinat Med* 2012; 40: 511–520.
12. Coustan DR, Lowe LP, Metzger BE, et al. The Hyperglycemia and Adverse Pregnancy Outcome (HAPO) study: paving the way for new diagnostic criteria for gestational diabetes mellitus. *Am J Obstet Gynecol* 2010; 202: 654.e1–6.

13. International Association of Diabetes and Pregnancy Study Groups Consensus Panel. International Association of Diabetes and Pregnancy Study Groups recommendations on the diagnosis and classification of hyperglycemia in pregnancy. *Diabetes Care* 2010; 33: 676–682.

14. Dorf A, Ballintine EJ, Bennett PH, et al. Retinopathy in Pima Indians: Relationships to glucose level, duration of diabetes, age at diagnosis and age at examination in a population with a high prevalence of diabetes mellitus. *Diabetes* 1976; 25: 554–560.

15. McCance DR, Hanson RL, Charles MA, et al. Comparison of tests for glycated hemoglobin and two hour plasma glucose concentrations as diagnostic methods for diabetes. *BMJ* 1994; 308: 1323–1328.

16. Enelgau MM, Thompson TJ, Herman WH, et al. Comparison of fasting and 2-hour glucose and HbA1c levels for diagnosing diabetes: diagnostic criteria and performance revisited. *Diabetes Care* 1997; 20: 785–791.

17. American Diabetes Association. Diagnosis and classification of diabetes mellitus. *Diabetes Care* 2010; 33 (suppl 1): S62–S69.

18. International Expert Committee. International Expert Committee report on the role of the A1c assay in the diagnosis of diabetes. *Diabetes Care* 2009; 32: 1327–1334.

19. American College of Obstetricians and Gynecologists. Screening and diagnosis of gestational diabetes mellitus. Committee Opinion No. 504. *Obstet Gynecol* 2011; 118: 751–753.

20. HAPO Study Cooperative Research Group, Metzger BE, Lowe LP, Dyer AR, et al. Hyperglycemia and Adverse Pregnancy Outcome (HAPO) Study Cooperative Research Group. Hyperglycemia and adverse pregnancy outcomes. *N Engl J Med* 2008; 358: 1991–2002.

21. Pettitt DJ, Knowler WC, Baird HR, et al. Gestational diabetes: Infant and maternal complications of pregnancy in relation to third-trimester glucose tolerance in the Pima Indians. *Diabetes Care* 1980; 3: 458–464.

22. Pettitt DJ, Baird HR, Aleck KA, et al. Excessive obesity in offspring of Pima Indian women with diabetes during pregnancy. *New Engl J Med* 1983; 308: 242–245.

23. Pettitt DJ, Bennett PH, Knowler WC, et al. Gestational diabetes and impaired glucose tolerance during pregnancy: Long-term effects on obesity and glucose tolerance in the offspring. *Diabetes* 1985; 34 (suppl 2): 119–122

24. Pettitt DJ, Bennett PH, Saad MF, et al. Abnormal glucose tolerance during pregnancy in Pima Indian women: Long-term effects on offspring. *Diabetes* 1991; 40 suppl 2: 126–130.

25. Alberti KG, Zimmet PZ. Definition, diagnosis and classification of diabetes mellitus and its complications. Part 1: diagnosis and classification of diabetes mellitus provisional report of a WHO consultation. *Diabet Med* 1998; 15: 539–553.

26. American Diabetes Association. Standards of medical care in diabetes—2013. *Diabetes Care* 2013; 36 (suppl 1): S11–S66.

27. Groop L, Pociot F. Genetics of diabetes—Are we missing the genes or the disease? *Mol Cell Endocrinol* 2013 (Published ahead of print online April 13, 2013).

28. Ntzani EE, Kavvoura FK. Genetic risk factors for type 2 diabetes: Insights from the emerging genomic evidence. *Curr Vasc Pharmacol* 2012; 10: 147–155.

29. Morris AP, Voight BF, Teslovich TM, et al. Large-scale association analysis provides insights into the genetic architecture and pathophysiology of type 2 diabetes. *Nat Genet* 2012; 44: 981–990.

30. Todd JA, Knip M, Mathieu C. Strategies for the prevention of autoimmune type 1 diabetes. *Diabet Med* 2011; 28: 1141–1143.

31. Walsh J, Roberts R, Vigersky RA, et al. New criteria for assessing the accuracy of blood glucose monitors meeting, October 28, 2011. *J Diabetes Sci Technol* 2012; 6: 466–74.

32. Thrower SL, Bingley PJ. Prevention of type 1 diabetes. *Br Med Bull* 2011; 99: 73–88.

33. Tuomilehto J, Lindström J, Eriksson JG, et al., for the Finnish Diabetes Prevention Study Group. Prevention of type 2 diabetes mellitus by changes in lifestyle among subjects with impaired glucose tolerance. *New Engl J Med* 2001; 344: 1343–1350.
34. Knowler WC, Barrett-Conner E, Fowler SE, et al., for the Diabetes Prevention Program Research Group. Reduction in the incidence of type 2 diabetes with lifestyle intervention or metformin. *New Engl J Med* 2002; 346: 393–403.
35. Buchanan TA, Xiang AH, Peters RK, et al. Preservation of pancreatic β-cell function and prevention of type 2 diabetes by pharmacological treatment of insulin resistance in high-risk Hispanic women. *Diabetes* 2002; 51: 2796–2803.
36. Knowler WC, Hamman RF, Edelstein SL, et al., for the Diabetes Prevention Program Research Group. Prevention of type 2 diabetes with troglitazone in the Diabetes Prevention Program. *Diabetes* 2005; 54: 1150–1156.
37. Xiang AH, Peters RK, Kjos SL, et al. Effect of pioglitazone on pancreatic β-cell function and diabetes risk in Hispanic women with prior gestational diabetes. *Diabetes* 2006; 55: 517–522.
38. DeFronzo RA, Tripathy D, Schwenke DC, et al. Pioglitazone for diabetes prevention in impaired glucose tolerance. *New Engl J Med* 2011; 364: 1104–1115.
39. The DREAM (Diabetes REduction Assessment with ramipril and rosiglitazone Medication) Trial Investigators. Effect of rosiglitazone on the frequency of diabetes in patients with impaired glucose tolerance or impaired fasting glucose: a randomised controlled trial. *Lancet* 2008; 368: 1096–1105.
40. Torgerson JS, Hauptman J, Boldrin MN, et al. XENical in the prevention of diabetes in obese subjects (XENDOS) study: a randomized study of orlistat as an adjunct to lifestyle changes for the prevention of type 2 diabetes in obese patients. *Diabetes Care* 2004; 27: 155–161.
41. Chiasson JL, Josse RG, Gomis R, et al., for the STOP-NIDDM Trial Research Group. Acarbose for prevention of type 2 diabetes mellitus: the STOP-NIDDM randomized trial. *Lancet* 2002; 359: 2072–2077.
42. Lewis JD, Ferrara A, Peng T, et al. Risk of bladder cancer among diabetic patients treated with pitolgitazone: interim report of a longitudinal cohort study. *Diabetes Care* 2011; 34: 916–922.
43. Nissen SE, Wolski K. Effect of rosiglitazone on the risk of myocardial infarction and death from cardiovascular causes. *New Engl J Med* 2007; 356: 2457–2471.
44. Carlsson LMS, Peltonen M, Ahlin S, et al. Bariatric surgery and prevention of type 2 diabetes in Swedish obese subjects. *New Engl J Med* 2012; 367: 695–704.
45. Gastrointestinal surgery for severe obesity: national Institutes of Health consensus development conference statement. *Am J Clin Nutr* 1992; 55: 615S–619S.
46. Sjöholm K, Anveden Å, Peltonen M, et al. Evaluation of current eligibility criteria for bariatric surgery: Diabetes prevention and risk factor changes in the Swedish Obese Subjects (SOS) study. *Diabetes Care* 2013; 36: 1335–1340.
47. Knowler WC, Pettitt DJ, Saad MF, et al. Diabetes mellitus in the Pima Indians: incidence, risk factors, and pathogenesis. *Diabetes/Metabolism Rev* 1990; 6: 1–27.
48. Dabelea D, Knowler WC, Pettitt DJ. Effect of diabetes in pregnancy on offspring: follow-up research in the Pima Indians. *J Maternal Fetal Med* 2000; 9: 83–88.
49. Terranova L, Busetto L, Vestri A, et al. Bariatric surgery: cost-effectiveness and budget impact. *Obes Surg* 2012; 22: 646–653.

## Chapter 3

# Medical complications of diabetes mellitus

*Lewis W. Johnson, MD and Ruth S. Weinstock, MD, PhD*

## Introduction

Medical complications of diabetes are largely responsible for the increased morbidity, premature mortality, and economic burden associated with the disease. The total estimated cost of diabetes in the United States in 2012 was $245 billion, 43% of which was for hospital inpatient care and 18% of which was for prescription medications to treat the complications of diabetes [1]. There were $176 billion in direct medical costs and $69 billion in reduced productivity [1].

Acute serious medical complications can be immediately life-threatening and include diabetic ketoacidosis (DKA), the hyperglycemic hyperosmolar state (HHS), severe hypoglycemia, and acute infections. These are important to recognize and treat promptly because they can be fatal if left untreated [2–4]. Chronic complications are primarily classified as microvascular (retinopathy, nephropathy, and neuropathy) or macrovascular (coronary heart disease, cerebrovascular disease, and peripheral arterial disease). Additional medical conditions are also more frequently seen in people with type 1 and/or type 2 diabetes and are described below. Recommendations for the evaluation, management, and prevention of complications in people with diabetes are discussed in this chapter.

## Acute complications

### Diabetic ketoacidosis

DKA most frequently occurs in type 1 diabetes but occasionally develops in individuals with type 2 diabetes. It may be the first presentation of type 1 diabetes. In type 1 diabetes, DKA can be precipitated by omission of insulin or by any major stress such as infection or myocardial infarction. Because myocardial infarction can be silent, an electrocardiogram is indicated in all adults with DKA. Nausea, vomiting, abdominal pain, increased urination, and increased thirst are common presenting symptoms. The person may have a rapid respiratory rate and the fruity odor of ketones on the breath. Osmotic diuresis promotes loss of multiple minerals and electrolytes, including sodium, potassium, phosphate,

Table 3.1   Hyperglycemic emergencies. Features of diabetic ketoacidosis (DKA) and the hyperglycemic hyperosmolar state (HHS).

|  | DKA | HHS |
|---|---|---|
| Age | <40 years | >60 years |
| Duration of symptoms | <2 days | >5 days |
| Plasma glucose | 250–600 mg/dL | >600 mg/dL |
| Serum sodium | 125–135 meq/L (normal to ↓) | >135 meq/L (normal to ↑) |
| Serum potassium | Normal to ↑ | Normal |
| Serum bicarbonate | <15 meq/L | >15 meq/L |
| Ketones (urine or blood) | Strongly elevated | Elevated or absent |
| Arterial pH | 6.8–7.3 | >7.3 |
| Arterial pCO2 | 20–30 mm Hg | Normal |
| Serum osmolality | 300–320 mOsm/ml | >330 mOsm/ml |
| Mortality | 3–5% | 10–20% |

calcium, magnesium, and chloride, all of which need to be replaced. A timely diagnosis is crucial because if untreated, DKA can progress to coma and death. Immediate hospitalization and treatment with insulin and intravenous hydration with electrolyte replacement are required. Most important in prevention of DKA is that the patient be appropriately educated in sick day care including continuing insulin therapy, intensifying glucose monitoring, checking urine or blood for ketones, and prompt consultation with his or her health care team whenever he or she has persistent hyperglycemia, ketonuria, or ketonemia.

### Hyperglycemic hyperosmolar state

HHS most commonly occurs in older individuals with type 2 diabetes. There is almost always a precipitating event such as infection, myocardial infarction, or stroke. The patient usually presents with a history of polyuria, weight loss, and diminished oral intake that may result in mental confusion, lethargy, or coma. Abnormal thirst sensation or limited access to fluids facilitates the development of this syndrome. In contrast to DKA, the insulin deficiency is less severe and marked ketosis or severe acidosis is absent (Table 3.1). The plasma glucose is frequently greater than 1,000 mg/dl and the individual is severely dehydrated. As with DKA, hospitalization and intensive hydration are required. The precipitating event should be determined and treated as soon as possible. Even with proper treatment the mortality is high.

### Hypoglycemia

Hypoglycemia, the most common acute complication in diabetes, is discussed in Chapter 4.

### Infections

There is increased frequency and severity of bacterial and fungal infections with diabetes. Predisposing factors are hyperglycemic-related impairment of the immune response, vascular insufficiency, peripheral neuropathy, autonomic neuropathy, urinary dysmotility, and skin and mucosal colonization with pathogens such as *Staphylococcus aureus* and *Candida* species. Vaccine efficiency is adequate in most patients but those with type 1 diabetes and high HbA1c levels are most likely to exhibit hypo-responsiveness [5, 6]. Acute deterioration of glycemic control should trigger evaluation for possible infection. Diabetes and hyperglycemia are strong independent risk factors for hospitalization as a result of pneumonia, urinary tract infection, and skin infection [7].

### Respiratory infections

The most frequent respiratory infections associated with diabetes are due to *Streptococcus pneumoniae* (pneumococcal pneumonia) and the influenza virus. People with diabetes are six times more likely to need hospitalization during influenza epidemics and develop serious complications [6]. Patients with diabetes have a high incidence of nasal carriage of *Staphylococcus aureus*. To reduce hospitalizations, death, and medical expenses, influenza and pneumococcal vaccination are recommended for all patients with diabetes [2]. Patients with diabetes are at higher risk of contracting tuberculosis than individuals without diabetes. Routine screening of patients with tuberculosis for diabetes and patients with diabetes for tuberculosis are also recommended [5, 8].

### Genitourinary infections

Although women with diabetes have greater prevalence of asymptomatic bacteriuria, the routine use of antibiotic therapy remains controversial [5]. Urinary tract infections are more prevalent and can evolve into more serious conditions. Acute pyelonephritis is four to five times more common in individuals with diabetes, and is more frequently bilateral. Additionally, people with diabetes are at increased risk for complications such as perinephric and/or renal abscesses. More than 90% of cases of emphysematous pyelonephritis occur in patients with diabetes. This entity can be diagnosed with a plain film of the abdomen and has a high mortality. Failure of fever to resolve after three to four days of treatment of a urinary tract infection in a patient with diabetes should arouse suspicion about the possibility of this uncommon complication. In addition to intravenous antibiotics, surgical drainage is usually required [9].

Mucosal colonization with *Candida albicans* is also common in people with diabetes who are overweight or are taking antibiotics. These infections can cause extreme discomfort and result in breakdown of the skin, which allows entry of more virulent organisms. Good glycemic control and local antifungal treatment usually resolve the problem. Women with diabetes who have poor glycemic control are prone to vulvovaginal candidiasis [4].

### Gastrointestinal and liver infections

Patients with diabetes may develop yeast infections in the gastrointestinal (GI) tract, especially when glycemic control is poor. The most common agent is *Candida albicans*. Yeast infection in the mouth (thrush) is characterized by a thick white coating of the tongue and throat. If the infection extends further, esophagitis results, which may cause intestinal bleeding, pain, and difficulty swallowing. Oral *Candida* can be diagnosed by physical examination, but esophagitis usually requires endoscopy. Treatment is with topical and/or systemic antifungal medication.

Emphysematous cholecystitis may be clinically similar to acute cholecystitis, but the proportion of males is higher, gangrene of the gallbladder and perforation are more frequent, and the overall mortality is higher. The diagnosis is established by radiographic demonstration of gas on X-ray or by abdominal computed tomography (CT). Emergency cholecystectomy, in addition to broad-spectrum antibiotics, is necessary [9, 10].

Patients with hepatitis C (HCV) are three times more likely to develop diabetes than individuals who are HCV negative. Patients with HCV who develop type 2 diabetes have more severe liver disease and increased fibrosis compared to those who do not have diabetes [5, 11]. Hepatitis B virus (HBV) infections have been reported among patients who shared blood glucose meters [12]. Acute HBV infection is twice as high among adults with diabetes. In 2012 the Centers for Disease Control and Prevention recommended HBV vaccination to adults with diabetes under 60 years of age [13].

## Head and neck infections

The two most serious head and neck infections are invasive external otitis and rhinocerebral mucormycosis. Dental infections will be discussed in Chapters 6 and 8.

Invasive external otitis is an uncommon infection of the ear canal that can extend to the skull and adjacent regions. It often affects the elderly, and the etiologic agent is usually *Pseudomonas aeruginosa*. The patient has severe pain, discharge from the ear canal, and hearing loss. Skull base osteomyelitis and cranial nerve involvement may occur. The best diagnostic method is magnetic resonance imaging. Treatment includes repeated debridement and antibiotic therapy [5, 10].

Rhinocerebral mucormycosis is a rare fungal infection of the nasal sinuses and brain. Approximately 50% of cases have diabetes. Ketoacidosis is the most important risk factor. Early manifestations include facial or ocular pain and nasal stuffiness. Diagnosis is established by biopsy and culture of necrotic tissue from the nasal passages or the palate. Surgical debridement of infected tissue and drainage of infected sinuses are key elements in achieving a cure. Control of diabetes and institution of amphotericin B are crucial [5, 10].

## Skin and soft tissue infections

Furunculosis and subcutaneous abscesses are more common in diabetes and are usually due to staphylococcus infection. Treatment includes application of warm compresses and may require drainage and administration of antibiotics.

Foot infections are the most common soft tissue infections in people with diabetes. All people with diabetes should be educated about proper foot care, inspect their feet daily, and seek medical attention immediately with signs of infection. Potential complications include osteomyelitis, which may result in amputation. The most common organisms are staphylococci, although they are frequently polymicrobial infections. Methacillin-resistant *Staphylococcus aureus* (MRSA) has begun to be increasingly important. Outpatient management of infected foot ulcers begins with surgical removal of the necrotic tissue and administration of antibiotics [5]. A multidisciplinary approach to treatment including surgical or podiatric consultation is recommended.

Necrotizing fasciitis is a life threatening infection that starts in the subcutaneous space and spreads along fascial planes. The most common locations are the arms, legs, and abdominal wall. The degree of pain is disproportionate to the findings on physical examination. Marked signs of systemic toxicity are usually present. In diabetes, fasciitis is typically polymicrobial. The associated mortality is approximately 40%. Prompt, aggressive surgical debridement is crucial in decreasing mortality [10].

### Surgical site infections

An association between diabetes and an increased risk of surgical site infections has been well established. Postoperative hyperglycemia is significantly associated with the development of surgical site infections [14]. One of the most devastating complications of cardiac surgery in patients with diabetes is deep sternal wound infection. The incidence of this complication is decreased by keeping the postoperative blood glucose below 200 mg/dl [15–17].

### Human immunodeficiency virus

There is an increased risk of developing type 2 diabetes in people with human immunodeficiency virus (HIV). The increased risk of diabetes is related to the HIV itself or its treatment. Insulin resistance is the main mechanism implicated in the pathogenesis of diabetes in HIV patients; protease inhibitors also cause insulin resistance [5]. Patients with HIV should be screened for diabetes at diagnosis and during drug therapy.

## Chronic complications

Chronic complications are responsible for most of the long-term morbidity and mortality associated with diabetes mellitus. The risk of developing both microvascular and macrovascular complications has been shown to be closely associated with the degree and duration of hyperglycemia. As the HbA1c increases from 5.5% to 9.5% there is a 10-fold increase in microvascular disease and about a two-fold increase in macrovascular disease. Reduction in chronic hyperglycemia prevents or delays the progression of retinopathy, nephropathy, and neuropathy but the evidence for this effect is less clear for macrovascular disease [18–22]. Other factors including hypertension, dyslipidemia, and cigarette smoking play major roles in the development and treatment of macrovascular complications.

### Mechanisms of development of chronic complications

An emerging theory is that hyperglycemia leads to epigenetic changes and damage to the microvasculature of the retina, kidney, and nervous system. Specific cell types such as the capillary endothelial cells in the retina, mesangial cells in the renal glomerulus, and the vasa vasorum of peripheral nerves are prone to develop the tissue-damaging changes associated with hyperglycemia because they cannot limit the entry of glucose. Other cells, such as smooth-muscle cells, when exposed to hyperglycemia reduce glucose transport so that their internal glucose concentration remains constant.

There are at least five pathways that may explain how hyperglycemia causes the chronic complications of diabetes [23]:

1 Elevated production of sorbitol through the polyol pathway, leading to low levels of reduced glutathione, an important antioxidant, increasing oxidative stress
2 Increased production of advanced glycation end products (AGEs) causing the modification of intracellular proteins, and increasing levels of inflammatory cytokines and growth factors
3 Increased expression of the receptor for AGEs and its activating ligands
4 Activation of protein kinase C altering the transcription of genes and decreasing the vasodilator endothelial nitrous oxide which is related to the production of abnormal collagen and extracellular matrix proteins
5 Increased flux through the hexosamine pathway altering glycosylation of proteins such as nitrous oxide synthase

The mechanisms underlying macrovascular disease are less clear but are associated with insulin resistance and elevated levels of circulating free fatty acids as well as hyperglycemia. Approximately 85% of people with type 2 diabetes have the metabolic syndrome which, in addition to insulin resistance, includes abdominal obesity, hypertension, and an atherogenic dyslipidemia, all of which are independent accelerating factors in the development of chronic complications.

Genetic factors are also involved in the development of chronic diabetes-related complications. The Joslin 50–Year Medalist Study enrolled individuals who have had type 1 diabetes for more than fifty years without developing any significant complications. These patients are being actively evaluated in an attempt to identify possible reasons for this protection [24].

### Microvascular complications

For each complication the following will be discussed: (1) the importance of the complication, (2) screening recommendations, (3) treatment goals, and (4) means of prevention (Table 3.2).

### Retinopathy

In the United States, diabetes is the leading cause of blindness in people between 20 and 74 years of age. There is a higher risk of retinopathy in type 1 diabetes but because type 2 is more common it accounts for more individuals with visual loss.

Diabetic retinopathy is associated with progressive changes in the retinal microvasculature leading to areas of nonperfusion, increased vascular permeability, and the proliferation of new pathologic vessels. Diabetic eye disease is classified as nonproliferative retinopathy (NPDR), proliferative retinopathy (PDR), and macular edema. NPDR is

Table 3.2   Chronic microvascular complications of diabetes mellitus. Screening recommendations.

| Complication | Screening Recommendations |
|---|---|
| Eye disease<br>  Retinopathy<br>  Macular edema<br>  Glaucoma<br>  Cataracts | Annual dilated eye exam (If excellent glycemic control and no retinopathy, this can be every two years) |
| Nephropathy<br>  Albuminuria<br>  Decreased GFR<br>  End-stage renal disease | Annual spot urine for albumin/creatinine ratio<br>Annual serum creatinine and calculation of GFR* |
| Neuropathy<br>  Distal symmetric polyneuropathy<br>  Autonomic neuropathy | Annual exam for loss of protective sensation<br>Careful history at each office visit |

*GFR: Glomerular filtration rate (ml/min/1.73 m²).

usually asymptomatic and marked by microaneurysms, blot hemorrhages, and exudates. It is present in many if not most individuals who have had diabetes for more than 20 years, particularly if their glycemic control has been suboptimal. NPDR can be progressive and lead to retinal ischemia which is a potent inducer of angiogenic growth factors such as vascular endothelial growth factor (VEGF). PDR is characterized by neovascularization leading to vitreous hemorrhage, fibrosis, and retinal detachment. Other eye diseases including cataracts and glaucoma occur earlier and more commonly in people with diabetes. In poorly controlled diabetes, high blood glucose levels can cause osmotic lens swelling resulting in blurred vision. Corrective lenses should not be prescribed until the glycemic control has improved.

Routine non-dilated retinal examinations performed by a primary care provider or diabetes specialist may not detect retinopathy and are therefore inadequate. Guidelines [2] recommend that adults and children with type 1 diabetes have a dilated eye examination by an ophthalmologist or optometrist within five years of the onset of diabetes. People with type 2 diabetes should have a dilated exam shortly after diagnosis because the duration of their disease is unknown. In the United Kingdom Prospective Diabetes Study (UKPDS) of type 2 diabetes, 35% of females and 39% of males had diabetic retinopathy at the time diabetes was diagnosed [25]. Patients with both type 1 and type 2 diabetes generally should have lifelong annual comprehensive eye exams by a qualified eye specialist. If retinopathy is present, close follow-up by an ophthalmologist experienced in the management of diabetic retinopathy is indicated.

Pregnancy can cause retinopathy to progress rapidly [26]. Women with known diabetes who are planning pregnancy should have a dilated eye exam before conception and then be followed closely by an ophthalmologist during pregnancy and for one year after delivery. Gestational diabetes does not place the mother at increased risk for developing retinopathy.

Serious retinopathy, if detected early, can be successfully treated with laser therapy [27, 28]. Newer therapies, including intraocular injection of a monoclonal antibody to

VEGF and glucocorticoids, may halt the progression of neovascularization and macular edema, improve vision, and reduce the need for laser therapy in some patients [29].

Factors that favor the development and progression of diabetic retinopathy are duration of diabetes, poor glycemic control, nephropathy, and hypertension. To reduce the risk of developing or to slow the progression of retinopathy, glycemic and blood pressure control should be optimized [18, 19, 21, 22, 30]. The presence of retinopathy is not a contraindication to the use of aspirin for cardioprotection when indicated.

## Nephropathy

Diabetic nephropathy occurs in 20–40% of people with diabetes and is the leading cause of end-stage renal disease (ESRD) in the United States. Nephropathy appears to be more common in type 1 diabetes, but because of the increasing number people with type 2 diabetes, more than 80% of people in renal replacement programs have type 2 diabetes. People with diabetic nephropathy commonly also have retinopathy.

Like other microvascular complications, the pathogenesis of diabetic nephropathy is related to chronic hyperglycemia, but hypertension plays a major role in its development and progression. The classic progression of diabetic nephropathy begins with microalbuminuria (30–299 mg/gm creatinine), then macroalbuminuria (equal to or greater than 300 mg/gm creatinine), followed by a decrease in the glomerular filtration rate (GFR). Microalbuminuria is a marker not only for the development of nephropathy, but also for increased cardiovascular risk [31].

Screening recommendations are to perform an annual urine albumin: creatinine ratio in type 1 diabetes of equal to or greater than five year's duration and in all type 2 patients starting at diagnosis [2]. In all adults with diabetes, the serum creatinine should be measured at least annually to calculate the GFR. The National Kidney Foundation classifies chronic kidney disease based on the calculated GFR (ml/min/$1.73 m^2$):

- Stage 1: equal to or greater than 90
- Stage 2: 60–89
- Stage 3: 30–59
- Stage 4: 15–29
- Stage 5 (ESRD): less than 15 or on dialysis

Renal dysfunction can occur in the absence of albuminuria, particularly in individuals with type 2 diabetes and hypertension. Nephrology consultation should be considered if the etiology of renal disease is uncertain (e.g., proteinuria in the absence of retinopathy) and for worsening renal function.

Glycemic and blood pressure control are the cornerstones for preventing and treating diabetic nephropathy. The importance of better glycemic control for forestalling or preventing nephropathy in type 1 diabetes was shown in the Diabetes Control and Complications Trial (DCCT) and its follow-up epidemiologic study (DCCT/EDIC) [19, 32]. The UKPDS and its 10-year follow-up showed similar results in type 2 diabetes [21, 22]. The more recent Action in Diabetes and Vascular disease: PreterAx and DiamicroN Modified Release Controlled Evaluation (ADVANCE) trial demonstrated that greater improvement in the HbA1c (to 6.5%) in type 2 diabetes was associated with further reduction in renal events [33].

Blood pressure control appears to be the most important single intervention to prevent progressive nephropathy in both type 1 and type 2 diabetes. For example, in the UKPDS, a reduction in systolic blood pressure from 154 to 144 mmHg was associated with a 30% reduction in microalbuminuria [30]. Although guidelines suggest specific targets for blood pressure, there does not appear to be any threshold for renal protection. Agents that interrupt the renin-angiotensin system such as angiotensin converting enzyme inhibitors (ACEI) and angiotensin receptor blockers (ARBs) provide a benefit over other antihypertensive agents and are recommended if microalbuminuria is documented. Most patients require two or more drugs for blood pressure control.

The role of lipid-lowering agents to prevent nephropathy is less clear but most individuals with diabetic nephropathy take a statin to prevent cardiovascular disease events. To date there is no evidence to suggest that statins reduce cardiovascular events in individuals who are on dialysis [34]. Fibrates are prescribed primarily to lower triglyceride levels in patients with hypertriglyceridemia. In a study of the effect of fenofibrate therapy on cardiovascular events in type 2 diabetes there was less albuminuria progression and less retinopathy needing laser treatment in the fenofibrate group [35].

Renal function can be worsened by the use of many drugs including over-the-counter nonsteroidal anti-inflammatory agents. Many medications require dose adjustments in the presence of renal dysfunction. Radiographic contrast agents can worsen renal function. Risk factors for contrast-induced nephrotoxicity are underlying renal disease and dehydration. It is recommended that metformin be discontinued before any procedure using contrast agents to prevent life threatening lactic acidosis and that the drug be resumed only when it has been ascertained that the creatinine has returned to baseline. Smoking can hasten the progression of renal dysfunction and cessation needs to be stressed.

## Neuropathy

Diabetic neuropathy is one of the most common long-term complications of diabetes, affecting more than 50% of individuals during the course of their disease [36, 37]. The major morbidity of neuropathy is foot ulceration, the precursor to gangrene and amputation. Early diagnosis is important because diabetes is the leading cause of nontraumatic lower extremity amputation in the United States. The major risk factors for developing neuropathy are duration of diabetes, poor glycemic control, and inadequate foot care. The importance of glycemic control has been documented for both type 1 [18, 19] and type 2 [21, 22] diabetes.

Diabetic neuropathy is classified as: (1) distal symmetric polyneuropathy (DSPN); (2) autonomic neuropathy; (3) focal mononeuropathy; and (4) proximal motor neuropathy. Focal mononeuropathies are frequently associated with pain and their course is usually self limiting. Proximal motor neuropathy is less common and primarily affects the elderly.

DSPN, the most common form of diabetic neuropathy, can usually be diagnosed by history and physical examination without need for nerve conduction studies. Symptoms may be absent but when present include loss of feeling, pain, numbness, tingling, sharpness, or burning in the feet that progress proximally in a "stocking-and-glove" distribution. Symptoms are often exacerbated at night. Physical examination reveals reduced or loss of sensation to a 10-gram monofilament, loss of pain, and vibratory sensation and decreased/absent ankle reflexes. Approximately 10% of neuropathies in people with diabetes are not due to diabetes [37]. Before attributing the neuropathy to diabetes other etiologies such as alcohol abuse, drug toxicity, renal disease, vasculitis, or vitamin B12 deficiency (may be related to metformin use) should be considered.

Autonomic neuropathy can cause dysfunction of every part of the body including cardiovascular, gastrointestinal, genitourinary, sudomotor (increased or decreased sweating), and metabolic systems. Diabetic autonomic neuropathy often goes unrecognized by both patients and physicians because of its insidious onset and multiple organ involvement. Cardiac autonomic neuropathy may present as a resting tachycardia, exercise intolerance, or orthostatic hypotension and may be related to the increased incidence of silent myocardial infarction in patients with diabetes. Gastrointestinal autonomic neuropathy may present as esophageal dysfunction, delayed gastric emptying (gastroparesis), diarrhea, or constipation. Gastroparesis can be problematic not only because of its associated symptoms (bloating, nausea, vomiting, and discomfort) but also because it may interfere with glycemic control and be a cause of unexpected hypoglycemia. The major complaint in genitourinary autonomic neuropathy in men is erectile dysfunction. Patients can also experience recurrent urinary tract infections. Sudomotor neuropathy causes dry skin of the feet which may predispose to infection. Finally, autonomic neuropathy may reduce the counter regulatory response to hypoglycemia, especially catecholamine release predisposing to hypoglycemic unawareness.

It is recommended that all patients be screened for DSPN and signs and symptoms of cardiovascular autonomic neuropathy starting at diagnosis for type 2 diabetes, five years after the diagnosis of type 1 diabetes, and at least annually thereafter [2]. Specialized testing is rarely needed.

Prevention of diabetic neuropathy involves good glycemic control. A multifactorial approach to therapy including lifestyle modification provides added benefit [38]. There are no medications to prevent or reverse diabetic neuropathy. Some antidepressants and anti-seizure medications are moderately effective for symptom relief of DSPN. Improved glycemic control may modestly slow progression but not reverse neuronal loss.

## *Diabetic foot*

Of all the complications of diabetes, foot problems are the most preventable. It is important that the patient be educated about daily self examination and the use of proper footwear. A focused comprehensive foot evaluation should be performed at least annually, although the feet should be examined at each office visit. The components of the comprehensive foot evaluation include [39, 40]:

1  Vascular: Ask about smoking and symptoms suggestive of intermittent claudication. Inspect the feet for discoloration and the presence of hair on the toes. Palpate for pedal pulses and a temperature difference between feet.
2  Neurologic: Ask about tingling, burning, or pins-and-needles sensation. Check for loss of protective sensation using a Semmes-Weinstein 10-gram monofilament, an inexpensive tool with excellent sensitivity for identifying people at risk for foot ulcers [41, 42]; vibration sensation can also be assessed.

3 Musculoskeletal: Identify deformities such as hammertoes, bunions, calluses due to abnormal pressure, evidence of Charcot foot.
4 Dermatologic: Examine for discoloration, redness, white discoloration between the toes, maceration, wetness, toenail fungus, and thickening and discoloration of the toenails.
5 Footwear: Check for poorly-fitting shoes (may promote callus formation) and ulcerations. Patients at high risk should be referred to a podiatrist. Management of foot ulcers is multidisciplinary and may include a podiatrist, vascular surgeon, and wound care specialist.

## Macrovascular complications

Macrovascular complications of diabetes are due to atherosclerotic cardiovascular disease (CVD) and are classified as coronary heart disease (CHD), cerebrovascular disease, and peripheral arterial disease (PAD). As many as 80% of patients with type 2 diabetes develop and possibly die of complications of CVD [43]. The Framingham Study showed that the incidence of CVD in people with diabetes was two to three times that in those without diabetes [44]. As with microvascular complications, the following will be discussed: (1) the importance of the complication, (2) screening recommendations, (3) treatment goals, and (4) means of prevention (Table 3.3). For CVD, prevention includes lifestyle modification as well as management of risk factors such as hyperglycemia, hypertension, dyslipidemia, smoking, and the hypercoagulable state.

### Coronary heart disease

There is a predisposition to premature and accelerated CHD. Women lose the premenopausal cardioprotection observed in those without diabetes. Guidelines have designated diabetes as a "CHD equivalent" indicating that an individual with diabetes without documented CHD has the same level of risk of having a cardiovascular event as a person without diabetes but with documented CHD [45].

Table 3.3   Chronic macrovascular complications of diabetes mellitus. Screening recommendations.

| Complication | Screening Recommendations |
|---|---|
| Coronary heart disease | Careful cardiac history at each office visit<br>Recent resting EKG in medical record<br>Low threshold for advanced cardiac evaluation if any symptoms suggestive of cardiac disease |
| Cerebrovascular disease | Careful history of any symptoms of TIA or stroke at each office visit<br>Listen for carotid bruits at each office visit |
| Peripheral arterial disease | Careful history for symptoms of intermittent claudication at each office visit<br>Examine legs, palpate foot pulses |

People with diabetes have a higher incidence of atypical angina and silent myocardial infarction and should have a baseline electrocardiogram (EKG). At every office visit patients should be questioned about chest pain or tightness, shortness of breath, or decreased exercise tolerance. Symptoms of angina may be atypical, possibly related to cardiac autonomic neuropathy, and there should be a high level of suspicion of CHD. Indications for performing an exercise stress test are: (1) an abnormal resting EKG, especially if it is suggestive of previous myocardial infarction, (2) typical or atypical symptoms suggestive of angina. Routine screening for CHD in asymptomatic patients is not recommended [2].

The prevention of CHD in patients with both type 1 and type 2 diabetes involves the management of CVD risk factors. The following factors will be discussed individually: hyperglycemia, blood pressure, dyslipidemia, smoking, and the use of antiplatelet agents.

## Glycemic control

The DCCT (type 1 diabetes) enrolled patients without significant chronic complications and UKPDS (type 2 diabetes) studied patients with new onset diabetes. They both showed an increase in microvascular and macrovascular complications with higher HbA1c values [18, 21]. The long-term follow-up of both studies also documented a decrease in CHD events with early intense (HbA1c goal 7%) vs. conventional glycemic control. During subsequent long-term follow-up, when the HbA1c levels were similar in the two groups, these benefits persisted, suggesting "metabolic memory"—the so called "legacy effect" [20, 22].

Because epidemiologic studies have indicated that lower HbA1c values were associated with fewer complications, several studies tested this theory by further lowering the goal HbA1c to 6–6.5%. Enrolled patients were older, had diabetes of longer duration, and many either had or were at high risk for CVD. CVD events were not decreased and in some studies mortality was higher with more intense glycemic control [46]. It is possible that unrecognized hypoglycemia played a role. These studies support the current recommendation that glycemic goals be individualized (Chapter 4).

## Blood pressure control

Hypertension is common, especially in type 2 diabetes. It is a risk factor for both microvascular and macrovascular disease. Blood pressure should be carefully measured at each office visit using an appropriately sized cuff located at heart level, with the patient relaxed, and the arm supported. In diabetes a blood pressure equal to or greater than 140/80 mm Hg is considered to represent hypertension. If the blood pressure remains elevated on a second day, treatment is indicated. Lifestyle modification including weight reduction if overweight, increased physical activity, and a low-sodium diet should be encouraged. If not contraindicated, inhibitors of the renin-angiotensin system (ACEI or ARBs) are the first-line drugs. Many if not most patients require two or more medications for blood pressure control. ACEI and ARBs are contraindicated during pregnancy.

In epidemiological studies blood pressure values as low as 115 mmHg systolic are associated with decreased CVD risk. In the ACCORD trial [47], which enrolled older adults with long duration diabetes and high CVD risk, targeting blood pressure to a systolic less than 120 mmHg compared with less than 140 mmHg did not reduce the total incidence of fatal and nonfatal CVD events, although stroke was reduced. The target blood pressure goal in diabetes has been changed from equal to or less than 130/80 mmHg to equal to or less than 140/80 mmHg [2]. However, the goal needs to be individualized and lower or higher targets may be appropriate.

## Dyslipidemia

Patients with diabetes have an increased prevalence of dyslipidemias. Any type of dyslipidemia can occur, but the most common type associated with type 2 diabetes is related to insulin resistance and elevated triglyceride (TG) and reduced HDL cholesterol (HDL-C) levels. Although the LDL cholesterol (LDL-C) levels may not be elevated, the LDL particles are smaller, dense, and more atherogenic.

In most adult patients a fasting lipid panel (total cholesterol, LDL-C, HDL-C, and TG) should be obtained annually. The primary therapeutic target is the LDL-C because there is good evidence that lowering LDL-C with statin drugs decreases CVD events [48, 49]. Guidelines recommend statin therapy for patients with documented CVD and for those without CVD who are over 40 years of age with one or more additional risk factors [2]. For patients without CVD the LDL-C goal is less than 100 mg/dL with an option of less than 70 mg/dL in those with known CVD. The American College of Cardiology (ACC) and the American Heart Association (AHA), in collaboration with the National Heart, Lung, and Blood Institute, released a new 2013 ACC/AHA Guideline on the treatment of blood cholesterol to reduce atherosclerotic cardiovascular risk in adults. The new guidelines recommend statin therapy for all adults age 40–75 years with type 1 or 2 diabetes with an LDL-C of 70 mg/dl or higher. The intensity of statin treatment is determined by calculation of 10-year risk of having a cardiovascular event (fatal or nonfatal heart attack or stroke) using a new calculator. There is some controversy about these new guidelines and at the present time they have not been endorsed by the American Association of Clinical Endocrinologists or by the National Lipid Association [50]. After statin therapy many patients continue to have increased residual risk for CVD events. The routine additions of fibrates or niacin have been disappointing in their ability to further reduce risk [35, 51, 52]. Statin drugs are contraindicated in pregnancy.

A TG greater than 1,000 mg/dL is associated with pancreatitis. In addition to appropriate medications (usually starting with fibrate therapy), diet and improved glycemic control are very important in the treatment of hypertriglyceridemia. Individuals with hypertriglyceridemia should be screened for thyroid disease and alcohol use, and should avoid drugs such as estrogen that can exacerbate this disorder.

## Smoking

Smoking is a major risk factor for both microvascular disease and CVD and should be addressed in all patients with diabetes. If the person is motivated to stop smoking, counseling and associated forms of treatment should be offered.

## Antiplatelet agents

Low-dose aspirin is recommended for secondary prevention in those with diabetes and a previous cardiovascular event. Current guidelines recommend aspirin for primary prevention for those individuals with type 1 or type 2 diabetes at increased cardiovascular risk (10-year risk greater than 10%). This includes most men over 50 years of age or women over 60 years of age who have at least one additional major risk factor (family history of CVD, hypertension, smoking, dyslipidemia, or albuminuria). Aspirin is no longer recommended for low-risk patients because the risk of bleeding is felt to be greater than the benefit. If the individual is allergic to aspirin, clopidogrel can be substituted. Use of aspirin in individuals under the age of 21 years is contraindicated due to the associated risk of Reye's syndrome.

## Multifactorial approach to the management of CHD

Although the evaluation and management of risk factors have been discussed individually, given the multifactorial nature of atherogenic disease, all contributory factors need to be treated for optimal results. The value of this approach was tested in the Steno-2 study, in which patients with type 2 diabetes and microalbuminuria were randomized to receive either conventional treatment or intensive therapy that included behavior modification, targeted pharmacotherapy for hyperglycemia, hypertension, dyslipidemia, and microalbuminuria and aspirin. Patients receiving the intensive therapy had a significantly lower incidence of cardiovascular disease, nephropathy, retinopathy, and autonomic neuropathy. Overall, long-term intensive treatment of risk factors reduced the risk of cardiovascular mortality by about 50% [38, 53, 54]. Table 3.4 summarizes the common treatment goals for lifestyle modification, HbA1c, blood pressure, LDL-C, and the use of anti-platelet agents.

Table 3.4   Treatment goals for individuals with diabetes.

| |
|---|
| • Weight loss if overweight or obese<br>• Moderate exercise: 150 minutes/week<br>• Smoking cessation<br>• Antiplatelet agents*<br>• HbA1c <7%**<br>• Blood pressure <140/80 mm Hg***<br>• LDL-C <100 mg/dL****<br>Consider statin therapy for those with a history of MI or over 40 years old with other risk factors. |

*Unless contraindicated, 81–162 mg aspirin to those with type 1 or type 2 diabetes and documented CVD (secondary prevention) and to high risk individuals without known CVD (primary prevention). High risk includes most men over 50 years old and women over 60 years old with at least one other major CVD risk factor (family history of CVD, hypertension, smoking, dyslipidemia, or albuminuria).
**More or less stringent glycemic goals may be appropriate for individual patients. Goals should be individualized based on duration of diabetes, age/life expectancy, comorbid conditions, known CVD or advanced microvascular complications, hypoglycemic unawareness, and individual patient considerations.
***Based upon patient characteristics and response to therapy, lower systolic blood pressure targets may be appropriate.
****In individuals with overt CVD, a lower LDL-C goal of less than 70 mg/dL using a high dose statin is an option.

## Cardiomyopathy in diabetes

Diabetes is associated with a four-fold increase in the risk of heart failure. The etiology may involve coronary artery disease with previous myocardial infarction and left ventricular hypertrophy related to hypertension. Diabetes can also affect cardiac structure and function in the absence of coronary artery disease or hypertension, called diabetic cardiomyopathy [55]. The patient can develop both systolic (impaired emptying) and diastolic (impaired filling) left ventricular dysfunction resulting in signs and symptoms of left ventricular failure. The diagnosis is made noninvasively by echocardiography. A stress test may be necessary to help determine if coronary artery disease is present. Early recognition of left ventricular dysfunction and treatment with evidence-based therapies may prevent the development of overt heart failure.

### Cerebrovascular disease

Individuals with diabetes are at least two times more likely to have a stroke than those without diabetes. The outcome after stroke is worse in patients with diabetes, with higher mortality and slower and less complete recovery. The etiology of stroke in diabetes may be cerebrovascular atherosclerosis involving small and large vessels, cardiac thromboembolism, or clotting abnormalities [56]. There is more involvement of small cerebral vessels in diabetes producing lacunar infarcts in the thalamic and subthalamic areas. Thromboemboli may be related to underlying atrial fibrillation or originate from the left ventricle in a patient with a previous myocardial infarction or cardiomyopathy. The risk factors are the same as in CHD: advancing age, duration of diabetes, smoking, hypertension, and dyslipidemia. People with diabetes also have platelet dysfunction, a hypercoagulable state, and impaired thrombolysis.

   Primary prevention is recommended in a person with diabetes and at least one other major risk factor or atrial fibrillation. Secondary prevention is recommended for anyone who has had a stroke or transient ischemic attack (TIA). Both primary and secondary prevention include optimal glycemic and blood pressure control, statin therapy [48, 49], smoking cessation, and weight reduction if overweight or obese. The LDL-C goal in a person with diabetes and a previous stroke is less than 70 mg/dl.

### Peripheral arterial disease

PAD generally refers to atherosclerotic narrowing of the arteries to the legs. In patients with diabetes, the arterial disease is diffuse and more frequently located below the knee. Intermittent claudication, the classic symptom of PAD, refers to a pain, ache, or other discomfort in the affected leg that comes on with exertion and is relieved by rest. Because most patients with diabetes do not have typical symptoms of claudication, PAD is underdiagnosed and undertreated [57]. Symptoms may be particularly difficult to evaluate in the person with associated neuropathy.

   The major risk factors for PAD are advanced age, cigarette smoking, diabetes, dyslipidemia, and hypertension. The risk of developing PAD is increased two-to four-fold in diabetes. PAD not only interferes with quality of life but correlates strongly with major cardiovascular events, because it frequently associates with coronary and cerebral athero-sclerosis. The evaluation for PAD begins with a careful history and palpation of pedal pulses. The ankle brachial index (ABI) is a noninvasive test performed in the office to diagnose and quantitate the severity of PAD. An ABI should be done in patients with symptoms suggestive of claudication, and is recommended on all patients with diabetes over age 50 [2].

NCEP ATP III guidelines have classified PAD as a CHD equivalent [45]. The person with diabetes and PAD is at very high risk for having a cardiovascular event. Careful attention to glycemic, lipid, and blood pressure goals and antiplatelet therapy is indicated. Smoking cessation and a supervised exercise program are most effective in improving symptoms.

## Other conditions frequently associated with diabetes

### Autoimmune diseases

People with type 1 diabetes are at increased risk for other autoimmune conditions (Table 3.5). Fifteen to 30% of subjects with type 1 diabetes have autoimmune thyroid disease (hypothyroid or hyperthyroid), 4–9% have celiac disease (CD), and 0.5% have Addison's disease (primary adrenal insufficiency). These conditions are associated with organ-specific autoantibodies: thyroid peroxidase and thyroglobulin with autoimmune thyroid disease, endomysial and tissue transglutaminase autoantibodies with CD, and 21-hydroxylase autoantibodies with Addison's disease [58]. Current recommendations are to screen for thyroid disease on an annual basis using a serum TSH [2]. At diagnosis of type 1 diabetes, CD-associated autoantibodies should be obtained and repeated if symptoms suggest CD. There are no general recommendations for screening for adrenal autoimmunity but an adrenal evaluation should be performed for suspected insufficiency. Other autoimmune diseases observed more frequently in type 1 diabetes include vitiligo, pernicious anemia, Sjögren's syndrome, lupus, myasthenia gravis, and rheumatoid arthritis. Routine testing is not recommended, but the health care provider should have a high index of suspicion for the development of these diseases.

Table 3.5   Common comorbidities associated with diabetes.

* Other autoimmune disease (celiac disease, autoimmune thyroid disease, Addison's disease, vitiligo, pernicious anemia, Sjögren's syndrome, lupus, rheumatoid arthritis, myasthenia gravis)*
* Obstructive sleep apnea
* Non-alcoholic fatty liver disease
* Low testosterone in men
* Erectile dysfunction
* Certain cancers (liver, pancreas, endometrial, colon/rectal, breast, and bladder)
* Depression and anxiety
* Musculoskeletal problems (adhesive capsulitis, trigger finger, Dupuytren's contracture, carpal tunnel syndrome)
* Fractures
* Skin disease (diabetic dermopathy, necrobiosis lipoidica, acanthosis nigricans, eruptive xanthomas)
* Hearing impairment

*Associated with autoimmune type 1 diabetes only.

## Obstructive sleep apnea

In patients with diabetes, the prevalence of obstructive sleep apnea (OSA) is about 23% [59] but in those with type 2 diabetes and obesity it may be as high as 86% [60]. In OSA there is sympathetic nervous system activation, hypothalamic-pituitary dysfunction, systemic inflammation, high leptin levels, and low adiponectin levels, all of which are related to insulin resistance. OSA is also associated with hypertension and an increased risk of cardiovascular events and death. Benefits of treatment include improved quality of life and blood pressure control.

## Fatty liver disease

Non-alcoholic fatty liver disease includes a spectrum of liver damage, from simple steatosis to steatohepatitis (non-alcoholic steatohepatitis or NASH) to cirrhosis. The pathogenesis is related to increased free fatty acid transport to the liver leading to triglyceride deposition, inflammation, and fibrosis. The diagnosis is generally considered when there are elevated liver enzymes and supported by the presence of excessive fat on imaging of the liver. Other etiologies such as alcohol, viral hepatitis, autoimmune hepatitis, hemochromatosis, α1-antitrypsin deficiency, and Wilson's disease should be excluded. Liver biopsy is the gold standard for diagnosis but is usually not necessary [61].

Patients with NASH tend to consume excess carbohydrates and fat. Dietary modification including weight reduction and good glycemic control are central to management. The Look AHEAD study demonstrated that intensive lifestyle modification with calorie restriction and exercise reversed radiographic evidence of steatosis [62].

## Sexual dysfunction

In men the most common problem is erectile dysfunction (ED), which has been found in more than half of all men in the United States with diabetes. Many patients have a multifactorial basis for their ED. Pathophysiology can include neuropathy, psychogenic factors, atherosclerotic narrowing of the blood vessels supplying the penis, and hypogonadism. Many drugs are associated with the development of ED [63]. The clinician should ask about ED in all male patients with diabetes. Oral pharmacological agents are available that are effective for some patients.

Testosterone levels are lower in men with diabetes compared with age-matched men without diabetes. Obesity, OSA, and insulin resistance are all associated with low testosterone levels. It is not recommended that all men with diabetes be tested but if the patient complains of ED or symptoms of hypogonadism, the investigation should include an assessment of serum testosterone. If the testosterone level is low, implementation of lifestyle measures such as weight loss and exercise, if successful, can raise serum testosterone concentrations and provide multiple health benefits. Indications for testosterone therapy should be reserved for clinical androgen deficiency with sustained, unequivocally low testosterone after appropriate diagnostic workup. In general, testosterone should not be given to men with diabetes and low-normal testosterone levels [64, 65]. If testosterone is given, it is imperative to assess for prostatic disease and polycythemia.

The prevalence of sexual dysfunction in women with diabetes remains uncertain. Although men typically complain of ED, women complain of inadequate enjoyment or interest which affects the quality of their relationship. It is important to ask women about sexual problems and the inquiry should include a history of new medications and signs or symptoms of depression. A clinical examination should be performed to exclude vaginal infections [61].

## Cancer

Several cancers (liver, pancreas, endometrium, colon and rectum, breast, and bladder) have been consistently associated with diabetes [66]. There is a reduced risk of prostate cancer. The pathogenesis is not clear but hyperinsulinemia, hyperglycemia, and inflammation are proposed contributory factors. Some epidemiologic studies suggested that the use of glargine insulin was related to an increase in cancer [67, 68], but this was refuted in a large randomized trial [69]. Metformin may protect against the development of certain cancers and may improve prognosis in patients with cancer [61, 66]. Patients with diabetes should be encouraged to undergo age and sex-appropriate screenings and to reduce their modifiable cancer risk factors [2].

## Mental illness

Diabetes is associated with an increased prevalence of depression and anxiety disorders. Not only do these conditions cause distress and reduced quality of life but also affect diabetes management and outcomes. People with diabetes should be screened regularly for depression and anxiety and receive appropriate pharmacological and psychological treatments. Diabetes is also more common in people with severe mental illnesses, such as schizophrenia and bipolar affective disorder. Antidepressant and antipsychotic medications can induce weight gain, and some second generation antipsychotic drugs such as clozapine and olanzapine increase glucose levels even without significant weight gain [70]. Weight reduction, smoking cessation, and exercise programs can be successful in people with severe mental illness and may be better options than trying to change or discontinue antipsychotic medication [61].

## Musculoskeletal complications

Musculoskeletal and rheumatologic symptoms are common. The pathophysiology may involve the formation of advanced glycation end products that impair the structure and function of connective tissue. Syndromes more common in diabetes are adhesive capsulitis (frozen shoulder), limited mobility of the small joints of the hands, trigger finger, Dupuytren's contracture, and carpal tunnel syndrome. It is important to provide supportive care, symptom relief, and optimization of glycemic control [61].

## Bone disease

Individuals with type 1 diabetes can have reduced bone mass and increased risk of fragility fracture, while those with type 2 diabetes, despite having normal or above-normal bone mineral density (BMD), are subject to low-trauma fractures, especially hip fractures. Risk factors for fracture should be thoroughly evaluated in both men and women with diabetes and BMD testing recommended if appropriate. For at-risk patients it is reasonable to consider standard primary or secondary prevention strategies (fall prevention, adequate calcium and vitamin D intake, and avoidance of medications that adversely affect bone). Pharmacotherapy with bisphosphonates is considered for high-risk patients [2].

Osteonecrosis of the jaw (ONJ) is a rare complication of bisphosphonate therapy in which localized bone necrosis of the mandible or maxillary alveolar ridge appears, usually after an oral surgical procedure such as tooth extraction, root canal, or placement of implants. The hallmark of ONJ is failure of the surgical site to heal accompanied by localized jaw pain and the appearance of exposed necrotic bone. The vast majority of ONJ cases reported are in patients with myeloma or solid malignant tumors treated with large doses of intravenous bisphosphonates. Only 4–5% of ONJ cases have occurred in patients taking oral bisphosphonates for osteoporosis. The incidence in patients being treated for osteoporosis is estimated to be one per 100,000 cases [71]. One report suggested that diabetes may be a risk factor for ONJ in patients receiving mostly intravenous bisphosphonates for cancer treatment [72]. A recent statement from the American Dental Association lists age older than 65 years, periodontitis, prolonged use of bisphosphonates (greater than two years), smoking, denture wearing, and diabetes as being associated with an increase risk of antiresorptive agent-induced ONJ. At the present time there is not good evidence for stopping bisphosphonates prior to dental surgery [73]. The long duration of action of these drugs probably makes discontinuing them before dental work ineffective. If possible, patients should have dental work performed prior to starting therapy.

### Skin diseases

Non-infection-related skin lesions that are more common in diabetes [61, 74] are shown in Figure 3.1. Diabetic dermopathy is characterized by reddish-brown, round, scaly patches on the shins. Necrobiosis lipoidica commonly affects the shins and presents as atrophic yellowish-red plaques with prominent telangiectasias. This may precede the diagnosis of diabetes. Eruptive xanthomas are reddish-yellow papules, frequently on the buttocks, associated with hypertriglyceridemia. Acanthosis nigricans, a velvety dark brown thickening of the skin on the back of the neck and in the axillae, and skin tags are associated with insulin resistance. Vitiligo, or skin depigmentation, occurs more often in type 1 diabetes patients. Individuals on insulin can develop areas of lipoatrophy and lipohypertrophy at injection sites. It is important to recognize these conditions and advise the patient to avoid injecting in these areas because insulin absorption may be irregular.

### Hearing impairment

Hearing impairment is twice as frequent in people with diabetes [75]. Diabetes-related hearing loss is likely related to microvascular disease and neuropathy involving the inner ear. High-frequency loss is associated with history of CHD and peripheral neuropathy, whereas low-/medium-frequency loss is associated with low HDL and poor reported health status [76]. Hearing aids can be helpful.

(A)    (B)

(C)    (D)

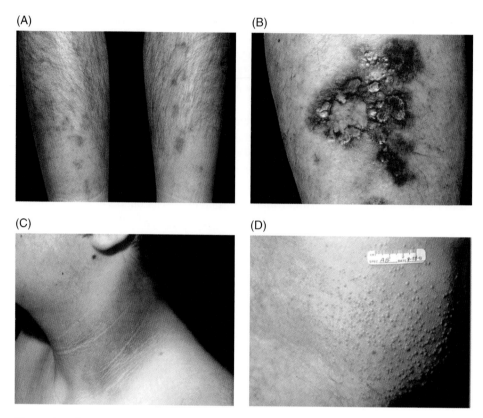

Figure 3.1    Dermatologic Lesions Associated with Diabetes. (A) Diabetic dermopathy: These are circumscribed, atrophic, slightly depressed lesions on the anterior lower legs that are asymptomatic. They arise in crops and generally resolve, but new lesions occur and may ulcerate. (B) Necrobiosis lipoidica diabeticorum: The lesions are distinctive, sharply circumscribed, multicolored plaques occurring on the anterior surfaces of the lower legs. The lesions may ulcerate. (C) Acanthosis nigricans: Velvety, brownish thickening of the skin with prominent skin creases, often associated with insulin resistance. (D) Eruptive xanthomas: Reddish-yellow papules on the buttocks and extensor surfaces of the extremities. Although generally asymptomatic, there is often an underlying severe hyper triglyceridemia (greater than 1,000 mg/dL) and potentially undiagnosed diabetes. *Fitzpatrick's Dermatology in General Medicine, 8th Edition*, with permission from McGraw-Hill Companies.

## Summary

With improved treatment of diabetes, people are living longer and the acute complications of DKA or HHS are less common. The major focus of care is prevention of hypoglycemia and chronic complications. It has been conclusively shown that early intensive glycemic control can delay or prevent many complications. A multifactorial approach including lifestyle modification; glycemic, blood pressure, and lipid control; smoking cessation; social and psychological support; and appropriate use of antiplatelet agents are all important. In addition to micro- and macrovascular complications, sleep apnea, fatty liver disease, erectile dysfunction, anxiety, depression, and certain cancers are more common. For type 1 diabetes, other autoimmune diseases may be present. Timely recognition and treatment of diabetes-related conditions can significantly improve patient outcomes and has the potential to reduce the cost of health care.

## References

1. American Diabetes Association. Economic costs of diabetes in the U.S. in 2012. *Diabetes Care* 2013; 36: 1033–1046.
2. American Diabetes Association: Standards of medical care in diabetes—2013. *Diabetes Care* 2013; 36 (Suppl. 1):S11–S66.
3. Kaufman FR, Ed. *Medical Management of Type 1 Diabetes*, 6th ed. American Diabetes Association, 2012.
4. Burant CF, Young LA, Eds. *Medical Management of Type 2 Diabetes*, 7th ed. American Diabetes Association, 2012.
5. Casqueiro J, Casqueiro J, Alves C. Infections in patients with diabetes mellitus: A review of pathogenesis. *Indian J Endocrinol Metab* 2012; 16(Suppl 1): S27–S36.
6. Peleg AY, Weerarathna T, McCarthy JS, et al. Common infections in diabetes: pathogenesis, management and relationship to glycemic control. *Diabetes Metab Res Rev* 2007; 23(1): 3–13.
7. Benfield T, Jensen JS, Nordestgaard BG. Influence of diabetes and hyperglycemia on infectious disease hospitalization and outcome. *Diabetologia* 2007; 50(3): 549–554.
8. Dooley KE, Chaisson RE. Tuberculosis and diabetes mellitus: convergence of two epidemics. *Lancet Infect Dis* 2009; 9(12): 737–746.
9. Paauw DS. Infectious emergencies in patients with diabetes. *Clinical Diabetes* 2000; 18(3): 102–105.
10. Joshi N, Caputo GM, Weitekamp MR, et al. Infections in patients with diabetes mellitus. *N Engl J Med* 1999; 341: 1906–1912.
11. Negro F, Alaei M. Hepatitis C virus and type 2 diabetes. *World J Gastroenterol* 2009; 15: 1537–1547.
12. Thomson ND, Perez JF. Eliminating the blood: ongoing outbreaks of hepatitis B virus infection and the need for innovative glucose monitoring technologies. *J Diabetes Sci Technol* 2009; 3: 283–288.
13. Centers for Disease Control and Prevention. Use of hepatitis B vaccination for adults with diabetes mellitus: recommendations of the Advisory Committee on Immunization Practices (ACIP). *MMWR* 2012; 60: 1709–1711.
14. Ata A, Lee J, Bestle SL, et al. Postoperative hyperglycemia and surgical site infection in general surgery patients. *Arch Surg* 2010; 145:858–864.
15. Latham R, Lancaster AD, Covington JF, et al. The association of diabetes and glucose control with surgical-site infections among cardiothoracic surgery patients. *Infect Control Hosp Epidemiol* 2001; 22: 607–612.
16. Zerr KJ, Furnary AP, Grunkemeier GL, et al. Glucose control lowers the risk of wound infection in diabetics after open heart operations. *Ann Thorac Surg* 1997; 63(2): 356–361.
17. Furnary AP, Zerr KJ, Grunkemeier GL, et al. Continuous intravenous insulin infusion reduces the incidence of deep sternal wound infection in diabetic patients after cardiac surgical procedures. *Ann Thorac Surg* 1999; 67(2): 352–362.
18. The DCCT Research Group. The effect of intensive treatment of diabetes on the development and progression of long-term complications in insulin-dependent diabetes mellitus. *N Engl J Med* 1993; 329: 977–986.

19. The DCCT/EDIC Research Group. Effect of intensive therapy on the microvascular complications of type 1 diabetes mellitus. *JAMA* 2002; 287: 2563–2569.
20. The DCCT/EDIC Research Group. Intensive diabetes treatment and cardiovascular disease in patients with type 1 diabetes. *N Engl J Med* 2005; 353: 2643–2653.
21. UK Prospective Diabetes Study (UKPDS) Group. Intensive blood-glucose control with sulphonylureas or insulin compared with conventional treatment and risk of complications in patients with type 2 diabetes (UKPDS 33). *Lancet* 1998; 352: 837–853.
22. Holman RR, Paul SK, Bethel MA, et al. 10-year follow-up of intensive glucose control in type 2 diabetes. *N Engl J Med* 2008; 359: 1577–1589.
23. Giacco F, Brownlee M. Oxidative stress and diabetic complications. *Circ Res* 2010; 107: 1058–1070.
24. Sun JK, Keenan HA, Cavallerano JD, et al. Protection from retinopathy and other complications in patients with type 1 diabetes of extreme duration: The Joslin 50-Year Medalist Study. *Diabetes Care* 2011; 34: 968–974.
25. Kohner EM, Aldington SJ, Stratton IM, et al. for the United Kingdom Prospective Diabetes Study. United Kingdom Prospective Diabetes Study, 30: Diabetic retinopathy at diagnosis of non-insulin-dependent diabetes mellitus and associated risk factors. *Arch Ophthalmol* 1998; 116: 297–303.
26. Diabetes Control and Complications Trial Research Group. Effect of pregnancy on microvascular complications in the diabetes control and complications trial. *Diabetes Care* 2000; 23: 1084–1091.
27. The Diabetic Retinopathy Study Research Group. Preliminary report on the effects of photocoagulation therapy. *Am J Ophthalmol* 1976; 81: 383–396.
28. Early Treatment Diabetic Retinopathy Study. Photocoagulation for diabetic macular edema. Early Treatment Diabetic Retinopathy Study report number 1. *Arch Ophthalmol* 1985; 102: 1796–1806.
29. Nguyen QD, Brown DM, Boyer DS, et al. RISE and RIDE Research Group. Ranibizumab for diabetic macular edema: results from 2 phase III randomized trials: RISE and RIDE. *Ophthalmology* 2012; 119: 789–801.
30. UK Prospective Diabetes Study Group. Tight blood pressure control and risk of macrovascular and microvascular complications in type 2 diabetes: UKPDS 38. *BMJ* 1998; 317: 703–713.
31. Garg JP, Bakris GL. Microalbuminuria: marker of vascular dysfunction, risk factor for cardiovascular disease. *Vasc Med* 2002; 7: 35–43.
32. Diabetes Control and Complications Trial/Epidemiology of Diabetes Interventions and Complications Research Group. Retinopathy and nephropathy in patients with type 1 diabetes four years after a trial of intensive therapy. *N Engl J Med* 2000; 342: 381–389.
33. Patel A, MacMahon S, Chambers J, et al. The ADVANCE Collaborative Group. Intensive blood glucose control and vascular outcomes in patients with type 2 diabetes. *N Engl J Med* 2008; 358: 2560–2572.
34. Fellerstrom BC, Jardine AG, Schmieder RE et al. Rosuvastatin and cardiovascular events in patients undergoing hemodialysis. *N Engl J Med* 2009; 360: 1395–1407.
35. Keech A, Simes RJ, Barter P, et al.: FIELD study investigators. Effects of long-term fenofibrate therapy on cardiovascular events in 9795 people with type 2 diabetes mellitus (the FIELD study): randomized controlled trial. *Lancet* 2005; 366: 1849–1861.
36. Tesfaye S, Boulton AJ, Dyck PJ, et al: Toronto Diabetic Neuropathy Expert Group. Diabetic neuropathies: update on definitions, diagnostic criteria, estimation of severity, and treatments. *Diabetes Care* 2010; 33: 2285–2293.
37. Dyck PJ, Kratz KM, Karnes JL, et al. The prevalence by staged severity of various types of diabetic neuropathy, retinopathy, and nephropathy in a population-based cohort: The Rochester Diabetic Neuropathy Study. *Neurology* 1993; 43: 817–824.

38. Gaede P, Vedel P, Parving HH, et al. Intensified multifactorial intervention in patients with type 2 diabetes mellitus and microalbuninuria: the Steno type 2 randomised study. *Lancet* 1999; 353: 617–622.
39. Rothenberg G. Avoiding foot complications. *Diabetes Insight* 2012; Volume 3: Issue 22 November 6, 2012.
40. Boulton AJ, Armstrong DG, Albert SF, et al. Comprehensive foot examination and risk assessment: a report of the Task Force of the Foot Care Interest Group of the American Diabetes Association, with endorsement by the American Association of Clinical Endocrinologists. *Diabetes Care* 2008; 31: 1679–1685.
41. Armstrong DG, Lavery LA, Vela SA, et al. Choosing a practical screening instrument to identify patients at risk for diabetic foot ulceration. *Arch Intern Med* 1998; 158: 289–292.
42. Mayfield JA, Sugarman JR. The use of the Semmes-Weinstein monofilament and other threshold tests for preventing foot ulceration and amputation in persons with diabetes. *J Fam Pract* 2000; 49: S17–29.
43. Buse JB, Ginsberg HN, Bakris GL, et al. Primary Prevention of Cardiovascular Diseases in People with Diabetes Mellitus: A scientific statement from the American Heart Association and the American Diabetes Association. *Diabetes Care* 2007; 30: 162–172.
44. Kannel WB, McGee DL. Diabetes and cardiovascular risk: the Framingham study. *Circulation* 1979; 59: 8–13.
45. Expert Panel on Detection, Evaluation, and Treatment of High Blood Cholesterol in Adults. Executive summary of the Third Report of the National Cholesterol Education Program (NCEP) Expert Panel on Detection, Evaluation, and Treatment of High Blood Cholesterol in Adults (Adult Treatment Panel III). *JAMA* 2001; 285: 2486–2497.
46. Gerstein HC, Miller ME, Byington RP, et al. The Action to Control Cardiovascular Risk in Diabetes Study Group. Effects of intensive glucose lowering in type 2 diabetes. *N Engl J Med* 2008; 358: 2545–2559.
47. Cushman WC, Evans GW, Byington RP, et al. ACCORD Study Group. Effects of intensive blood pressure control in type 2 diabetes mellitus. *N Engl J Med* 2010; 362: 1575–1585.
48. Collins R, Armitage J, Parish S, et al. Heart Protection Study Collaborative Group. MRC/BHF Heart Protection Study of cholesterol-lowering with simvastatin in 5963 people with diabetes: a randomised placebo-controlled trial. *Lancet* 2003; 361: 2005–2016.
49. Colhoun HM, Betteridge DJ, Durrington PN, et al. Primary prevention of cardiovascular disease with atorvastatin in type 2 diabetes in the Collaborative Atorvastatin Diabetes Study (CARDS): multicentre randomised placebo-controlled trial. *Lancet* 2004; 364: 685–696.
50. Stone NJ, Robinson J, Lichtenstein AH, et al. 2013 ACC/AHA guideline on the treatment of blood cholesterol to reduce atherosclerotic cardiovascular risk in adults: a report of the American College of Cardiology/American Heart Association Task Force on Practice Guidelines. *J Am Coll Cardiol* 2013; published online November 13.
51. Ginsberg HN, Elam MB, Lovato LC, et al. The ACCORD Study Group. Effects of combination lipid therapy in type 2 diabetes mellitus. *N Engl J Med* 2010; 362: 1563–1574.
52. Boden WE, Probstfield JL, Anderson T, et al. The AIM-HIGH Investigators. Niacin in patients with low HDL cholesterol levels receiving intensive statin therapy. *N Engl J Med* 2011; 365: 2255–2267.
53. Gaede P, Vedel P, Larsen N, et al. Multifactorial intervention and cardiovascular disease in patients with type 2 diabetes. *N Engl J Med* 2003; 348: 383–393.
54. Gaede P, Lund-Andersen H, Parving HH, et al. Effect of a multifactorial intervention on mortality in type 2 diabetes. *N Engl J Med* 2008; 358: 580–591.
55. Boudina S, Abel D. Diabetic cardiomyopathy revisited. *Circulation* 2007; 115: 3213–3223.
56. Biller J, Love BB. Diabetes and stroke. *The Medical Clinics of North America* 1993; 77(1): 95–110.

57. Hirsch AT, Criqui MH, Treat-Jacobson D, et al. Peripheral arterial disease detection, awareness, and treatment in primary care. *JAMA* 2001; 286: 1317–1324.
58. Barker JM. Clinical review: Type 1 diabetes-associated autoimmunity: Natural history, genetic associations, and screening. *J Clin Endocrinol Metab* 2006; 91: 1210–1217.
59. Shaw JE, Punjabi NM, Wilding JP, et al. Sleep-disordered breathing and type 2 diabetes: A report from the International Diabetes Federation Taskforce on Epidemiology and Prevention. *Diabetes Res Clin Pract* 2008; 81: 2–12.
60. Foster GD, Sanders MH, Millman R, et al for the Sleep AHEAD Research Group. Obstructive sleep apnea among obese patients with type 2 diabetes. *Diabetes Care* 2009; 32: 1017–1019.
61. Shaw KM, Cummings MH, Eds. Diabetes: *Chronic Complications*, 3rd ed. 2012. Wiley-Blackwell, West Sussex, UK.
62. Lazo M, Solga SF, Horska A, et al for the Fatty Liver Subgroup of the Look AHEAD Research Group. Effect of a 12-month intensive lifestyle intervention on hepatic steatosis in adults with type 2 diabetes. *Diabetes Care* 2010; 33: 2156–2163.
63. Selvin E, Burnett AL, Platz EA. Prevalence and risk factors for erectile dysfunction in the U.S. *American Journal of Medicine* 2007; 120: 151–157.
64. Bhasin S, Cunningham GR, Hayes FJ, et al. Testosterone therapy in men with androgen deficiency syndromes: an Endocrine Society clinical practice guideline. *J Clin Endocrinol Metab* 2010; 95: 2536–2559.
65. Grossman M. Low testosterone in men with type 2 diabetes: Significance and treatment. *J Clin Endocrinol Metab* 2011; 96: 2341–2353.
66. Giovannucci E, Harlan DM, Archer MC, et al. Diabetes and cancer: A consensus report. *Diabetes Care* 2010 33: 1674–1685.
67. Smith U, Gale EA. Does diabetes therapy influence the risk of cancer? *Diabetologia* 2009; 52: 1699–1708.
68. Currie CJ, Johnson JA. The safety profile of exogenous insulin in people with type 2 diabetes: justification for concern. *Diabetes Obes Metabolism* 2012; 14: 1–4.
69. The ORIGIN Trial Investigators. Basal insulin and cardiovascular and other outcomes in dysglycemia. *N Engl J Med* 2012; 367: 319–328.
70. American Diabetes Association, American Psychiatric Association, American Association of Clinical Endocrinologists, North American Association for the Study of Obesity. Consensus Development Conference on Antipsychotic Drugs and Obesity and Diabetes. *Diabetes Care* 2004; 27: 596–601.
71. Favus MJ. Editorial: Diabetes and the risk of osteonecrosis of the jaw. *J Clin Endocrinol Metab* 2007; 92: 817–818.
72. Khamaisi M, Regev E, Yarom N, et al. Possible association between diabetes and bisphosphonate-related jaw osteonecrosis. *J Clin Endocrinol Metab* 2007; 92: 1172–1175.
73. Hellstein JW, Adler RA, Edwards B, et al. Managing the care of patients receiving antiresorptive therapy for the treatment of osteoporosis: Executive summary of recommendations from the American Dental Association Council on Scientific Affairs. *JADA* 2011; 142(11): 1243–1251.
74. VanHattem S, Bootsma AH, Bing Thio H. Skin manifestations of diabetes. *Cleveland Clinic Journal of Medicine* 2008; 75: 772–787.
75. Bainbridge KE, Hoffman HJ, Cowie CC. Diabetes and hearing impairment in the United States: audiometric evidence from the National Health and Nutrition Examination Survey, 1999 to 2004. *Ann Intern Med* 2008; 149: 1–10.
76. Bainbridge KE, Hoffman HJ, Cowie CC. Risk factors for hearing impairment among U.S adults with diabetes: National Health and Nutrition Examination Survey, 1999 to 2004. *Diabetes Care* 2011; 34: 1540–1545.

# Chapter 4

# Glycemic treatment of diabetes mellitus

*Harpreet Kaur, MD and Ruth S. Weinstock, MD, PhD*

## Introduction

It has been well demonstrated that good blood glucose control can help prevent or slow the development of diabetes complications [1–5]. The approach to achieving glycemic goals and the pharmacological therapy used need to be individualized, and vary depending upon the type of diabetes, age, life expectancy, degree of hypoglycemic awareness, and presence of diabetes-related complications and other co-morbidities [6, 7]. Different treatment options are described, and their potential benefits and risks discussed in this chapter.

## Team approach

Diabetes, more than any other chronic disease, requires daily self management. Lifestyle change is often recommended. A multidisciplinary team approach, providing comprehensive education and training as well as pharmacological therapy, can be particularly effective [8–13]. Team members may include, but are not limited to, physicians, dentists, physician extenders, dietitians, nurse educators, podiatrists, pharmacists, eye care providers, health coaches, social workers, and mental health professionals. Other specialists such as cardiologists, nephrologists, and neurologists may be required to assist with management of diabetes-related complications. Support from family, friends, and community can be especially helpful in attaining lifestyle change goals. To obtain the necessary instruction, people with diabetes and their family and friends should be referred to certified diabetes educators (CDEs) and/or comprehensive diabetes education programs that meet the National Standards for Diabetes Self-Management Education and Support [14]. Programs are certified by the American Diabetes Association (http://professional. diabetes.org/Recognition.aspx?typ=15&cid=84040) or the American Association of Diabetes Educators (http://www.diabeteseducator.org/ProfessionalResources/accred). Reimbursement can be available from Medicare and other insurers if the individual is referred to a certified program. Health care professionals interested in becoming CDEs

*Diabetes Mellitus and Oral Health: An Interprofessional Approach*, First Edition. Edited by Ira B. Lamster.
© 2014 John Wiley & Sons, Inc. Published 2014 by John Wiley & Sons, Inc.

are referred to the website of the National Certification Board for Diabetes Educators (http://www.ncbde.org/).


## Glycemic goals

### *Assessments of glycemic control*

Every person with diabetes should have an individualized glycemic goal [6, 7, 15, 16]. Goals are defined by results from the following methods for assessing glycemic control: home self-monitoring of blood glucose (SMBG), continuous glucose monitoring (CGM), and hemoglobin A1c (HbA1c) levels.

Home blood glucose monitoring devices, which use a small drop of blood to measure blood glucose levels, are readily available. Frequency and timing of SMBG is individualized and vary with different insulin regimens, taking into consideration patient-specific factors such as history of hypoglycemia and hypoglycemic unawareness. SMBG should be performed by all individuals who use insulin therapy.

The use of SMBG for people with type 2 diabetes who are not treated with insulin is controversial [17–21]. Potential benefits include the detection of severe hypoglycemia (relatively rare in non-insulin-treated patients) and a better understanding of glycemic excursions which alert patients to the need to modify their diet and/or medical regimen. Patients should have the skills and the ability to work collaboratively with their health care team to use the information from SMBG to improve their glycemic status [18]. The arguments against using SMBG in non-insulin-treated patients with type 2 diabetes primarily concern the expense, inconvenience, and paucity of evidence directly linking SMBG with improved glycemic control [17, 19, 20].

Continuous glucose monitoring systems use subcutaneous electrochemical sensors to measure interstitial glucose levels every few minutes, 24 hours/day. Glucose values are sent wirelessly to a receiver (a separate external device or an insulin pump). Individual values and trend arrows and graphs are displayed on the receiver, and alarms are used to warn users of serious hypoglycemia and hyperglycemia. By displaying glucose levels and trends every few minutes, patients are provided with important information that allows them to make better decisions regarding insulin dosing, carbohydrate intake, and physical activity. CGM systems need to be calibrated daily with SMBG and are not as accurate as SMBG, and values may lag behind SMBG when glucose concentrations change rapidly. Candidates for personal CGM systems are motivated individuals using intensive insulin regimens, primarily adults with type 1 diabetes who are willing and able to use the CGM system regularly as directed and make changes based on the CGM data [22–24]. CGM may particularly help people with a history of severe hypoglycemia, nocturnal hypoglycemia, or hypoglycemic unawareness [25]. Professional CGM systems are also available. These systems are purchased by the physician's office, and are given to patients to wear for several days. Unlike the personal CGM systems, the patients cannot see their glucose levels in real time. When the devices are returned to the physician's office, the CGM data are downloaded and reviewed. Changes in pharmacologic as well as non-pharmacologic therapies are often recommended based upon this information.

Table 4.1    Correlation of A1c with average glucose (AG).

| A1c (%) | Mean plasma glucose | |
|---|---|---|
| | mg/dL | mmol/L |
| 6 | 126 | 7.0 |
| 7 | 154 | 8.6 |
| 8 | 183 | 10.2 |
| 9 | 212 | 11.8 |
| 10 | 240 | 13.4 |
| 11 | 269 | 14.9 |
| 12 | 298 | 16.5 |

These estimates are based on ADAG data of approximately 2,700 glucose measurements over three months per A1c measurement in 507 adults with type 1, type 2, and no diabetes. The correlation between A1c and average glucose was 0.92 [99]. A calculator for converting A1c results into eAG, in either mg/dL or mmol/L, is available at http://professional.diabetes.org/eAG.

With permission from The American Diabetes Association. Standards of Medical Care in Diabetes 2013. *Diabetes Care*. 2013; 36 (Suppl 1): S19

The A1c test measures glycated hemoglobin, an indicator of the average blood glucose level over the past two to three months (Table 4.1). Higher A1c levels are associated with the development of more diabetes-related complications [1–5]. The standard of care is to obtain this test two to four times annually [6]. Blood samples can be sent to a certified clinical laboratory, or the test can be performed in the office using a small drop of blood in a point-of-care device.

## Setting glycemic goals

Establishing individualized goals requires the consideration of many factors, including the patient's age, type of diabetes, duration of diabetes, presence of co-morbidities including microvascular and macrovascular diseases, degree of hypoglycemic awareness, life expectancy, financial constraints, and psychosocial issues (Figure 4.1) [6, 7, 15, 16]. The 2013 Standards of Medical Care in Diabetes, published by the American Diabetes Association recommend the following [6]:

1  For healthy nonpregnant adults with new onset or short duration diabetes, in general, a "reasonable" A1c goal is around or below 7% (fasting glucose 70–130 mg/dl; peak post-prandial glucose lower than 180 mg/dl) if this can be achieved without serious or frequent hypoglycemia. This is based upon the evidence from large randomized clinical trials in type 1 and type 2 diabetes demonstrating reduced microvascular and macrovascular disease at these A1c levels [1–5]. Lower A1c levels (e.g., A1c less than 6.5%) may be appropriate in some adults with long life expectancy in the absence of significant cardiovascular disease and other serious co-morbidities.

Approach to management
of hyperglycemia:

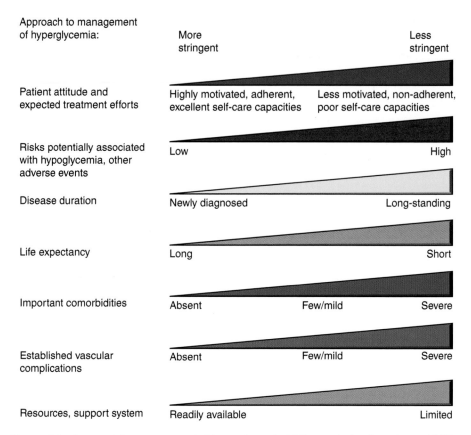

Figure 4.1    Approach to management of hyperglycemia. With permission from: Inzucchi SE, Bergenstal RM, Buse JB, Diamant M, et al. Management of hyperglycemia in type 2 diabetes: a patient-centered approach. Position statement of the American Diabetes Association (ADA) and the European Association for the Study of Diabetes (EASD). *Diabetes Care 2012*. 35:1366

2  An A1c goal of less than 8% should be considered for non-pregnant adults with serious co-morbidities, reduced life expectancy, advanced age, long-duration diabetes, cardiovascular disease, multiple cardiac risk factors, history of severe hypoglycemia or hypoglycemic unawareness, frailty, psycho-social problems (e.g., poor social support), and/or difficulty achieving A1c of 7% despite diabetes self-management education and support and use of appropriate monitoring and therapies. This is based, in part, upon the evidence from large randomized clinical trials demonstrating either limited or no cardio-vascular benefit or increased mortality with intensive therapy in patients with longstanding type 2 diabetes and cardiovascular disease and/or cardiovascular risk factors [26, 27].

3  For children with type 1 diabetes, in general, the following goals are used: ages 0–6 years, A1c less than 8.5%, pre-meal glucose 100–180 mg/dl, and bedtime/overnight glucose 110–200 mg/dl; ages 6–12 years, A1c less than 8%, pre-meal glucose 90–180 mg/dl, bedtime/overnight glucose 100–180 mg/dl; ages 13–19 years, A1c less than 7.5%, pre-meal glucose 90–130 mg/dl, bedtime/overnight glucose 90–150 mg/dl. Lower goals can be used if they can be achieved without excessive hypoglycemia, taking into account the ability of the child to detect and appropriately respond to hypoglycemia.

4 For hospitalized adults who are critically ill, insulin therapy is recommended, with the goal glucose 140–180 mg/dl. For non-critically ill hospitalized patients, pre-meal glucose less than 140 mg/dl and random glucose less than 180 mg/dl are recommended. These goals should be adjusted based upon the presence or absence of severe co-morbidities and hypoglycemia.

5 In pregnancy, more stringent glycemic goals are recommended to prevent fetal malformations and other adverse fetal and maternal outcomes. For women with diabetes pre-conception, the A1c goal is less than 6%; pre-meal, bedtime, and overnight glucose 60–99 mg/dl, and peak post-prandial glucose levels 100–129 mg/dl [28]. In gestational diabetes, the pre-prandial glucose goal is less than or equal to 95 mg/dl and either one-hour post meal less than or equal to 140 or two-hour post meal less than or equal to 120 mg/dl.

## Glycemic management of type 1 diabetes mellitus

People with type 1 diabetes have an absolute deficiency of insulin production and depend upon insulin therapy. This usually involves self-administration of at least 4 subcutaneous insulin injections daily (one to two injections of a basal insulin and mealtime injections of rapid-acting insulin; Figure 4.2A), or use of an insulin pump which is also referred to as continuous subcutaneous insulin infusion (CSII). If insulin therapy is interrupted or suspended in people with type 1 diabetes for a significant amount of time, they are at risk for developing life-threatening diabetic ketoacidosis.

### Lifestyle

Medical nutrition therapy (MNT; individualized nutrition counseling) is an essential aspect of management because specific diet-related behaviors influence glycemic control [29]. The mealtime insulin dosing depends in part on the carbohydrate content of that meal. Patients are taught carbohydrate monitoring (use of carbohydrate-consistent diets, experience-based carbohydrate estimations, or counting grams of carbohydrate). Nutritional recommendations are also based upon personal, social, cultural, and psychological factors; weight management considerations; and nutritional needs. In general, low-saturated fat (less than 7% of calories) and limited trans fat in the diet are recommended [6] to help reduce cardiovascular risk. Reimbursement of MNT by Medicare and many insurers is possible when provided by a registered dietitian.

Regular physical activity (at least 150 minutes/week of aerobic exercise and twice/week resistance training) is recommended for people with diabetes who feel well and are not ketotic [6]. People with good glycemic control usually experience a fall in glucose levels with exercise, but glucose concentrations can rise in patients with uncontrolled diabetes (glucose greater than 250 mg/dL). The glucose response to exercise depends on the type, intensity, and duration of exercise; the serum glucose and insulin concentrations at the time of exercise; and the time, type, dose, and site of the recent insulin injections. Adjustments of insulin dosing and administration of carbohydrate-containing snacks are generally needed, particularly with long-term exercise [30]. Healthy individuals need to be educated in ways of avoiding hypoglycemia (reducing insulin dosing or adding carbohydrate before, during, and/or after exercise) prior to starting a new exercise regimen. Patients with cardiac disease, uncontrolled hypertension, severe neuropathy, untreated proliferative retinopathy, and other serious co-morbid conditions or cardiovascular risk factors should not begin an exercise program before consulting with their physician.

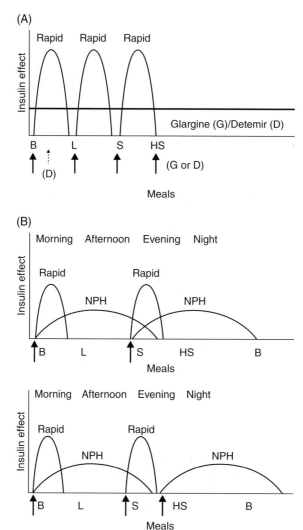

**Figure 4.2** (A) Schematic representation of idealized insulin effect provided by three daily injections with rapid-acting insulin at meals and once-daily insulin glargine or detemir at bedtime. Detemir sometimes is given twice daily (dashed arrow). B=breakfast, L=lunch, S=supper, HS=bedtime, arrow=time of insulin injection before meals. (B) Schematic representation of idealized insulin effect provided by "split-mixed" insulin regimen consisting of two daily injections of rapid- and intermediate-acting insulin given before breakfast and supper (upper panel) and three daily injections with rapid- and intermediate-acting insulin before breakfast, rapid-acting insulin at supper, and intermediate-acting insulin at bedtime (lower panel). B=breakfast, L=lunch, S=supper, HS=bedtime, arrow=time of insulin injection before meals.

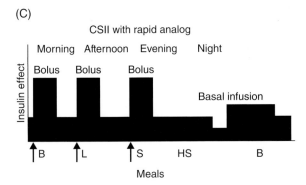

Figure 4.2 (*Continued*) (C) Schematic representation of idealized insulin effect provided by continuous subcutaneous insulin infusion (insulin pump) with rapid analog. B=breakfast, L=lunch, S=supper, HS=bedtime, arrow=time of insulin injection before meals. With permission from the American Diabetes Association [100].

## Home glucose monitoring

SMBG is essential in the management of type 1 diabetes to help prevent serious hypoglycemia and hyperglycemia. It is recommended that people with type 1 diabetes self-monitor before meals and snacks; prior to, during, and after exercise; at bedtime; before driving or performing other potentially dangerous tasks; when under stress; when hypoglycemia or hyperglycemia are suspected; and occasionally after meals. Patients are taught to modify the timing and/or dosage of insulin and the timing and/or content of meals and snacks based on these glucose results. CGM can also be helpful in selected individuals.

## Insulin therapy

Individuals with type 1 diabetes require basal (continuous) insulin to keep glucose levels normal when not eating, and bolus (rapidly acting) insulin with meals to prevent postprandial hyperglycemia. Bolus insulin is also used to correct hyperglycemia. The basal and prandial insulin requirements typically comprise 40–50% and 50–60%, respectively, of the total daily dose. This is accomplished with subcutaneous insulin injection therapy (usually at least four injections daily) or insulin pump therapy. Insulin therapy is adjusted for multiple factors, the most important of which are carbohydrate intake, physical activity, stress, and use of concomitant medications known to increase glucose levels (e.g., glucocorticoids).

Insulin injections are administered using either a needle and syringe or an insulin pen. Injection therapy with insulin syringes requires drawing the amount of insulin needed from the vial into the syringe accurately. Because insulin is needed for meals and most snacks, a major limitation in the use of insulin vials, needles, and syringes is the inconvenience of carrying these items throughout the day. Insulin pens are pre-filled with insulin and may be either disposable or reusable. They are portable, easy to use, provide accurate dosing, may be particularly helpful for people with difficulties with vision and/or dexterity, and are associated with higher patient satisfaction compared to use of vials

Table 4.2   Insulin preparations available for subcutaneous use.

| Insulin | | | |
|---|---|---|---|
| **Human insulins** | **Onset of action** | **Peak action** | **Duration of action** |
| Rapidly acting: Lispro (Humalog) Aspart (Novolog) Glulisine (Apidra) | 5–30 minutes | 0.5–3 hours | 3–5 hours |
| Short acting: Regular (R) | 30–60 minutes | 1–5 hours | 6–8 hours |
| Intermediate acting: | 1–4 hours | 4–10 hours | 14–24 hours |
| NPH, NPL, NPA | 3–4 hours | 4–8 hours | 6–24 hours |
| Detemir (Levemir) | | (modest) | |
| Long acting: Glargine (Lantus) | 2–3 hours | none | 24–30 hours |

| Premixed insulins | | | | |
|---|---|---|---|---|
| **Insulin** | **Components** | **Onset** | **Peak** | **Duration** |
| Human 70/30 (Humulin-70/30 Novolin-70/30) | 30% Regular 70% NPH | 30 minutes | 2–4 hours | 8–24 hours |
| NovoLog Mix 70/30 | 30% aspart 70% aspart protamine | 15 minutes | 1–4 hours (mean 60 minutes) | 8–24 hours |
| Humalog Mix 75/25 | 25% lispro 75% lispro protamine | 15 minutes | 1–4 hours (mean 60 minutes) | 8–24 hours |
| Human 50/50 (Humulin 50/50) | 50% Regular 50% NPH | 30 minutes | 2–4 hours | 8–24 hours |

Note: The pharmacokinetics of insulin preparations vary in different individuals and can change depending upon site of injection, dose, and other factors.

and syringes [31–33]. Insulin administration using syringes, however, is less expensive than using insulin pens.

Insulin preparations are classified by duration of action: rapid-, short-, intermediate–, and long-acting (Table 4.2). Regular and neutral protamine hagedorn (NPH) insulin are the least expensive. They have the same amino acid sequence as human insulin. All other insulin preparations are insulin analogs, in which the insulin molecule has been modified to change its onset and duration of action. The pre-mixed insulins (Table 4.2) may be useful in selected patients with type 2 diabetes.

Only regular insulin should be given intravenously. This is usually needed in hospital settings for the treatment of diabetic ketoacidosis, or for use in insulin infusions in inpatients who require insulin therapy and are not eating.

### Basal insulin preparations

Insulin glargine is a long-acting insulin analog that has the amino acid sequence of human insulin except for a substitution of glycine for asparagine in position A21 and the addition of two arginine molecules at the C-terminus of the B-chain of the insulin molecule.

Because of these modifications, the insulin (in the vial or pen) needs to be at a lower pH to remain in solution. After injection into the subcutaneous tissue (neutral pH), microprecipitates form and small amounts of insulin are slowly released. This results in a prolonged duration of action with no pronounced peak effect. Insulin glargine is usually self-administered once daily (Figure 4.2A).

Insulin detemir is a long-acting insulin analog that has duration of action that is partially dose-related, lasting longer when higher amounts are used. This analog differs from human insulin by the lack of threonine at position B30 and the addition of a fatty acid side chain at B29. Release from the subcutaneous tissue is slowed by self-association and albumin binding. A randomized trial comparing insulin glargine with insulin detemir for basal coverage in type 1 diabetes concluded that each provided similar effects on glycemic control (A1c levels) and risk of hypoglycemia, and there was no difference in tolerability [34]. Patients with type 1 diabetes require one to two injections of detemir daily for basal coverage (Figure 4.2A), and may require a higher dose of detemir compared to glargine.

NPH (neutral protamine Hagedorn) insulin is an intermediate-acting insulin. It is neutral regular crystalline zinc insulin complexed to protamine; Hagedorn's laboratory was the first to use protamine to prolong insulin action. NPH insulin is less expensive than the basal insulin analogs. NPH insulin needs to be used at least twice daily to provide 24-hour basal coverage, and has a significant peak activity, usually 6–8 hours after injection (Table 4.2, Figure 4.2B). Care is needed to avoid hypoglycemia during times of peak activity, which for morning dosing would occur in the afternoon, and for evening dosing could happen in the middle of the night. Administering NPH insulin at bedtime instead of before dinner can reduce the likelihood of middle-of-the-night hypoglycemia. The basal insulin analogs have been shown to be more effective than NPH in lowering fasting glucose levels in type 1 diabetes [35, 36]. Other intermediate-acting insulin preparations, primarily used in insulin mixtures, are shown in Table 4.2.

### Bolus insulin preparations

Regular insulin has the same amino acid sequence as human insulin. It is complexed with zinc and self-associates into hexamers after injection. The hexamers need to dissociate into dimers and monomers to be absorbed into the bloodstream, prolonging its time of onset and duration of action (Table 4.2). Regular insulin is the least expensive short-acting insulin, but has the disadvantage that, when injected subcutaneously, has a slower onset of action and longer duration of action when compared to the rapidly acting insulin analogs. For this reason it should be injected at least 30 minutes before the meal and can cause hypoglycemia several hours after eating.

There are three rapidly acting insulin analogs: aspart (aspartic acid at B28), lispro (proline B28 and lysine B29 are reversed), and glulisine (lysine at B3, glutamine acid at B29). These modifications result in faster absorption from the subcutaneous tissue resulting in a shorter duration of action (Table 4.2). The rapidly acting insulin analogs are routinely used for mealtime coverage in insulin injection therapy (Figure 4.2A). They are usually self-administered at the start of the meal or within 5–15 minutes of the start of the meal, with peak activity usually within one to two hours. In specific circumstances, such as when carbohydrate intake is uncertain, rapidly acting insulin is given right after the meal to avoid giving too much insulin, which would result in hypoglycemia. Some studies have shown better prandial glycemic control and lower risk of hypoglycemia with the use of insulin analogs [36]. The rapidly-acting insulin analogs are preferred for use in insulin pumps [37, 38]. Their higher cost (compared to regular insulin) is a disadvantage of the insulin analogs.

### Insulin pump therapy (continuous subcutaneous insulin infusion)

Insulin pumps are widely used as an alternative method of delivering insulin in type 1 diabetes. The pump is an external device that contains rapidly acting insulin. CSII devices accurately deliver insulin, especially small doses, because fractions of a unit can be administered. The insulin is delivered subcutaneously through a disposable small catheter (infusion set) that is typically changed every two to three days by the patient. In most commercially available pumps, the catheter is connected by tubing to the pump which controls the rate of insulin delivery. The pump is typically placed in a clothing pocket or pouch. Alternatively, there are "tubing-free" CSII systems in which the insulin is placed in a "pod." The pod is taped to the skin and directly delivers insulin subcutaneously through a small integrated canula. In the latter case, the device controlling the insulin infusion delivery communicates wirelessly with the pod. Some models of insulin pumps can receive SMBG and CGM values wirelessly.

Insulin pumps deliver insulin every few minutes to provide basal insulin coverage. The basal insulin infusion rate(s) can be programmed either to deliver insulin at a constant rate over the 24-hour period or, commonly, to vary infusions rates at different times over the 24-hour period for patients who have different basal insulin requirements during the day or night (Figure 4.2C). Patients can also temporarily alter their basal rates. For example, during times of physical activity, basal rates can be reduced to avoid hypoglycemia.

CSII devices can receive input (glucose levels and anticipated carbohydrate intake), and contain calculators that help patients determine their bolus doses. To control post-prandial hyperglycemia, boluses of insulin are delivered in proportion to the anticipated carbohydrate intake, typically using insulin:carbohydrate ratios. A bolus can also be used to correct hyperglycemia. To help determine the "correction dose," the calculator uses the following insulin pump settings: glucose target, insulin on board (duration of active insulin), and "sensitivity factors" or "correction factors." The latter are the glucose-lowering effect of one unit of insulin for that patient (e.g., one unit may lower glucose levels by 40 mg/dl). Pump systems also warn patients of insulin "stacking" (i.e., taking correction doses of insulin too close to each other which can results in later hypoglycemia).

CSII is considered more flexible and convenient than injection therapy because patients do not have to carry insulin vials and syringes or insulin pens. A meta-analysis concluded that CSII, especially CGM (sensor)-augmented pump therapy, is associated with better glycemic control in adults with type 1 diabetes compared to SMBG with injection therapy [39]. In adults, quality of life was better with CSII, and in children, treatment satisfaction was higher with CSII treatment [39].

Disadvantages of insulin pump therapy are the following: The costs of the pump and pump supplies are higher than those of supplies needed for injection therapy. There is a small risk of infection at the insulin infusion site, especially if the infusion sets are not changed every three days. In addition, because only rapid-acting insulin is used in CSII, pump failure as a result of mechanical malfunction or catheter occlusion can quickly result in severe hyperglycemia and ketoacidosis. Patients treated with CSII must be motivated and properly trained to use pump therapy, should monitor their glucose levels frequently, and must always be prepared for the possibility of failure of the infusion system.

### Pramlintide therapy

Amylin, co-secreted with insulin by the pancreatic β cells, lowers post-prandial glucose levels. It reduces post-prandial glucagon secretion, slows gastric emptying time, and promotes satiety through centrally mediated appetite suppression. The amylin response to food intake is absent in type 1 diabetes and diminished in type 2 diabetes [40]. Pramlintide is a subcutaneously administered amylin analog approved for mealtime use in type 1 and type 2 diabetes using prandial insulin therapy. Modest improvements in glycemic control have been reported [41]. It may also assist with weight management [40, 41]. Hypoglycemia has been reported, especially when pramlintide treatment was started without reducing the pre-meal insulin dosages. It is recommended to decrease meal-time insulin dose by 20–50% when starting pramlintide and to perform SMBG more often initially. The most commonly reported side effect from pramlintide is mild to moderate nausea. This generally dissipates by four weeks and can be minimized by slow dose titration. Pramlintide therapy is expensive, requires an additional injection before meals, and should not be used in patients with gastroparesis or who have hypoglycemic unawareness.

## Glycemic management of type 2 diabetes mellitus

Type 2 diabetes is primarily characterized by impaired insulin secretion and hepatic and peripheral insulin resistance. The insulin secretory defect commonly worsens over time, at a rate that varies in different individuals. The progressive failure of the pancreatic β cells necessitates intensification of therapy and, for many individuals, treatment with insulin. The insulin resistance is manifest primarily as an inappropriate production of glucose from the liver and impaired glucose uptake in skeletal muscle. Glucagon-like peptide-1 (GLP-1) secretion is also reduced in type 2 diabetes. This incretin hormone, produced in intestinal L cells and secreted in response to nutrients, affects glucose control by increasing glucose-dependent insulin secretion, reducing postprandial glucagon secretion, slowing gastric emptying, and decreasing food intake by suppressing appetite. Drugs are available that target the defects in insulin secretion, insulin resistance, and GLP-1 concentrations.

### Lifestyle

Lifestyle modifications, including weight management (diet and physical activity), play important roles in the achievement of glycemic goals. Obesity, especially visceral adiposity, is associated with increased insulin resistance. For individuals with type 2 diabetes who are overweight or obese (the majority of people with type 2 diabetes), weight loss is of great benefit. Meal plans should be individualized and guided by factors such as age, lifestyle, body weight, medication regimen, motivation, finances, and cultural and social issues. For those individuals using basal/bolus insulin therapy, MNT is similar to that described above for type 1 diabetes.

Regular exercise improves insulin sensitivity, glycemic control, cardiovascular risk status (blood pressure, triglyceride levels, waist circumference), and quality of life, and helps maintain weight loss [42–44]. At least 150 minutes/week of aerobic physical activity and resistance training at least twice weekly is recommended [6, 43]. These beneficial effects persist with maintenance of the exercise regimen. However, many individuals with type 2 diabetes have limited capacity to exercise due to advanced age, obesity-related complications (e.g., arthritis), and diabetes-related co-morbidities such as cardiovascular disease (including subclinical left ventricular dysfunction) and autonomic dysfunction, [6, 45]. Individuals with these conditions as well as uncontrolled hypertension and severe retinopathy or neuropathy should consult with their physicians before starting an exercise program. An exercise specialist or physical therapist may be helpful in selected cases.

## Pharmacological therapy

Oral as well as non-insulin injectable agents are available for the treatment of type 2 diabetes (Table 4.3) [7, 46–49]. These drugs can be used alone or in combination. In general, metformin is the initial medication prescribed [7, 48, 49]. If metformin monotherapy is insufficient for attainment of glycemic goals or cannot be given because of contraindications or intolerance, other oral or injectable medications can be added or substituted. For patients who present with severe hyperglycemia or who cannot tolerate or achieve glycemic goals with these medications, insulin therapy is used.

### Metformin

Metformin is the most commonly used first -ine agent for the treatment of type 2 diabetes due to its efficacy, safety, and low cost. Its main mechanism of action is activation of AMP-kinase and reduction of hepatic glucose production. It does not cause hypoglycemia and is weight neutral. A systematic review of 29 trials concluded that metformin was associated with decreased all-cause mortality and rate of myocardial infarction in obese and overweight patients [50].

The most common side effects of metformin are gastrointestinal, including nausea, abdominal discomfort, and diarrhea. These can be minimized by the gradual titration of the metformin dose. Metformin also reduces intestinal absorption of vitamin $B_{12}$ in up to 30% of patients. The risk of developing vitamin $B_{12}$ deficiency depends on the dose and duration of therapy. Lactic acidosis is considered an extremely rare side effect of metformin. Pooled data from 347 comparative trials and cohort studies failed to demonstrate any cases of fatal or nonfatal lactic acidosis in 70,490 patient-years of metformin use [51]. Renal insufficiency is considered a risk factor for the development of lactic acidosis with metformin. Metformin should be discontinued in patients who are about to receive intravenous iodinated contrast material or undergo a surgical procedure. It can be resumed after 48 hours or once patients have stable renal function.

Table 4.3  Medications commonly used to treat type 2 diabetes.

| Medication class | Medication | Major mechanisms/ action | Benefits | Disadvantages/side effects | Cost |
|---|---|---|---|---|---|
| Biguanide (oral) | Metformin (Glucophage, Glumetza, Riomet, Fortamet) | Activate hepatic AMP-kinase; decrease hepatic glucose production | First line therapy<br>Weight neutral<br>No hypoglycemia<br>Possibly fewer CVD events and cancer<br>Generics available | GI: diarrhea (usually but not always transient), abdominal discomfort, nausea, vomiting, anorexia<br>Rare lactic acidosis<br>Vitamin $B_{12}$ deficiency | Low |
| Sulfonylurea (oral) | Glyburide (DiaBeta, Micronas, Glynase)<br>Glipizide (Glucotrol)<br>Glimepiride (Amaryl) | Closes $K_{ATP}$ channels on pancreatic β-cells; stimulation of insulin secretion | Generics available | Hypoglycemia<br>Weight gain<br>May adversely affect ischemic preconditioning | Low |
| Meglitinides (oral) | Repaglinide (Prandin)<br>Nateglinide (Starlix) | Closes $K_{ATP}$ channels on pancreatic β-cells<br>Stimulates insulin secretion | Short acting | Hypoglycemia (less than sulfonylureas)<br>Weight gain<br>Dose before each meal | Medium |
| Thiazolidinediones (oral) | Pioglitazone (Actos)<br>Rosiglitazone (Avandia) | Activates transcription factor PPAR-gamma<br>Alters transcription of specific genes<br>Decreases insulin resistance | No hypoglycemia<br>Possible decrease in myocardial infarctions | Weight gain<br>Edema, Congestive heart failure, ↑ MI (Avandia)<br>Bone fractures<br>Macular edema<br>↑ bladder cancer (Actos) | High |
| Alpha-glucosidase inhibitors (oral) | Acarbose (Precose)<br>Miglitol (Glyset) | Competitively inhibit α-glucosidase in intestines<br>Delays carbohydrate absorption<br>Reduction in post prandial glucose levels | No hypoglycemia<br>Weight neutral<br>Moderate efficacy in lowering postprandial glucose levels | GI: flatulence, diarrhea, abdominal fullness and discomfort<br>Take with each carbohydrate-containing meal | Medium |

(Continued)

Table 4.3 (Continued)

| Medication class | Medication | Major mechanisms/action | Benefits | Disadvantages/side effects | Cost |
|---|---|---|---|---|---|
| GLP-1 receptor agonists (subcutaneous injection) | Exenatide (Byetta, Bydureon) Liraglutide (Victoza) | Activate GLP-1 receptor; increase glucose-stimulated insulin secretion, decrease glucagon secretion, slow gastric motility, increase satiety | Promote weight loss | Risk of pancreatitis GI: nausea, vomiting, diarrhea Hypoglycemia (less than sulfonylureas) Caution with renal insufficiency Inject subcutaneously (Byetta twice daily, Bydureon once weekly, Victoza once daily) | High |
| DPP-4 inhibitors (oral) | Sitagliptin (Januvia) Saxagliptin (Onglyza) Linagliptin (Trajenta) Alogliptin (Nesina) | Inhibit metabolism of GLP-1 | Weight neutral | Risk of pancreatitis Possible runny nose, URIs, headache Hypoglycemia: rare | High |
| SGLT2 inhibitors (oral) | Canagliflozin (Invokana) Dapagliflozin (Farxiga) | Reduce glucose reabsorption in the kidney Increases urinary glucose excretion | Weight loss possible, no hypoglycemia | Genital mycotic infections, urinary tract infections, hypotension, impaired renal function, hyperkalemia, hypersensitivity, increased LDL-cholesterol | High |

## Sulfonylurea drugs

Sulfonylurea drugs are inexpensive insulin secretagogues. They bind to the sulfonylurea receptor (SUR) on the pancreatic β cell, causing inhibition of ATP-dependent potassium channels, calcium influx, and stimulation of insulin secretion. Sulfonylureas are usually well tolerated but can be associated with weight gain. The most common side effect is hypoglycemia, which is more common in the elderly, in the presence of reduced renal and hepatic function, and with long-acting sulfonylureas such as glyburide. Glipizide (extended-release) and glimepiride are preferred because they can be given once daily in most patients and are associated with a lower risk of hypoglycemia. Some studies have linked sulfonylurea use with poorer outcomes after myocardial infarction due to adverse effects on ischemic preconditioning [52], but data supporting this are inconclusive.

## Meglitinides

Repaglinide and nateglinide are short-acting insulin secretagogues that are taken orally with each meal. They are pharmacologically and structurally distinct from sulfonylureas but act similarly by closing ATP-dependent potassium channels, causing release of insulin. Both drugs have a lower risk for weight gain and hypoglycemia but are more expensive than sulfonylurea drugs. They also need to be taken several times daily (with each meal). Nateglinide should not be used in the presence of renal insufficiency because of risk of hypoglycemia. Repaglinide is principally metabolized by the liver, with less than 10% excreted by the kidneys. No dose adjustment is necessary with repaglinide use in patients with renal insufficiency.

## GLP-1 receptor agonists

GLP-1 receptor agonists are effective in improving glycemic control. They are self administered by subcutaneous injection, can assist with weight loss, and are associated with low risk of hypoglycemia. There are three GLP-1 receptor agonists: once-daily liraglutide, twice-daily exenatide, and once-weekly exenatide extended release (exenatide ER). All use pen devices. Side effects are mainly gastrointestinal. Nausea and vomiting are common, but usually wane with increased duration of therapy and reduced dosing [53]. Disadvantages include cost and risk of pancreatitis. In general, these drugs should be used with caution in patients with moderate renal impairment and they are not recommended with severe renal insufficiency due to reports of acute renal failure. Thyroid C-cell hyperplasia and tumors have been reported in rodents, but not in humans. Long-term safety is unknown.

## Dipeptidyl peptidase-4 inhibitors

Endogenous GLP-1 has a short half life due to rapid metabolism by dipeptidyl peptidase-4 (DPP-4). Oral DPP-4 inhibitors, which increase endogenous GLP-1 levels, include sitagliptin, saxagliptin, linagliptin, and alogliptin. These drugs are administered once daily, are well-tolerated, and are weight neutral. They do not cause hypoglycemia. Their efficacy in lowering A1c is less than that observed with the GLP-1 receptor agonists and they do not cause weight loss, possibly due to the fact that they do not raise GLP-1 levels as high or for as long as the GLP-1 receptor agonists [54]. Disadvantages include cost and risk of pancreatitis. Long-term safety is unknown.

### Thiazolidinediones

The thiazolidinedione drug pioglitazone is a peroxisome proliferator–activated receptor γ activator that improves insulin sensitivity by changing the transcription of specific genes. It does not cause hypoglycemia. Pioglitazone was associated with decreased mortality, non-fatal myocardial infarctions, and stroke in a large trial involving patients at high risk for macrovascular disease [55]. Disadvantages are cost, weight gain, fluid retention (edema and/or heart failure), increased risk of bone fractures, and bladder cancer [56, 57].

### α-glucosidase inhibitors

The α-glucosidase inhibitors acarbose and miglitol competitively inhibit the gastrointestinal α-glucosidases, slowing carbohydrate breakdown resulting in a delayed rise and reduced peak in post-prandial blood glucose concentrations. These drugs are given orally with meals, and their glucose-lowering effects are modest [58]. They are weight neutral and do not cause hypoglycemia. The major side effects are flatulence and diarrhea.

### Sodium-glucose cotransporter 2 inhibitors

Sodium-glucose cotransporter 2 (SGLT2) regulates approximately 90% of glucose reabsorption in the proximal tubules of the kidney. The oral inhibitors of SGLT2, canaglifloxin, and dapagliflozin, improves glycemic control by increasing urinary glucose excretion. Weight loss is possible, and it does not cause hypoglycemia. Potential side effects include increased genital mycotic infections and urinary tract infections, polyuria with volume depletion including possible hypotension and impaired renal function, hyperkalemia, and increased LDL-cholesterol concentrations. Long-term side effects are unknown.

### Other noninsulin medications

The bile acid sequestrant colesevelam, primarily used to lower LDL-cholesterol levels, has a modest effect on improving glycemic control. It does not cause hypoglycemia. Side effects include constipation and elevation of triglyceride concentrations. It is expensive and can interfere with the absorption of other medications.

Use of the dopamine-2 agonist bromocriptine is associated with improvement in insulin sensitivity. There is no hypoglycemia, but the effect on A1c is modest. Side effects include nausea, fatigue, dizziness, syncope, and rhinitis.

### Insulin

Patients who do not reach glycemic goals despite non-insulin monotherapy or combination therapy or cannot tolerate the medications described above require insulin therapy. Use of insulin should never be used as a threat or referred to as a treatment of last resort in type 2 diabetes, because it is appropriate therapy in a variety of circumstances. Insulin can be added to oral glycemic control drugs or the oral medication(s) can be discontinued and insulin used alone.

The A1c level and results of SMBG direct the intensity of insulin therapy in type 2 diabetes, taking into consideration individualized glycemic goals. When fasting glucose levels are elevated, basal insulin can be added to the oral or non-insulin injectable therapy, with titration of the dose of basal insulin to the fasting glucose level. The use of bedtime insulin glargine is associated with less nocturnal hypoglycemia than bedtime NPH [59]. Insulin glargine and insulin detemir have similar efficacy and safety in type 2 diabetes, with insulin detemir more likely to be administered twice daily and with higher doses, and insulin glargine administered once daily and with more weight gain [60].

When the addition of basal insulin to oral therapy is insufficient, meal-time rapidly acting insulin is added. Metformin therapy is usually continued, and may help prevent weight gain and higher insulin doses. Oral insulin secretagogue therapy is stopped when bolus insulin therapy is used. The general principles involved in the use of basal-bolus insulin therapy in type 2 diabetes are similar to that discussed for type 1 diabetes.

In selected patients, premixed "biphasic insulin" preparations, typically administered before breakfast and dinner, can be used (Table 4.2, Figure 4.2B upper panel). They are simple to use, convenient, and may be associated with fewer dosing errors. Unlike basal-bolus therapy, in which the mealtime insulin dose can be increased for higher carbohydrate content of meals or to correct hyperglycemia, premixed insulin contain fixed amounts of both short and intermediate acting insulins, so a higher dose will not only cover the meal but will also increase insulin levels many hours later. It is therefore more difficult to treat short-term high and low glucose levels with pre-mixed insulins, and there can be a greater risk of hypoglycemia. Glycemic control is better with basal-bolus regimens than with biphasic insulin therapy [61].

Achieving glycemic goals in patients with severe insulin resistance is particularly challenging. For those who require more than 200 units of insulin daily, the delivery of sufficient insulin can be a problem. In these circumstances, a concentrated formulation of regular insulin (U-500 regular insulin, 500 units/cc) can be helpful. This insulin preparation is five times as concentrated as regular (U-100, 100 units/cc) insulin, and its pharmacokinetics are similar to a mixture of regular and NPH insulin, with a delay in peak effect compared to regular insulin [62].

## Hypoglycemia

Hypoglycemia is most common with insulin therapy. It is also observed with insulin secretagogues, especially sulfonylurea drugs. Hypoglycemia is particularly common in people with long-duration type 1 diabetes [63], but also occurs in type 2 diabetes. It is a major barrier to achieving optimal glycemic control [64, 65]. Nocturnal hypoglycemia is a significant problem for many patients with long-standing insulin-requiring diabetes. Fear of hypoglycemia can be a limiting factor in glycemic management as well. A history of severe hypoglycemic episodes has been associated with more cognitive impairment/dementia, cardiac ischemia, and cardiac arrhythmias and stroke, and can cause seizures, coma, and even death [66–72]. Risk is higher during and after physical activity and with advanced age, increased duration of diabetes, impaired hypoglycemic unawareness, impaired release of glucose counter-regulatory hormones (glucagon, cortisol, epinephrine), renal insufficiency, liver disease, sepsis, use of intensive insulin therapies, and poor nutritional status. Alcohol and the use of drugs such as pentamidine, quinine, and quinolones are also associated with the development of hypoglycemia.

Symptoms of hypoglycemia include anxiety; extreme hunger; sweating; mood/behavior changes; nervousness; headache; confusion; palpitations; tremor; tingling of hands, lips, or tongue; vision change; slurred speech; pallor; poor coordination; dizziness; seizures; and loss of consciousness. Some people with type 1 diabetes and long-standing type 2 diabetes have hypoglycemia-associated autonomic failure. This condition is related to repeated episodes of hypoglycemia and is associated with poor hypoglycemic awareness and defective glucose counter regulation. It can reverse with avoidance of hypoglycemia for several weeks [73, 74].

### Treatment of hypoglycemia

Patients, family members, co-workers, and friends should be educated on the recognition and treatment of hypoglycemia. When SMBG indicates glucose at or below 70 mg/dl or at or below 80 mg/dl with symptoms in a conscious individual, fast-acting carbohydrate (15–20 grams) should be ingested. If the glucose level is less than 50 mg/dl, a 30-gram carbohydrate snack should be eaten. Blood glucose levels should be retested after 10–15 minutes. For individuals prone to hypoglycemia, SMBG should be performed before exercise, driving, or engaging in any other potentially dangerous activity, and fast-acting carbohydrate should be readily available. Many individuals with diabetes carry glucose tablets for this purpose. After the initial treatment, a meal or snack containing carbohydrate and protein should be given so that the hypoglycemia does not recur. Depending upon the cause of the hypoglycemia, consideration should be given to providing follow-up education, adjusting the treatment regimen, and/or raising the glycemic goals.

Insulin users should be prescribed glucagon and a family member, partner, or other close associate should be trained in how to reconstitute and inject it. When the person with diabetes is unable to swallow or is unconscious, the local emergency response team (e.g., 911) should be called and glucagon given. When glucagon is administered, the patient should be on his/her side because nausea and vomiting can occur. In hospital settings, intravenous dextrose is administered for severe hypoglycemia. This is commonly followed by an intravenous dextrose infusion or ingestion of food if the patient is able to eat.

## Medications that commonly raise glucose levels

Glucocorticoid administration, which increases insulin resistance and causes impairment of pancreatic $\beta$ cell function, is commonly associated with elevations in glucose concentrations [75]. Higher doses of steroid hormones cause greater hyperglycemia [76]. For patients with diabetes, glycemic treatment usually requires intensification when these drugs (e.g., prednisone, hydrocortisone, prednisolone, methlyprednisolone, dexamethasone) are initiated or doses increased. Megestrol acetate has also been reported to raise glucose levels.

The presence of psychosis and the use of anti-psychotic medications are associated with an increase in diabetes and obesity [77, 78]. In some studies, the use of second generation "atypical" anti-psychotic medications (e.g., clozapine, olanzapine) is more likely to produce hyperglycemia. This has led to the recommendation that people treated with antipsychotic drugs receive regular monitoring of weight, glucose levels, and other cardiovascular risk factors.

Antiretroviral drugs have also been associated with the development of hyperglycemia [77]. Patients with HIV receiving treatment with protease inhibitors as well as people taking immunosuppressant drugs should have their glycemic status monitored.

## Sick day management

Any stress, including the presence of an acute illness such as an infection, can increase insulin requirements in people with diabetes. Concentrations of counter-regulatory hormones, such as epinephrine and cortisol, may be elevated and contribute to increased insulin resistance. In addition, mealtime insulin requirements may be altered if there is diminished oral intake of carbohydrates related to decreased appetite, nausea, vomiting, or other factors. To avoid significant hyperglycemia and ketoacidosis as well as hypoglycemia during acute illnesses, people with diabetes and their caretakers must understand general "sick day rules," perform more frequent SMBG, and contact their physician.

During an acute illness, the following "rules" are particularly important for individuals with type 1 diabetes or long-standing insulin-requiring type 2 diabetes. Patients need to perform SMBG more frequently (every two to three hours or more often if necessary). Urine or blood ketone levels should be measured at home every three to four hours in the presence of severe hyperglycemia or nausea and vomiting, diarrhea, or fever. Basal insulin administration must always be continued and oral hydration maintained. Supplemental doses of short-acting or rapidly acting insulin should be used for elevated glucose levels and/or ketosis. If food intake is poor, fluids containing carbohydrates and electrolytes should be ingested. If sufficient oral intake is not possible (e.g., persistent vomiting), intravenous hydration should be administered at an appropriate facility. The development of diabetic ketoacidosis requires intensive therapy with intravenous fluids and insulin, and should be managed in a hospital.

## Surgery

When elective outpatient surgery is being considered, including oral surgery and periodontal surgery, individuals with diabetes should consult with their diabetes care team to optimize their glycemic control and discuss pre-operative medication adjustments and instructions [79]. Surgery should be scheduled as early as possible in the morning. The stress of surgery, anesthesia, and post-operative pain can lead to the release of counter-regulatory hormones (epinephrine, glucagon, cortisol) and increased insulin resistance. The degree of the stress response and perioperative management vary in people and are affected by the type and duration of surgery and anesthesia, and additional factors such as presence of infection, nutritional status, ability to eat after surgery, and use of glucose-containing intravenous fluids and medications that raise glucose levels such as steroids. Because it is difficult to predict insulin requirements and glycemic responses, frequent SMBG is recommended.

Patients with type 1 diabetes mellitus have absolute insulin deficiency and require continuous insulin therapy. If insulin is withheld, they can quickly develop hyperglycemia and ketoacidosis. The insulin secretory capacity of people with type 2 diabetes is diminished but more variable. These patients can also become hyperglycemic and ketotic with the stress of surgery. In general, for people with type 1 diabetes, basal insulin analogs are continued at 80–100% of the home dose. For patients with type 2 diabetes using basal insulin therapy, a greater reduction in dose is sometimes suggested for the morning of surgery, particularly if the individual is using NPH insulin. If food is held, mealtime rapidly acting doses of insulin are not given until food is restarted post-operatively. In type 2 diabetes, oral hypoglycemic medications should not be taken on the morning of surgery. Oral and non-insulin injectable drugs are restarted after eating resumes. Metformin should be held up to 48 hours after surgery if there is risk of dehydration and renal injury.

Patients scheduled for long, complicated surgery should be placed on intraveneous insulin and glucose infusions perioperatively and have frequent glucose monitoring with titration of infusion rates to achieve and maintain glycemic goals [79]. Non-insulin glycemic control medications are discontinued during this time. Subcutaneous insulin is usually restarted when the patient begins eating again.

# Prevention of diabetes

### Type 1 diabetes

Research in the prevention of type 1 diabetes has focused on the use of therapies to arrest or reverse the autoimmune destruction of pancreatic β cells. Results to date have been disappointing [80–85]. There are ongoing and planned studies using immunomodulatory drugs that are promising, but currently there are no treatments that are approved for clinical practice.

### Type 2 diabetes

Lifestyle change interventions that focus on weight reduction and increased physical activity in people at high risk of developing diabetes can prevent or slow the progression to type 2 diabetes [86–92]. The Diabetes Prevention Program (DPP), a randomized clinical trial that enrolled adults in the United States at high risk for developing diabetes, demonstrated that an intensive lifestyle intervention was more effective in preventing diabetes than metformin, and both demonstrated benefit when compared to placebo [86, 91]. These interventions, particularly lifestyle, were cost-effective over 10 years of follow-up [92]. The Diabetes Prevention Lifestyle Program was costly and was conducted through academic medical centers. Since publication of these results, efforts have been made to translate this program into community settings in a less expensive manner. Several studies have shown that adaptations of the DPP can be delivered through community centers, YMCAs, and faith-based organizations [93–96]. The DPP intensive lifestyle intervention can also be delivered successfully by telephone, with greater weight loss observed in individuals who participated in group sessions (conference calls) compared to solo calls [97]. The American Diabetes Association recommends that people with pre-diabetes (fasting glucose 100–125 mg/dl, 2-hour glucose 140–199 mg/dl in a 75-gm oral glucose tolerance test, or A1c 5.7–6.4%) participate in a lifestyle program with the goal of weight loss of 7% of body weight and moderate physical activity (e.g., walking) of at least 150 minutes/week [6]. Metformin therapy can also be used in patients with pre-diabetes, especially for those with BMI greater than 35 kg/m², age under 60 years, and women with prior gestational diabetes [6].

## Future directions

The prevalence of diabetes is increasing at an alarming rate. To reduce the morbidity, mortality, and costs associated with this epidemic, better prevention and treatment approaches as well as earlier detection are needed. In addition to medical facilities, the dental office is a site where people with pre-diabetes, undiagnosed diabetes, or poorly controlled diabetes can be identified, as is discussed in Chapter 9 [98]. Improved communication and collaboration between medical and dental professionals could contribute to better diabetes care and outcomes.

For type 1 diabetes, more research is needed to develop safe and effective approaches for prevention. Technological advances, including efforts to develop an artificial pancreas, have made great progress and should improve the treatment of this disease in the future. Research in islet-cell transplantation and pancreatic beta cell regeneration also show promise. For type 2 diabetes, prevention efforts need to focus on lifestyle change. Preventing and treating obesity and encouraging physical activity are critical, and have become a major public health focus. New oral and injectable medications are also in development that could help better treat this disease. For all people with diabetes, prevention of complications involves not only glycemic control, but also management of blood pressure, lipid abnormalities, and other cardiovascular risk factors (Chapter 3). This comprehensive treatment approach has improved the lives of people with diabetes.

## References

1. The Diabetes Control and Complications Trial Research Group. The effect of intensive treatment of diabetes on the development and progression of long-term complications in insulin-dependent diabetes mellitus. *N Engl J Med* 1993; 329: 977–986.
2. The Diabetes Control and Complications Trial/Epidemiology of Diabetes Interventions and Complications Research Group. Effect of intensive therapy on the microvascular complications of type 1 diabetes mellitus. *JAMA* 2002; 287: 2563–2569.

3. The Diabetes Control and Complications Trial/Epidemiology of Diabetes Interventions and Complications Research Group. Intensive diabetes treatment and cardiovascular disease in patients with type 1 diabetes. *N Engl J Med* 2005; 353: 2643–2653.
4. UK Prospective Diabetes Study (UKPDS) Group. Intensive blood glucose control with sulphonylureas or insulin compared with conventional treatment and risk of complications in patients with type 2 diabetes (UKPDS 33). *Lancet* 1998; 352:837–853.
5. UK Prospective Diabetes Study (UKPDS) Group. Effect of intensive blood-glucose control with metformin on complications in overweight patients with type 2 diabetes (UKPDS 34). *Lancet* 1998; 352:854–865.
6. American Diabetes Association. Standards of medical care in diabetes—2013. *Diabetes Care* 2013; 36(Suppl 1):S11–S66.
7. Inzucchi SE, Bergenstal RM, Buse JB, et al. Management of hyperglycemia in type 2 diabetes: a patient-centered approach: position statement of the American Diabetes Association (ADA) and the European Association for the Study of Diabetes (EASD). *Diabetes Care* 2012; 35:1364–1379.
8. Renders CM, Valk GD, Griffin SJ, et al. Interventions to improve the management of diabetes in primary care, outpatient, and community settings: a systematic review. *Diabetes Care* 2001; 24:1821–1833.
9. Hogg W, Lemelin J, Dahrouge S, et al. Randomized controlled trial of anticipatory and preventive multidisciplinary team care for complex patients in a community-based primary care setting. *Can Fam Physician.* 2009; 55:e76–85.
10. Scanlon DP, Hollenbeak CS, Beich J, et al. Financial and clinical impact of team-based treatment for Medicaid enrollees with diabetes in a federally qualified health center. *Diabetes Care* 2008; 31:2160–2165.
11. Lin EHB, Von Korff M, Ciechanowski P, et al. Treatment adjustment and medication adherence for complex patients with diabetes, heart disease, and depression: a randomized controlled trial. *Ann Fam Med* 2012; 10:6–14.
12. Wagner EH. The role of patient care teams in chronic disease management. *BMJ* 2000; 320:569–572.
13. Glazier RH, Bajcar J, Kennie NR, et al. A systematic review of interventions to improve diabetes care in socially disadvantaged populations. *Diabetes Care* 2006; 29:1675–1688.
14. Haas L, Maryniuk M, Beck J, et al. National standards for diabetes self-management education and support. *Diabetes Care* 2013; 36(Suppl 1):S100–S108.
15. Qaseem A, Vijan S, Snow V, et al. Glycemic control and type 2 diabetes mellitus: the optimal hemoglobin A1c targets. A guidance statement from the American College of Physicians. *Ann Intern Med* 2007; 147:417–422.
16. Pogach LM, Tiwari A, Maney M, et al. Should mitigating comorbidities be considered in assessing healthcare plan performance in achieving optimal glycemic control?. *Am J Managed Care* 2007; 13:133–140.
17. Malanda UL, Bot SD, Nijpels G. Self-monitoring of blood glucose in noninsulin-using type 2 diabetic patients: it is time to face the evidence. *Diabetes Care* 2013; 36:176–178.
18. Polonsky, WH, Fisher L. Self-monitoring of blood glucose in noninsulin-using type 2 diabetic patients: right answer, but wrong question: self-monitoring of blood glucose can be clinically valuable for noninsulin users. *Diabetes Care* 2013; 36:179–182.
19. Malanda UL, Welschen LM, Riphagen II, et al. Self-monitoring of blood glucose in patients with type 2 diabetes mellitus who are not using insulin. *Cochrane Database Syst Rev* 2012; 1:CD005060

20. Davidson MB. Evaluation of self monitoring of blood glucose in non-insulin-treated diabetic patients by randomized controlled trials: little bang for the buck. *Rev Recent Clin Trials* 2010; 5: 138–142.
21. Polonsky WH, Fisher L, Schikman CH, et al. Structured self-monitoring of blood glucose significantly reduces A1c levels in poorly controlled, noninsulin-treated type 2 diabetes: results from the structured testing program study. *Diabetes Care* 2011; 34: 262–267.
22. Tamborlane WV, Beck RW, Bode BW, et al. Continuous glucose monitoring and intensive treatment of type 1 diabetes. *N Engl J Med* 2008; 359: 1464–1476.
23. Huang ES, O'Grady M, Basu A, et al. The cost-effectiveness of continuous glucose monitoring in type 1 diabetes. *Diabetes Care* 2010; 33: 1269–1274.
24. Bergenstal RM, Tamborlane WV, Ahmann A, et al. Effectiveness of sensor-augmented insulin-pump therapy in type 1 diabetes. *N Engl J Med* 2010; 363: 311–320.
25. The Juvenile Diabetes Research Foundation Continuous Glucose Monitoring Study Group. Sustained benefit of continuous glucose monitoring on A1c, glucose profiles, and hypoglycemia in adults with type 1 diabetes. *Diabetes Care* 2009; 32: 2047–2049.
26. Gerstein HC, Miller ME, Byington RP, et al. The Action to Control Cardiovascular Risk in Diabetes Study Group. Effects of intensive glucose lowering in type 2 diabetes. *N Engl J Med* 2008; 358: 2545–2559.
27. Duckworth W, Abraira C, Moritz T, et al. Glucose control and vascular complications in veterans with type 2 diabetes. *N Engl J Med* 2009; 360: 129–139.
28. Kitzmiller JL, Block JM, Brown FM, et al. Managing preexisting diabetes for pregnancy: summary of evidence and consensus recommendations for care. *Diabetes Care* 2008; 31: 1060–1079.
29. Delahanty LM, Halford BN. The role of diet behaviors in achieving improved glycemic control in intensively treated patients in the Diabetes Control and Complications Trial. *Diabetes Care* 1993; 16: 1453–1458.
30. Koivisto VA, Sane T, Fyhrquist F, et al. Fuel and fluid homeostasis during long-term exercise in healthy subjects and type 1 diabetic patients. *Diabetes Care* 1992; 15: 1736–1741.
31. Korytkowski M, Bell D, Jacobsen C, et al. A multicenter, randomized, open-label, comparative, two-period crossover trial of preference, efficacy, and safety profiles of a prefilled, disposable pen and conventional vial/syringe for insulin injection in patients with type 1 or 2 diabetes mellitus. *Clin Ther* 2003; 25: 2836–2848.
32. Campos C, Lajara R, Deluzio T. Usability and preference assessment of a new prefilled insulin pen versus vial and syringe in people with diabetes, physicians and nurses. *Expert Opin Pharmacother* 2012; 13: 1837–1846.
33. Magwire ML. Addressing barriers to insulin therapy: The role of insulin pens. *Am J Ther* 2011; 18: 392–402.
34. Heller S, Koenen C, Bode B. Comparison of insulin detemir and insulin glargine in a basal-bolus regimen, with insulin aspart as the mealtime insulin, in patients with type 1 diabetes: a 52-week, multinational, randomized, open-label, parallel-group, treat-to-target noninferiority trial. *Clin Ther* 2009; 31: 2086–2097.
35. Rosenstock J, Park G, Zimmerman J, and U.S. Insulin Glargine Type 1 Diabetes Investigator Group. Basal insulin glargine versus NPH insulin in patients with type 1 diabetes on multiple daily insulin regimens. *Diabetes Care* 2000; 23: 1137–1142.
36. Home P, Bartley P, Russell-Jones D, et al. Study to Evaluate the Administration of Detemir Insulin Efficacy, Safety and Suitability (STEADINESS) Study Group. Insulin detemir offers improved glycemic control compared with NPH insulin in people with type 1 diabetes: a randomized clinical trial. *Diabetes Care* 2004; 27: 1081–1087.

37. Radermecker RP, Scheen AJ. Continuous subcutaneous insulin infusion with short-acting insulin analogues or human regular insulin: efficacy, safety, quality of life, and cost-effectiveness. *Diabetes Metab Res* 2004; 20: 178–188.
38. Colquitt J, Royle P, Waugh N. Are analogue insulins better than soluble in continuous subcutaneous insulin infusion? Results of a meta-analysis. *Diabet Med* 2003; 20: 863–866.
39. Yeh HC, Brown TT, Maruthur, N, et al. Comparative effectiveness and safety of methods of insulin delivery and glucose monitoring for diabetes mellitus: a systematic review and meta-analysis. *Ann Intern Med* 2012; 157: 336–347.
40. Younk LM, Mikeladze M, Davis SN. Pramlintide and the treatment of diabetes: a review of the data since its introduction. *Expert Opin Pharmacother* 2011; 12: 1439–1451.
41. Edelman S, Maier H, Wilhelm K. Pramlintide in the treatment of diabetes mellitus. *Biodrugs* 2008; 22: 375–386.
42. Chudyk A, Petrella RJ. Effects of exercise on cardiovascular risk factors in type 2 diabetes: a meta-analysis. *Diabetes Care* 2011; 34: 1228–1237.
43. Umpierre D, Ribeiro PA, Kramer CK, et al. Physical activity advice only or structured exercise training and association with HbA1c levels in type 2 diabetes: a systematic review and meta-analysis. *JAMA* 2011; 305: 1790–1799.
44. Myers VH, McVay MA, Bashear MM, et al. Exercise training and quality of life in individuals with type 2 diabetes: a randomized controlled trial. *Diabetes Care* 2013; 36:1884–1890.
45. Fang ZY, Sharman J, Prins JB, et al. Determinants of exercise capacity in patients with type 2 diabetes. *Diabetes Care* 2005; 28: 1643–1648.
46. Nathan DM, Buse JB, Davidson MB, et al. Medical management of hyperglycemia in type 2 diabetes: a consensus algorithm for the initiation and adjustment of therapy: a consensus statement of the American Diabetes Association and the European Association for the Study of Diabetes. *Diabetes Care* 2009; 32: 193–203.
47. Bolen S, Feldman L, Vassy J, et al. Systematic review: comparative effectiveness and safety of oral medications for type 2 diabetes mellitus. *Ann Intern Med* 2007; 147:386–399.
48. Qaseem A, Humphrey LL, Sweet DE, et al. Oral pharmacologic treatment of type 2 diabetes mellitus: a clinical practice guideline from the American College of Physicians. *Ann Intern Med* 2012; 156:218–231.
49. Ismail-Beigi F. Glycemic management of type 2 diabetes mellitus. *N Engl J Med* 2012; 366:1319–1327.
50. Saenz A, Fernandez-Esteban I, Mataix A, et al. Metformin monotherapy for type 2 diabetes mellitus. *Cochrane Database Syst Rev* 2005; 3:CD002966.
51. Salpeter SR, Greyber E, Pasternak GA, et al. Risk of fatal and nonfatal lactic acidosis with metformin use in type 2 diabetes mellitus. *Cochrane Database Syst Rev.* 2010; 4:CD002967.
52. Riddle MC. Sulfonylureas differ in effects on ischemic preconditioning—is it time to retire glyburide? *J Clin Endocrinol Metab* 2003; 88:528–530.
53. Shyangdan DS, Royle P, Clar C, et al. Glucagon-like peptide analogues for type 2 diabetes mellitus. *Cochrane Database Syst Rev.* 2011; 10:CD006423.
54. Drucker DJ, Sherman SI, Gorelick FS, et al. Incretin-based therapies for the treatment of type 2 diabetes: evaluation of the risks and benefits. *Diabetes Care* 2010; 33:428–433.
55. Dormandy JA, Charbonnel B, Eckland DJ, et al. Secondary prevention of macrovascular events in patients with type 2 diabetes in the PROactive study (PROspective pioglitAzone clinical trial in macroVascular events): a randomised controlled trial. *Lancet* 2005; 366:1279–1289.
56. Motola D, Piccinni C, Biagi C, et al. Cardiovascular, ocular and bone adverse reactions associated with thiazolidinediones. *Drug Safety* 2012; 35: 315–323.
57. Azoulay L, Yin H, Filion KB, et al. The use of pioglitazone and the risk of bladder cancer in people with type 2 diabetes: nested case-control study. *BMJ* 2012; 344: e3645.

58. Van de Laar FA, Lucassen PL, Akkermans RP, et al. Alpha-glucosidase inhibitors for patients with type 2 diabetes: results from a Cochrane systematic review and meta-analysis. *Diabetes Care* 2005; 28: 154–163.
59. Riddle MC, Rosenstock J, Gerich J. The treat-to-target trial: randomized addition of glargine or human NPH insulin to oral therapy of type 2 diabetic patients. *Diabetes Care* 2003; 26: 3080–3086.
60. Swinnen SG, Simon AC, Holleman F, et al. Insulin detemir versus insulin glargine for type 2 diabetes mellitus. *Cochrane Database Syst Rev* 2011; 7: CD006383.
61. Holman RR, Farmer AJ, Davies MJ, et al. Three-year efficacy of complex insulin regimens in type 2 diabetes. *N Engl J Med* 2009; 361: 1736–1747.
62. Reutrakul S, Wroblewski K, Brown RL. Clinical use of U-500 regular insulin: review and meta-analysis. *J Diabetes Sci Techol* 2012; 6: 412–420.
63. Weinstock RS, Xing D, Maahs DM, et al. Severe hypoglycemia and diabetic ketoacidosis in adults with type 1 diabetes: results from the T1D Exchange clinic registry. *J Clin Endocrinol Metab* 2013; 98: 3411–3419.
64. McCrimmon RJ, Sherwin RS. Hypoglycemia in type 1 diabetes. *Diabetes* 2010; 59: 2333–2339.
65. Frier, BM. The incidence and impact of hypoglycemia in type 1 and type 2 diabetes. *Int Diabetes Monitor* 2009; 21: 210–218.
66. Strachan MW, Reynolds RM, Marioni RE, et al. Cognitive function, dementia and type 2 diabetes mellitus in the elderly. *Nature Rev Endocrinol* 2011; 7: 108–114.
67. Zoungas S, Patel A, Chalmers J, et al. Severe hypoglycemia and risks of vascular events and death. *N Engl J Med* 2010; 363: 1410–1418.
68. Whitmer RA, Karter AJ, Yaffe K, et al. Hypoglycemic episodes and risk of dementia in older patients with type 2 diabetes mellitus. *JAMA* 2009; 301: 1565–1572.
69. Nordin C. The case for hypoglycaemia as a proarrhythmic event: basic and clinical evidence. *Diabetologia* 2010; 53: 1552–1561.
70. McCoy RG, Van Houten HK, Ziegenfuss JY, et al. Increased mortality of patients with diabetes reporting severe hypoglycemia. *Diabetes Care* 2012; 35: 1897–1901.
71. Snell-Bergeon JK, Wadwa RP. Hypoglycemia, diabetes, and cardiovascular disease. *Diabetes Technol Ther* 2012; 14(Suppl 1): S51–S58.
72. Gill GV, Woodward A, Casson IF, et al. Cardiac arrhythmia and nocturnal hypoglycaemia in type 1 diabetes—the 'dead in bed' syndrome revisited. *Diabetologia* 2009; 52: 42–45.
73. Cryer PE. The barrier of hypoglycemia in diabetes. *Diabetes* 2008; 57: 3169–3176.
74. Ramanathan R, Cryer PE. Adrenergic mediation of hypoglycemia-associated autonomic failure. *Diabetes* 2011; 60: 602–606.
75. Di Dalmazi G, Pagotto U, Pasquali R, et al. Glucocorticoids and type 2 diabetes: from physiology to pathology. *J Nutr Metab* 2012; 2012: 525093.
76. Gurwitz JH, Bohn RL, Glynn RJ, et al. Glucocorticoids and the risk for initiation of hypoglycemic therapy. *Arch Intern Med* 1994; 154: 97–101.
77. Luna B, Feinglos MN. Drug-induced hyperglycemia. *JAMA* 2001; 286: 1945–1948.
78. Lambert TJR, Chapman LH. Diabetes, psychotic disorders and antipsychotic therapy: a consensus statement. *Med J Aust* 2004; 181: 544–548.
79. DiNardo M, Donihi AC, Forte P, et al. Standardized glycemic management and perioperative glycemic outcomes in patients with diabetes mellitus who undergo same-day surgery. *Endocr Pract* 2011; 17: 404–411.
80. Silverstein J, Maclaren N, Riley W, et al. Immunosuppression with azathioprine and prednisone in recent-onset insulin-dependent diabetes mellitus. *N Engl J Med* 1988; 319: 599–604.

81. Gottlieb PA, Quinlan S, Krause-Steinrauf H, et al. Failure to preserve beta-cell function with mycophenolate mofetil and daclizumab combined therapy in patients with new onset type 1 diabetes. *Diabetes Care* 2010; 33: 826–832.

82. Christie MR, Molvig J, Hawkes CJ, et al. IA-2 antibody-negative status predicts remission and recovery of C-peptide levels in type 1 diabetic patients treated with cyclosporin. *Diabetes Care* 2002; 25: 1192–1197.

83. Pescovitz MD, Greenbaum CJ, Krause-Steinrauf H, et al. Rituxan, B-lymphocyte depletion, and preservation of beta-cell function. *N Eng J Med* 2009; 361: 2143–2152.

84. Ludvigsson J, Krisky D, Casas R, et al. GAD65 antigen therapy in recently diagnosed type 1 diabetes mellitus. *N Engl J Med* 2012; 366: 433–442.

85. Orban T, Bundy B, Becker DJ, et al. Co-stimulation modulation with abatacept in patients with recent-onset type 1 diabetes: a randomised, double-blind, placebo-controlled trial. *Lancet* 2011; 378: 412–419.

86. Knowler WC, Barrett-Connor E, Fowler SE, et al. Diabetes Prevention Program Research Group. Reduction in the incidence of type 2 diabetes with lifestyle intervention or metformin. *N Engl J Med* 2002; 346: 393–403.

87. Tuomilehto J, Lindström J, Eriksson JG, et al. Finnish Diabetes Prevention Study Group. Prevention of type 2 diabetes mellitus by changes in lifestyle among subjects with impaired glucose tolerance. *N Engl J Med* 2001; 344: 1343–1350.

88. Pan, X-R, Li G-W, Hu Y-H, et al. Effects of diet and exercise in preventing NIDDM in people with impaired glucose tolerance: the Da Qing IGT and Diabetes Study. *Diabetes Care* 1997; 20: 537–544.

89. Li G, Zhang P, Wang J, et al. The long-term effect of lifestyle interventions to prevent diabetes in the China Da Qing Diabetes Prevention Study: a 20-year follow-up study. *Lancet* 2008; 371: 1783–1789.

90. Lindström J, Ilanne-Parikka P, Peltonen M, et al. Sustained reduction in the incidence of type 2 diabetes by lifestyle intervention: follow-up of the Finnish Diabetes Prevention Study. *Lancet* 2006; 368: 1673–1679.

91. Knowler WC, Fowler SE, Hamman RF, et al. Diabetes Prevention Program Research Group. 10-year follow-up of diabetes incidence and weight loss in the Diabetes Prevention Program Outcomes Study. *Lancet* 2009; 374: 1677–1686.

92. The Diabetes Prevention Program Research Group. The 10-year cost effectiveness of lifestyle intervention or metformin for diabetes prevention: an intent-to-treat analysis of the DPP/DPPOS. *Diabetes Care* 2012; 35: 723–730.

93. Ali MK, Echouffo-Tcheugui JB, Williamson DF. How effective were lifestyle interventions in real-world settings that were modeled on the Diabetes Prevention Program? *Health Affairs* 2012; 31: 67–75.

94. Katula JA, Vitolins MZ, Rosenberger CS, et al. One-year results of a community-based translation of the Diabetes Prevention Program Healthy-living Partnerships to Prevent Diabetes (HELP PD) Project. *Diabetes Care* 2011; 34: 1451–1457.

95. Ackermann RT, Finch EA, Caffrey HM, et al. Long-term effects of a community-based lifestyle intervention to prevent type 2 diabetes: the DEPLOY extension pilot study. *Chronic Illness* 2011; 7: 279–290.

96. Boltri JM, Davis-Smith M, Okosun IS, et al. Translation of the National Institutes of Health Diabetes Prevention Program in African American churches. *J Natl Med Assoc* 2011; 103: 194–202.

97. Weinstock RS, Trief PM, Cibula D, et al. Weight loss success in metabolic syndrome by telephone interventions: results from the SHINE Study. *J Gen Intern Med* 2013; 28: 1620–1628.

98. Lalla E, Kunzel C, Burkett S, et al. Identification of unrecognized diabetes and pre-diabetes in a dental setting. *J Dent Res* 2011; 90: 855–860.

99. Nathan DM, Kuenen J, Borg R, et al. A1c-Derived Average Glucose Study Group. Translating the A1c assay into estimated average glucose values. *Diabetes Care* 2008; 31: 1473–1478.

100. Kaufman FR (ed). *Medical Management of Type 1 Diabetes*, 6th ed., American Diabetes Association, 2012; 69–72.

# Section 2

# Dental considerations

# Chapter 5

# Management of the patient with diabetes mellitus in the dental office

*Brian L. Mealey, DDS, MS*

Due to the high prevalence of diabetes mellitus in the population, it is common for people with diabetes, both diagnosed and undiagnosed, to seek care in the dental office. Patients with diabetes may require precautions before, during, and after dental treatment. Proper management of these patients in the dental office requires a thorough understanding of current diagnosis and medical treatment of diabetes. Laboratory tests used in the diagnosis and management of diabetes are discussed in Chapter 2, while Chapter 4 contains a thorough review of currently available medications used in diabetes. The purpose of this chapter is to provide clinical pathways of care for use in the dental office.

## Outcomes of periodontal and dental implant therapy in patients with diabetes

### Results of periodontal therapy

Many studies reviewed in other chapters in this text have examined the impact of diabetes on periodontal health and the potential impact of periodontal therapy on metabolic control of diabetes. However, there is much less research examining the outcomes of periodontal therapy in periodontitis patients with diabetes compared to those without diabetes. In many of the studies of the effects of periodontal therapy in patients with diabetes, the average changes in probing depth and attachment level seen following scaling and root planing are similar in magnitude to studies of scaling and root planing performed in people without diabetes. However, these are not controlled trials of periodontal treatment in individuals with and without diabetes and therefore provide only low-level evidence that patients with diabetes as a group respond well to periodontal therapy.

In a comparison of periodontitis patients without diabetes and those with well-controlled diabetes, the short-term clinical and microbiologic responses to scaling and root planing were similar three to four months after treatment [1, 2]. Whereas many patients with diabetes and chronic periodontitis show improvement in clinical periodontal parameters after scaling and root planing, patients with poor glycemic control may have a more rapid recurrence of deep pockets and a less favorable long-term response. In a study of patients with type 1 diabetes, four weeks after scaling and

*Diabetes Mellitus and Oral Health: An Interprofessional Approach*, First Edition. Edited by Ira B. Lamster.
© 2014 John Wiley & Sons, Inc. Published 2014 by John Wiley & Sons, Inc.

root planing, those with good glycemic control had similar reductions in probing depth, clinical attachment level, and bleeding on probing as patients without diabetes, and the improved parameters remained stable for 12 months. Conversely, those with poorly controlled diabetes showed initial improvement at four weeks but then had a greater recurrence of deep probing depths at 12 months than those with well-controlled diabetes or no diabetes [3]. Therefore, the short-term benefits of periodontal therapy may not be sustained in people with poorly controlled diabetes.

There are few long-term studies of periodontal therapy in patients with diabetes. In one small longitudinal study, 20 people with diabetes (types 1 and 2) and 20 without diabetes received scaling and root planing, modified Widman flap surgery at sites with residual probing depths greater than 5 mm, and regular periodontal maintenance therapy [4]. Five years after the baseline examination, both groups of subjects had a similar percentage of sites demonstrating gain, loss, or no change in clinical attachment. Most of the patients with diabetes in this study were well controlled or moderately controlled at baseline, so the study does not address those with poor glycemic control. However, it does suggest that people with relatively well controlled diabetes have a positive response to periodontal treatment that can be sustained over extended periods of time as long as regular periodontal maintenance is performed.

Progression of periodontitis and incident tooth loss were examined in 23 subjects with poorly controlled type 2 diabetes (mean glycated hemoglobin [HbA1c] = 9.1%), 23 with well-controlled type 2 diabetes (mean HbA1c = 6.1%) and 46 without diabetes [5]. Subjects were recalled for periodontal maintenance every four to six months following active periodontal treatment, which consisted of nonsurgical therapy with or without subsequent periodontal surgery. While there were no differences in clinical parameters between groups before treatment, at the five-year examination the subjects with poorly controlled diabetes had a higher mean probing depth, clinical attachment loss, bleeding on probing, and number of teeth lost compared to those with well-controlled diabetes or without diabetes. There were no differences between those with well-controlled diabetes and those without diabetes. Progression of periodontitis was defined as an increase of 3 mm or more in clinical attachment loss at two or more interproximal sites between study visits. After five years, the number of subjects with periodontitis progression was significantly greater in the poorly controlled diabetes group (39.2% of subjects) compared to either the well-controlled diabetes group (21.7% of subjects) or the group without diabetes (23.9% of subjects). Likewise, the percentage of sites with progressive attachment loss was significantly greater in poorly controlled diabetes (6.1% of sites) compared to either well-controlled diabetes (2.5% of sites) or no diabetes (2.8% of sites). Thus, the overall response to periodontal therapy may be less favorable in individuals with poorly controlled diabetes, whereas those with well-controlled diabetes appear to respond to periodontal therapy in a manner similar to patients without diabetes.

The studies mentioned above generally involve a small number of subjects and study results are based on means of subject groups. Because not all patients in clinical practice reflect the mean and standard deviation in clinical studies, clinicians are advised to evaluate each subject individually with an understanding that each patient may or may not have responses to therapy similar to the "mean subject" in any given study. Further longitudinal studies of various periodontal treatment modalities in larger subject populations are clearly needed to determine the periodontal healing response in individuals with diabetes compared to individuals without diabetes and to assess the impact of glycemic control on the results of treatment.

### Results of dental implant therapy

Diabetes affects bone metabolism via multiple different mechanisms that may impair bone healing and normal homeostatic bone turnover [6]. Elevated glucose levels may inhibit differentiation and proliferation of osteoblasts, with resulting decreased formation of bone matrix [6, 7]. Both type 1 and type 2 diabetes have been associated with increased risk of hip fracture, but HbA1c was not correlated with the rate of fractures [8]. Animal studies have shown that osseointegration is impaired in animals with chemically induced diabetes compared to animals without diabetes [9, 10]. However, human research on the impact of diabetes on dental implant failure or complications is equivocal. Some studies show that diabetes increases the risk of implant failure by two-fold to three-fold compared to patients without diabetes [11], while others show no difference in failure rates associated with diabetes [12–14]. Reviews of the overall body of evidence suggest that implant failures in patient with diabetes tend to occur early after placement; furthermore, the percentage of *patients* with diabetes who experience implant failures appears to be relatively high but the percentage of *implants* that fail is similar to that of patients without diabetes [15].

The impact of glycemic control on implant failures in people with diabetes is unclear. Most studies of implant therapy in diabetes fail to evaluate the level of glycemic control among the patients. The few studies that have gathered adequate HbA1c data on the patients with diabetes all had a small number of study subjects and included only subjects with type 2 diabetes [16–19]. Most of the studies report implant failure rates only in the short-term post-placement period [16, 18, 19]. There is little evidence from these studies that elevated HbA1c levels adversely affect short-term failure rates of dental implants, with the exception of patients with very poor glycemic control (HbA1c greater than 9%) [17]. Clinicians must recognize, however, that the evidence base is incomplete. Until further research is performed clinicians should proceed cautiously with implant therapy in diabetic patients having only moderate or poor levels of glycemic control. Further research on long-term implant outcomes in type 1 and type 2 diabetes is clearly needed.

## Evaluation and management of patients with diabetes: pathways of care

### The patient with undiagnosed diabetes

The U.S. Centers for Disease Control estimated in 2011 that approximately 25.8 million American have diabetes and that about 7 million of those individuals are undiagnosed [20]. Patients with undiagnosed diabetes are a major target population for the dental office, because signs and symptoms of diabetes may present initially in the oral cavity (chapters 6 and 8). Dentists and dental hygienists may be the first to recognize signs and symptoms such as advanced periodontal diseases or other infections, burning mouth, xerostomia, or parotid enlargement. The medical history must be reviewed thoroughly to determine if the patient has been previously diagnosed with diabetes or if the patient has risk factors for diabetes such as prediabetes, overweight/obesity, racial risk factors, family history of diabetes, history of gestational diabetes, or others discussed in Chapter 2.

Diabetes is associated with an increased prevalence and severity of gingivitis and periodontitis, with the greatest risk in individuals with poor glycemic control [6, 21, 22]. Poor glycemic control also increases the risk of periodontal disease progression over time [23]. Signs and symptoms of undiagnosed diabetes may also be present in individuals with diagnosed diabetes in whom glycemic control is poor. These findings should initiate a clinical pathway of care directed toward medical evaluation of the patient's diabetes condition. Interaction between the dentist and physician is a critical component of care.

During the initial oral evaluation, the dentist should assess the periodontium for signs of potential undiagnosed or poorly controlled diabetes such as extensive gingival bleeding, presence of multiple simultaneously occurring periodontal abscesses, localized or generalized gingival swelling that may be accompanied by tissue that appears to proliferate out of the periodontal pocket, rapid progression of bone loss and attachment loss that is inconsistent with the level of plaque and calculus, or a poor wound healing response after periodontal therapy (chapters 6 and 8).

If such signs are present, the dentist should thoroughly review the medical history again. This is a critical step that is often overlooked in the dental office. If the patient does not currently have a diagnosis of diabetes, the dentist needs to ask appropriate questions directed at those conditions commonly associated with undiagnosed diabetes [24] (Figure 5.1). It is best if these questions are part of the written medical history; if not, they should be asked verbally. It is important to first ask the patient directly, "Have you ever been diagnosed with diabetes?" If not, the dentist should ask whether the patient has any first degree relatives with diabetes; this includes the father, mother, sisters, or brothers. If the patient has first degree relatives with diabetes, there is an increased risk that the patient has diabetes. If the patient is female, the dentist should ask if she has ever been pregnant and, if so, whether or not she had gestational diabetes during any of her pregnancies. Also ask if the patient ever had a baby weighing more than 9 lbs. at birth. A positive history of gestational diabetes or birth of a child over 9 lbs. increases the risk of the patient developing type 2 diabetes later in life [21, 24]. In addition to questioning the patient for risk factors, the dentist should evaluate the patient's race and body morphotype. Ethnic groups with higher risk for diabetes include African American, Latino, Native American, Asian American, and Pacific Islander [24]. Increased body mass index (BMI) is clearly associated with risk for type 2 diabetes [24].

It is important to remember that "increased risk" does not necessarily mean "presence of disease"; that is, just because a given patient has one or more risk factors for diabetes does not mean that this given patient actually has diabetes. However, the dentist and dental hygienist play a major role in assessing risk factors for diabetes, because many individuals visit the dentist's office more frequently than they do the physician's office. In the presence of intraoral signs and symptoms of possible undiagnosed diabetes, patients with one or more risk factors for diabetes should receive further evaluation.

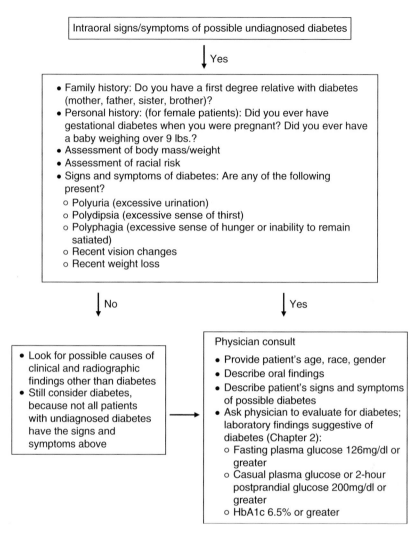

**Figure 5.1**   Clinical pathway of care: Patient without a diagnosis of diabetes (initial assessment).

Following the review of the medical history and assessment of the patient's physical features and race, the dentist should ask the patient about a history of polyuria (frequent urination), polydipsia (excessive sense of thirst) and polyphagia (excessive sense of hunger or inability to remain satiated after a meal), recent vision changes, or rapid weight loss (Figure 5.1). These are common signs and symptoms of undiagnosed diabetes. If the patient reports no such signs or symptoms, the dentist should look for other potential underlying medical conditions that might be associated with the oral findings noted in that patient; however, the dentist cannot rule out diabetes simply because these signs and symptoms are not present. Consultation with the patient's physician may be indicated.

Communication between dentist and physician offices is frequently poor, and patients may suffer due to the inability of dentists and physicians to communicate fully. A study of general dentists and periodontists demonstrated that 77% of periodontists and 44% of generalists always ask patients with diabetes what type of diabetes they have, and about 80% of periodontists and 56% of generalists ask about the patient's medical management regimen or level of glycemic control [25]. However, only 35% of periodontists and 14% of general dentists consistently communicate with the diabetic patient's physicians, and only 28% of periodontists and 14% of generalists objectively evaluate glycemic control by consulting the physician about laboratory test values such as the glycated hemoglobin (HbA1c) test, which is the gold standard for assessing the quality of glycemic control.

It is important that the medical consultation sent by the dentist be clear, informative, and precise. The consultation should provide the patient's age, gender, and race; a brief but clear description of the oral findings; and the specific signs and symptoms of possible diabetes noted for that patient (Figure 5.1). The dentist should then ask specifically what he or she wants the physician to do. For example, a consultation might say, "Mr. Smith is a patient of record in your office. He is a 57-year old African American male with a severe infection of the gum and bone tissues around his teeth (periodontitis) that is not consistent with the usual findings for such conditions. He reports a positive history of polyuria and polydipsia. He is significantly overweight. Mr. Smith reports that his mother and brother have type 2 diabetes. Please evaluate the patient for possible diabetes. I appreciate your evaluation of Mr. Smith and request that the results of your examination be sent to my office fax at 123-456-7890."

Such a consult does several things. First, it demonstrates for the physician that the dentist has evaluated the patient for risk factors such as race, body morphotype, and presence of known signs and symptoms of diabetes. Second, it provides to the physician the information about the patient's oral health that initiated the dentist's suspicion of undiagnosed diabetes in the first place. Finally, it makes a specific request of the physician to evaluate the patient for diabetes and to provide the results of that evaluation back to the dental office.

This consultation generally leads to ordering and evaluating laboratory tests to determine a diagnosis of diabetes. The following lab values are all suggestive of diabetes: fasting plasma glucose of 126 mg/dl or greater, casual plasma glucose of 200 mg/dl or greater, two-hour postprandial glucose of 200 mg/dl or greater, or HbA1c value of 6.5% or greater [24] (Figure 5.1). These tests are discussed in detail in Chapter 2.

### The patient with a diagnosis of diabetes

If the patient indicates on the medical history that he or she has been previously diagnosed with diabetes, the dentist must first determine which type of diabetes the patient has. Simply ask the patient, "What type of diabetes do you have?" (Figure 5.2). The patient who says, "I have had type 2 diabetes for 12 years, and I take a combination of metformin and sitagliptin every day" understands her disease much better than the patient who replies, "I don't know; is there more than one type of diabetes?" The purpose of the dentist's question about the patient's type of diabetes is designed to preliminarily assess the patient's own understanding of his or her diabetes.

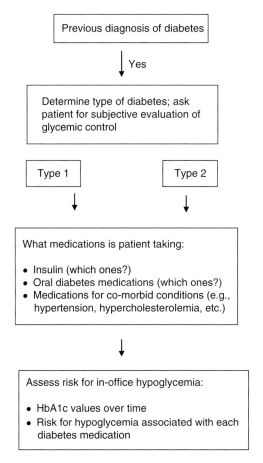

**Figure 5.2** Clinical pathway of care: Patient with a previous diagnosis of diabetes (initial assessment).

In addition, the clinician should ask the patient to describe the level of glycemic control by asking, "How well is your diabetes controlled?" Often, patients give a reply such as, "Pretty good." Conversely, a patient might say something like, "My control was good until two years ago when I lost my job, and it hasn't been very good since then." The purpose of asking the question is not to obtain an accurate evaluation of glycemic control from the patient. It is as inappropriate to use patient responses to definitively determine the level of glycemic control in patients with diabetes as it would be to use patient responses to accurately determine blood pressure levels in a patient with hypertension. Rather, these questions are used to assess the patient's knowledge of his own condition before the clinician begins a course of therapy that may require communication with the physician and alterations in the diabetes management plan, or may involve dental treatment with outcomes that depend in part on the patient's ability to maintain good glycemic control. An accurate determination of glycemic control will follow as part of the treatment planning process (see below).

The pathophysiology and medical treatment regimens vary between type 1 and type 2 diabetes, and dental management may differ as well. After determining what type of diabetes the patient has, the clinician must obtain an accurate and detailed understanding of the patient's medical management regimen. Simply asking the patient, "What medications do you take?" often elicits incomplete or inaccurate answers. The dentist can consult with the patient's physician about the medication regimens, but this is often made difficult by the presence of multiple physician providers prescribing different medications for a single patient. Instead, the dentist may simply ask the patient to bring all of his or her medications to the next dental appointment, with a reminder being given to the patient the day before the dental visit when confirming the appointment by telephone. Doing this allows the dentist to make a list of all current medications being taken by the patient by directly examining the prescriptions rather than relying on patient memory to provide an accurate medication list. Patients with type 1 diabetes all take insulin by injection or by subcutaneous insulin infusion pump. Individuals with type 2 diabetes may also take insulin but are often managed with oral medications or a combination of oral agents and insulin. Because some diabetes medications are associated with a significant risk for hypoglycemic emergency, it is critical that the dentist determine exactly which medications the patient takes [21, 26]. A detailed discussion of hypoglycemia and its relationship to diabetes medications is below.

## Treatment plan and therapy

After initial determination of the type of diabetes and medical management regimen, the dentist performs a thorough oral examination and develops a list of diagnoses. A preliminary treatment plan may also be formulated at this stage. If any acute lesions or conditions are found, they should be treated on an emergent basis (Figure 5.3). For example, if the patient has a periodontal abscess, it should be treated immediately in an appropriate fashion. The clinician should not delay treatment simply because the patient has diabetes. The presence of an acute infection may adversely influence glycemic control and should be treated as soon as it is recognized. The treatment done at this time is limited to managing the acute problem. To treat a periodontal abscess, the clinician may need to provide surgical or nonsurgical debridement of the defect, and systemic antibiotics may be indicated depending on the extent and severity of the infection. For routine dental treatment, there is little indication for routine use of prophylactic antibiotics in patients with diabetes. However, if an infection is present, antibiotics are generally indicated, especially if the patient's glycemic control is poor.

Once acute problems have been managed, or if no acute problems exist, the next step in the pathway of care involves accurately determining the patient's level of glycemic control over an extended period of time (Figure 5.3). This should be done before any definitive dental treatment. It is inappropriate to use individual blood glucose readings from the patient's glucometer as a means of determining glycemic control. The glucometer only provides a single point-in-time determination of capillary blood glucose levels, not a long-term assessment of glycemic control. Long-term glycemic control is evaluated by using the glycated hemoglobin test (HbA1c test) [24]. As glucose circulates in the bloodstream, it becomes irreversibly attached to a portion of the hemoglobin molecule on red blood cells and remains for the lifespan of the red blood cell, which is approximately $123 \pm 23$ days [27]. When blood glucose levels are high, a greater percentage of the

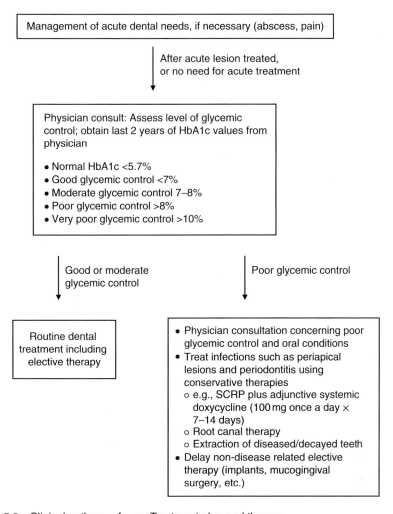

Figure 5.3   Clinical pathway of care: Treatment plan and therapy.

hemoglobin becomes glycated, and that percentage is measured using the HbA1c test. A normal HbA1c value is less than 5.7% [24]. The target goal for people with diabetes is to maintain glucose levels such that the HbA1c value is less than 7%. An HbA1c of greater than 8% is considered poor glycemic control and indicates a need for physician intervention to alter the management regimen.

The dentist should consult the patient's physician with a detailed request for information about the patient's glycemic control (Figure 5.3). Rather than asking a general question such as, "How well is the patient's diabetes controlled?", the dentist should find out the specific results of the HbA1c tests that have been ordered by the physician as part of the patient's medical care. In addition, the dentist needs to determine the level of glycemic control over the long term, not only the last time the HbA1c was performed. Just as the dentist would not try to determine how well controlled a hypertensive patient's blood pressure was by the results of a single blood pressure reading, the level of glycemic control over the long term cannot be determined by the results of a single HbA1c. Therefore, the consult to the physician should specifically ask for the results of the HbA1c tests for at least the past two years. As an example, a consultation might state, "Ms. Garcia is a patient of record in your office. She is a 64-year old Hispanic female who reports a positive history of type 2 diabetes for over 15 years. She has a significant infection of the gum and bone tissues around her teeth (severe chronic periodontitis), and I am in the process of developing a treatment plan for her. Could you please send the last two years of her HbA1c values to my office fax at 123-456-7890? I appreciate your help."

Such a consult demonstrates that the dentist has evaluated the patient's diabetes history, examined the patient and found significant oral disease, and needs the physician's assistance in determining an appropriate plan of care. The consult also makes a specific request of the physician to provide data to the dental office (two years of HbA1c values) that the dentist will use to determine and execute that plan of care.

This consult allows the dentist to objectively evaluate the glycemic control over an extended period of time (Figure 5.3). Over the past two years, has the patient's HbA1c consistently been relatively close to the normal range? For example, perhaps the HbA1c values have ranged from 6.2% to 6.9% over two years. If so, such good glycemic control is associated with a decreased risk of diabetes complications and possibly a better response to some forms of periodontal therapy. But it is also associated with a greater risk of hypoglycemic episodes. Or have the HbA1c values fluctuated widely or been consistently above 8% over the last two years, demonstrating poor glycemic control? If so, there may be a less favorable response to some forms of periodontal therapy or other oral treatment. The long-term glycemic control demonstrated by several years of HbA1c values may play a major role in determining the types of treatment the dentist will perform in managing the patient's oral health needs. The only accurate way to determine glycemic control is with the HbA1c values. Simply asking the patient, "How well controlled is your diabetes?" will lead to the same erroneous conclusions as asking a patient with hypertension, "How well is your blood pressure controlled?" Furthermore, the appropriate place to obtain HbA1c information is from the physician's office, not by asking the patient for those values.

Since 2010, many physicians have changed the way that they inform patients with diabetes about the level of glycemic control. Instead of providing the patient with the actual HbA1c value, that value is converted into an entity known as the estimated average glucose, or "eAG." Most patients with diabetes perform frequent self-monitoring of blood glucose with a glucometer. In the United States and many other countries, glucometer readings are given in mg/dl as the unit of measure; for example, 118 mg/dl. In some countries, glucometer values are presented in mmol/l as the unit of measure; for example, 6.6 mmol/l. In either case, people with diabetes are used to seeing blood glucose values on their glucometer in either mg/dl or mmol/l. When the patient sees a physician and is given an HbA1c value using a percentage as the unit of measure, the patient may not be able to "translate" that HbA1c percentage into values which the patient understands from daily glucometer testing.

Thus, a study of individuals with type 1 and type 2 diabetes was performed to determine the mathematical relationship between HbA1c values and average glucose levels over time [28]. HbA1c values were assessed at baseline and monthly for the next three months. The average glucose levels were determined using a continuous glucose monitoring

Table 5.1   Relationship between HbA1c values and estimated average glucose [24, 28].

| HbA1c (%) | Estimated average glucose (eAG) (mg/dl) | Estimated average glucose (eAG) (mmol/l) |
|---|---|---|
| 5 | 97 | 5.4 |
| 5.5 | 111 | 6.2 |
| 6 | 126 | 7.0 |
| 6.5 | 140 | 7.8 |
| 7 | 154 | 8.6 |
| 7.5 | 169 | 9.4 |
| 8 | 183 | 10.2 |
| 8.5 | 197 | 11.0 |
| 9 | 212 | 11.8 |
| 9.5 | 226 | 12.6 |
| 10 | 240 | 13.4 |
| 10.5 | 255 | 14.0 |
| 11 | 269 | 14.9 |
| 11.5 | 283 | 15.7 |
| 12 | 298 | 16.5 |

system that measured glucose levels every five minutes for at least two days and then every four weeks during the following three months. Linear regression analysis between the HbA1c and average glucose values revealed a consistent relationship and allowed determination of an estimated average glucose level using the formula: $eAG = 28.7 \times HbA1c - 46.7$. Table 5.1 demonstrates how HbA1c values and eAG values are associated across a range of glucose levels.

The estimated average glucose is not a laboratory test; it is a value determined from an HbA1c test by converting the HbA1c to an eAG using the formula above. It is important that the dentist can "speak the patient's language" when it comes to discussing glycemic control. Patients today may be more familiar with their estimated average glucose (measured in mg/dl) than they are with the HbA1c test values (measured in percent). Simple conversion calculators are readily available from web sites such as www.diabetes.org for converting HbA1c to eAG, or vice versa.

As routine dental therapy begins following completion of emergency treatment and assessment of long-term glycemic control via physician consultation, the dentist must consider the impact of diabetes on the treatment plan itself. There is some evidence, discussed previously in this chapter, that outcomes may be less favorable for some types of treatment in patients with poorly controlled diabetes relative to outcomes in patients without diabetes or with well-controlled diabetes. It is important that the dentist continue to monitor glycemic control throughout the course of therapy. This can be accomplished by frequent consultation with the physician to obtain the results of HbA1c tests or, more simply, by having the patient bring the printed laboratory results of each HbA1c test to the dental office at each visit, so that the results of the tests can be placed in the dental chart.

If the patient's glycemic control is determined to be relatively good and dental treatment is required, that treatment should be provided (Figure 5.3). Patients with well-controlled diabetes generally respond to periodontal therapy and dental implant therapy in a manner similar to patients without diabetes. If the patient's glycemic control is determined to be poor, the dentist should proceed cautiously with elective care. Treatment of inflammatory periodontal disease via scaling and root planing should be performed to reduce the bacterial bioburden and resultant inflammation. Reduction of inflammation may be associated with positive changes in glycemic control (discussed extensively in Chapter 7) [29]. An adjunctive antibiotic regimen may also be considered for patients with poor glycemic control. Research suggests that addition of a systemic tetracycline antibiotic to the scaling and root planing regimen may be beneficial for patients with diabetes [29–31]. Tetracyclines are effective in suppressing production of destructive host matrix metalloproteinase enzymes which are elevated in many patients with diabetes [6]. An adjunctive systemic antibiotic regimen commonly used in conjunction with scaling and root planing is doxycycline given at a dose of 100 mg orally per day for seven to 14 days (Figure 5.3). Ideally, scaling and root planing is completed during this seven- to 14-day course of antibiotics.

Periodontal re-evaluation should include an assessment of oral hygiene, changes in periodontal tissue health, and alterations in glycemic control. While the dentist may wish to perform periodontal re-evaluation at four to six weeks after scaling and root planing, an assessment of changes in HbA1c three months after scaling and root planing may provide valuable information. For this reason, some dentists prefer to wait about three months between completion of scaling and root planing and formal periodontal re-evaluation in patients with diabetes, at which time they not only evaluate the periodontal results of treatment but also request a new HbA1c test be done to determine any changes in glycemic control post treatment. Due to the long-term binding of glucose to hemoglobin, at least three months should be allowed between completion of scaling and root planing and the subsequent HbA1c test to allow changes to occur in the lab value. Many patients with diabetes show reduced HbA1c values after periodontal therapy, particularly when the periodontal inflammation and destruction were severe prior to treatment and when the glycemic control before treatment was poor [29–31]. However, the relationship between improvement in periodontal health and changes in glycemic control vary considerably between individual patients with diabetes and may differ between type 1 and type 2 diabetes [32]. For example, some research suggests that people with type 2 diabetes and periodontitis are more likely to have an improvement in glycemic control following periodontal therapy than are those with type 1 diabetes [33].

After scaling and root planing followed by re-evaluation, if the patient's glycemic control remains poor the dentist should generally postpone elective periodontal therapy. The patient can be placed on a schedule of frequent recall and periodontal maintenance intervals, performing needed debridement and oral hygiene reinforcement every two to three months for a year or longer. Over this course of time the periodontal status and glycemic control can be re-evaluated and a treatment plan determined based on the patient's periodontal needs, glycemic control, and compliance with oral hygiene and maintenance regimens.

## Evaluation and management of diabetes emergencies

Hyperglycemia generally does not result in emergencies in the dental office [21]. Sustained hyperglycemia is clearly a risk factor for long-term complications of diabetes. In addition, sustained hyperglycemia can lead to diabetic ketoacidosis or DKA, a life-threatening emergency. Fortunately, DKA generally does not occur in the dental office because it is not a condition that develops in minutes or hours. DKA is most common in people with type 1 diabetes, especially in children, but can occur in type 2 under conditions of significant physiologic stress. DKA occurs when there is an absolute or relative insulin deficiency, that is, a complete lack of insulin or insulin levels far below the patient's needs. Because those with type 1 diabetes no longer produce insulin, if they fail to take enough exogenous insulin to allow transport of glucose from the bloodstream into the tissues, the glucose in the bloodstream rises dramatically but the tissues are starved of needed glucose. Instead of glucose, the body begins to derive its energy from fat and protein. Breakdown of fat leads to elevated levels of free fatty acids and formation of ketone bodies in the bloodstream. The pH of blood decreases and the patient becomes acidotic. Ketones and glucose are excreted in the urine, drawing large quantities of water with them, resulting in dehydration and electrolyte imbalance. The combination of ketoacidosis and dehydration can be fatal, usually due to cerebral edema.

DKA is usually preceded by polyuria, polydipsia, fatigue, nausea, vomiting, and central nervous system depression and coma [21]. Patients may present with hyperventilation (called "Kussmaul breathing"), signs of dehydration, "fruity" breath odor, hypotension, tachycardia, and hypothermia. Treatment of DKA is done in the hospital and includes continuous intravenous infusion of short-acting insulin and rapid electrolyte and fluid replacement. Insulin infusion helps to correct the acidosis by reducing hyperglycemia, diminishing the transport of free fatty acids to the liver, and decreasing production of ketone bodies.

Unlike hyperglycemic emergencies, hypoglycemia is a much more likely cause of dental office emergency. Assessment of risk for an in-office hypoglycemic event should be part of the initial work-up for any dental patient with diabetes, because severe hypoglycemia may result in seizures or loss of consciousness [26]. The primary risk determinants for hypoglycemia associated with diabetes are the patient's level of metabolic control and the specific medication regimen used by the patient. The medical management of diabetes mellitus has changed significantly in the past 20 years since the publication of landmark studies in type 1 and type 2 diabetes showing marked reductions in the incidence and progression of diabetes complications in patients who improve their glycemic control [34, 35]. Intensive management regimens designed to lower blood glucose levels closer to the normal range have reduced diabetes complications such as neuropathy, nephropathy, retinopathy, and cardiovascular diseases. Physicians have changed the way in which they manage diabetes based on the results of such studies and on the development of new oral and injectable agents and insulin analogs that more closely mimic endogenous insulin secretion.

Patients with type 1 diabetes now come to the dental office on insulin regimens that involve three or four injections of insulin daily, or use of an insulin pump, instead of the single daily injection regimens of 20 years ago. Patients with type 2 diabetes are often taking multiple oral medications, sometimes in combination with insulin injections. While these intensive medication regimens reduce the risk of major long-term diabetes complications, they are not without their problems, especially as they relate to treatment in the dental office. The most common complication of insulin therapy is hypoglycemia, a medical emergency with significant potential for negative outcomes (Table 5.2). The incidence of hypoglycemia is highest in patients using insulin, but it can and does occur in patients using oral agents such as sulfonylureas and other medications (Tables 5.3 and 5.4). The incidence of severe hypoglycemia is markedly higher with intensive insulin regimens like those used today [36]. Hypoglycemia may result in a degree of neurologic

Table 5.2    Signs, symptoms, and treatment of hypoglycemia.

| Signs and symptoms | • Confusion<br>• Shakiness, tremors<br>• Agitation<br>• Anxiety<br>• Sweating<br>• Dizziness<br>• Tachycardia<br>• Feeling of "impending doom"<br>• Seizures<br>• Loss of consciousness |
|---|---|
| Blood glucose levels | Usually <60 mg/dl (but can be higher) |
| Treatment | • Discontinue dental treatment<br>• If patient can take food by mouth:<br>  ○ Give 15 grams of simple carbohydrate by mouth such as 4–6 oz. fruit juice, cola<br>• If patient is unconscious or cannot take food by mouth:<br>  ○ Give 30 ml of 50% dextrose (D50) IV or<br>  ○ Give 1 mg of glucagon IV, IM, subcutaneously, or submucosally |

Table 5.3    Risk for hypoglycemia associated with injectable diabetes medications.

| Agent | Risk of hypoglycemia | Action |
|---|---|---|
| Ultra short-acting insulins (lispro, aspart, glulisne) | Very high | Directly lower blood glucose (peak activity 30–90 minutes after injection) |
| Short-acting insulin (regular) | Very high | Directly lower blood glucose (peak activity two to three hours after injection) |
| Long-acting insulin (NPH) | High/moderate | Directly lower blood glucose (peak activity four to 10 hours after injection) |
| Ultra long-acting insulins (detemir, glargine) | Low | Maintain blood glucose levels similar to baseline pancreatic insulin secretion (no peak in activity; very slowly absorbed after injection) |
| Pramlintide (Symlin®) | High | Slows gastric emptying after meal, decreases postprandial glucose elevation; decreased hepatic glucose production |
| Incretin mimetics (exanatide, liraglutide) | Low | Stimulate insulin secretion only in response to increased blood glucose levels after a meal; slows insulin secretion as blood glucose approaches normal level |

Table 5.4   Risk for hypoglycemia associated with oral diabetes medications.

| Agent | Risk of hypoglycemia | Action |
|---|---|---|
| Sulfonylureas (glyburide, glipizide, glimepiride) | Moderate | Stimulate pancreatic insulin secretion immediately after a meal and then over several hours |
| Meglitinides (repaglinide, nateglinide) | Moderate | Stimulate rapid pancreatic insulin secretion after a meal |
| Biguanides (metformin) | Low | Block production of glucose by liver; improve tissue sensitivity to insulin |
| Thiazolidinediones (pioglitazone) | Low | Improve tissue sensitivity to insulin |
| α-glucosidase inhibitors (acarbose, miglitol) | Low | Slow absorption of carbohydrate from gut; decrease post-prandial peaks in glycemia |
| Dipeptidyl peptidase (DPP-4) inhibitors (sitagliptin, saxagliptin, linagliptin) | Low | Stimulate pancreatic insulin secretion only after a rise in glucose level following a meal; block hepatic glucose production |
| Combination agents (many oral agents are combined into single agent); examples: <br> • metformin + glyburide <br> • metformin + glipizide <br> • metformin + pioglitazone <br> • metformin + sitaglptin <br> • metformin + saxagliptin <br> • metformin + repaglinide <br> • glimepiride + pioglitazone | Depends on agents in combination | Combine actions from two different drug classes, as described above; level of risk for hypoglycemia depends on individual drugs in the combination agent |

impairment severe enough that the assistance of another person is required and if not treated immediately may lead to seizures or coma. Perhaps even more significant, severe hypoglycemic reactions often occur without warning symptoms for the patient, or warning symptoms may occur but fail to be perceived as such by the patient.

This risk for hypoglycemia must be recognized by dentists and dental hygienists as they treat patients with diabetes, especially those who are taking insulin (Figure 5.2). Each diabetes drug taken by the patient should be evaluated for its hypoglycemic risk prior to initiation of dental treatment (Tables 5.3 and 5.4). In addition, the HbA1c values are important in risk assessment. The risk for hypoglycemia is highest in patients with the best glycemic control. Thus, a patient with HbA1c values consistently between 6% and 7% is much more likely to experience hypoglycemic events than a patient with HbA1c values consistently near 10%, because the former patient has average daily glucose levels much lower than the latter. Symptoms of hypoglycemia usually occur when blood glucose levels drop below about 60 mg/dl, although they can occur at higher levels. Patients with consistently lower blood glucose values, such as those with HbA1c values under 7%, are more likely to fall below the threshold for hypoglycemia than those with consistently high blood glucose levels. The clinician must remember that while the risk of hypoglycemia is higher in patients with lower HbA1c values, even those with high HbA1c values can have rapid declines in blood glucose levels, resulting in signs and symptoms of hypoglycemia. During dental treatment, signs and symptoms of hypoglycemia must be recognized and treated immediately (Table 5.2). Hypoglycemia is a medical emergency and may result in seizures or unconsciousness. It is important that the dentist assess the risk of hypoglycemia for every patient with diabetes. Understanding the medications taken by the patient is foremost among risk assessment methods (Tables 5.3 and 5.4). The dentist should also ask how often the patient experiences hypoglycemia. Some people with diabetes develop a phenomenon known as hypoglycemia unawareness [37]. This is more common in those with type 1 diabetes, especially in individuals whose glycemic control is consistently good and who may experience more frequent episodes of hypoglycemia.

Recall that individuals with consistently good glycemic control tend to experience more hypoglycemic events than those whose glycemic control is consistently poor. For example, a patient with HbA1c values consistently around 6% has an estimated average glucose level of about 126 mg/dl. This is much closer to the common threshold for hypoglycemic symptoms of approximately 60 mg/dl than one would likely encounter in a patient whose HbA1c values are consistently around 9%, or an estimated average glucose level of 212 mg/dl, far from the 60 mg/dl hypoglycemia threshold.

While hypoglycemia unawareness is most common in type 1 diabetes, it may also be seen in type 2 diabetes [33]. Individuals with hypoglycemia unawareness often show none of the usual early symptoms of hypoglycemia such as tachycardia, sweating, dizziness, or anxiety before severe symptoms occur, including seizures or unconsciousness (Table 5.2). A patient with hypoglycemia unawareness may be acting normally one moment and the next moment begin to experience severe symptoms of hypoglycemia including seizures or unconsciousness. Thus, the dentist should ask patients with diabetes if they have hypoglycemia unawareness and be prepared for sudden onset of severe hypoglycemia in any individual with diabetes.

Prevention of hypoglycemia begins with knowing the patient's HbA1c levels over the past several years and assessing risk of hypoglycemia associated with their medications. In addition, the dentist should ensure that the patient has taken the usual medications and eaten the usual meals on the day of dental treatment. Perhaps the best means of avoiding hypoglycemia during the dental visit is to evaluate the patient's blood glucose level before treatment begins [26]. The most convenient means of doing so is to have all patients with diabetes bring their glucometer with them to the dental office. When the dental office establishes this process as a routine, patients often appreciate the dentist's concern about their well-being during dental treatment. The patient should check his glucose level using the glucometer, and the dentist should document the reading in the patient's dental chart. For example, a chart entry for the day's treatment might begin, "Pre-treatment glucose = 126 mg/dl by patient glucometer."

What does the dentist do with the information obtained from the pre-treatment glucometer reading? Obviously, a patient with a pre-treatment glucometer reading of 226 mg/dl is likely at lower risk of an intra-operative hypoglycemic event than one with a pre-treatment reading of 94 mg/dl because the former patient begins treatment at a glucose level much farther from the approximate 60 mg/dl hypoglycemia threshold than does the latter patient. However, glucose levels can change rapidly, especially in patients taking short-acting insulin. Therefore, in addition to the pre-treatment glucometer reading, the dentist must also consider the length of the procedure, the type and timing of the patient's medications, and recent meals or snacks. For longer appointments it may be useful to take another glucometer reading an hour or so after treatment begins to ensure the patient remains at relatively low risk for hypoglycemia. Again, the dentist must pay particular attention to those individuals taking medications with a high risk of hypoglycemia (Tables 5.3 and 5.4).

As an example, if a patient is scheduled for a 60-minute dental procedure and the pre-treatment glucose was less than 100 mg/dl, the dentist may wish to raise the glucose level by providing the patient with about 4 ounces of fruit juice. Fructose, abundant in fruit juices, is a monosaccharide and elevates blood glucose rapidly; therefore, providing fruit juice is an excellent way for the dentist to rapidly raise blood glucose levels. Depending on the type of juice, providing 4–6 ounces provides approximately 15 grams of carbohydrate. There is wide variability among patients with diabetes in the relationship between the number of grams of carbohydrate consumed and the degree of subsequent rise in blood glucose. As a general guideline, 1 gram of carbohydrate may raise blood glucose levels by 2–6 mg/dl. Therefore, providing 15 grams of carbohydrate before starting dental treatment, the blood glucose level may increase by 30–90 mg/dl. The patient should recheck the glucometer reading about 10–15 minutes later, before starting treatment, to ensure that the amount of fruit juice given was sufficient to raise the blood glucose by the desired amount. Furthermore, if the procedure is going to last longer than an hour, it may be prudent to have the patient recheck the glucose level with the glucometer about 60 minutes into treatment.

For some procedures, such as those involving certain forms of conscious sedation, patients are not able to take food by mouth prior to dental treatment (NPO). These patients must be managed carefully because the lack of food intake may dramatically increase the risk of an intraoperative hypoglycemic event. Physician consultation may be indicated to determine if changes are needed in medication regimens prior to dental treatment. For example, if the patient normally takes short-acting insulin prior to breakfast, she will not take this insulin dose on the morning of the procedure because she will not eat. Some oral medications, especially those associated with an increased risk for hypoglycemia, may also need to be modified on the day of the procedure. It is strongly recommended that NPO patients test their glucose level using their glucometer immediately prior to treatment in the dental office. If the dentist wishes to elevate the glucose level prior to treatment while maintaining the patient NPO, the dentist should use intravenous dextrose to do so. Solutions of 5% dextrose in water require large volumes of fluid to raise the glucose levels; therefore, the dentist may prefer use of 50% dextrose instead. Providing 15 grams of dextrose requires only 30 ml of 50% dextrose, which can be delivered in a matter of seconds, compared to 300 ml of 5% dextrose which takes much longer to administer intravenously.

If hypoglycemia occurs during dental treatment, that treatment should be terminated and all attention focused on managing the hypoglycemic event. If the patient is conscious and can take food by mouth, the dentist should provide approximately 15 grams of simple carbohydrates such as 4–6 ounces of fruit juice by mouth. Another glucometer reading should be done in 10–15 minutes. If symptoms do not resolve and the glucose level does not rise significantly within 10–15 minutes, another 15 grams of carbohydrate should be given and the glucose level rechecked in another 10–15 minutes. It is rare that giving 30 grams of simple carbohydrates does not raise the glucose level sufficiently to resolve hypoglycemia.

In hypoglycemic patients who cannot take food by mouth, perhaps due to loss of consciousness or onset of seizures, the dentist has two options. If an intravenous line (IV) has already been established, the dentist should rapidly give approximately 30 ml of 50% dextrose IV (15 grams of dextrose). It is not appropriate to use a 5% solution of IV dextrose as an emergency agent because it requires much longer to administer the 300 ml of fluid volume required to provide 15 grams of dextrose.

If an IV line has not been established, the drug of choice is glucagon. Glucagon is a hormone produced in the $\alpha$-cells of the pancreas which causes rapid release of endogenous glucose from the liver. Glucagon is available as an emergency drug in an injector kit. During hypoglycemic events in which the patient cannot take food by mouth and an IV line is not present, 1 mg of glucagon is given by subcutaneous, submucosal, or intramuscular injection. It does not matter where it is injected; it can be given under the skin, in a muscle, or intraorally under the mucosa. Glucagon is rapidly absorbed, causing immediate glucose release from the liver and thereby raising blood glucose levels promptly. It is important to note that nausea and vomiting may occur after administration of glucagon, so an unconscious patient should be placed in a position to avoid aspiration.

Some dentists consider having an office glucometer rather than relying on the patient to bring his or her glucometer. If the dental office has a glucometer for this purpose, the office must comply with the Clinical Laboratory Improvement Amendments (CLIA) of 1988 and their subsequent amended provisions. CLIA governs medical laboratories in the United States. If a dentist elects to keep an office glucometer, the dental office is considered a medical laboratory under CLIA. The same is true for other in-office medical tests a dentist may wish to perform such as a prothrombin test (International Normalized Ratio, or INR)or chair-side HbA1c test. Glucometer testing for the purposes described above is considered to be a CLIA-exempt procedure, meaning that a dental office using an office glucometer is considered a CLIA-waived medical laboratory. However, the dental office must still register with the government and receive a registration certificate. In addition CLIA requires documented evidence that the office glucometer is routinely monitored using control solutions specific to the glucometer, generally on a daily basis when the office glucometer is being used. The process for CLIA registration is administered through each state and the process is not burdensome. More information on CLIA may be found at www.cms.hhs.gov/clia.

### Timing of dental appointments

Appointment timing for patients with diabetes is important. Many older texts recommended treating patients with significant medical conditions in the early morning hours. That may or may not be appropriate for people with diabetes, depending primarily on the patient's medication regimen. The medications taken by the patient are the primary factor in deciding what time of day to treat the patient.

Ideally, dental treatment occurs at a time of day when blood glucose levels are higher rather than lower to reduce the risk of in-office hypoglycemia. This is determined by the patient's meal schedule and the medications being taken. As seen in Chapter 4, each medication that affects blood glucose levels does so with its own unique pharmacodynamic properties. For example, short-acting insulins reach peak activity only a few hours after injection (Table 5.2). Thus, if a patient takes short-acting insulin at 7:00 AM, the peak activity will likely occur around 9:00–10:00 AM. As insulin activity reaches its peak, blood glucose reaches its nadir shortly thereafter. Conversely, a longer acting insulin such as NPH insulin does not reach peak activity until 4–8 hours after injection. Thus, a patient injecting NPH insulin at 7:00 AM generally reaches the lowest level of blood glucose near lunch time. Each insulin formulation has its own unique profile of glucose-lowering activity and it is important that the dentist look up that information before deciding on an "appropriate" treatment time for the patient. The same holds true for oral agents which directly affect pancreatic insulin secretion, such as sulfonylureas (Table 5.3).

It is often not appropriate to simply treat the diabetic patient early in the morning. Many people with diabetes use complex medication regimens consisting of one or more drugs that directly lower blood glucose. The dentist must become familiar with each patient's regimen to determine the appropriate time of day for treatment to minimize risk for blood glucose levels falling to dangerous levels during the dental appointment. Again, use of the glucometer immediately before dental treatment provides a baseline glucose level from which the dentist can determine the likely direction of glucose fluctuation. If a patient ate his normal breakfast and took an injection of short-acting insulin at 7:00 AM, the carbohydrate from the meal will raise glucose levels over the next few hours while at the same time, the insulin injected will act to lower the blood glucose. If for some reason, the patient takes his normal amount of short-acting insulin at 7:00 AM but does not eat breakfast or eats less than usual, there will be an insufficient amount of glucose entering the blood stream to "counter" the glucose leaving the bloodstream due to the insulin action. This patient is likely to develop hypoglycemia during a dental appointment between 9:00 and 10:00 in the morning.

No matter the timing of the dental appointment, each visit should begin with several questions and actions:

1  What medications did you take today? Did you take the same amount of those medications that you would normally take?
2  What did you eat most recently? Was that the same type of food and same amount of food you normally eat at this time of day?
3  What is the baseline glucose level as determined by the patient's glucometer immediately prior to the dental procedure?

## Pain management

One important factor to consider in treating patients with diabetes is the possibility of postoperative pain. Diabetes management requires a delicate balance between carbohydrates being ingested by the patient, which raise blood glucose levels, and medications that are taken to lower blood glucose. Anything that interrupts this balance can lead to significant alterations in blood glucose dynamics. For people with diabetes, food is medicine. Therefore, if a patient is unable to eat following dental treatment, there is an increased risk of hypoglycemia unless the medications that lower blood glucose levels are also modified. It is generally best to limit the size of surgical fields when possible. For example, surgical therapy performed by quadrant or half-mouth is generally more appropriate in people with diabetes than full-mouth surgical treatment. This allows the patient to maintain appropriate nutrition following treatment.

## Conclusion

Dental management of patients with diabetes can be challenging. Working closely with the physician and understanding the patient's daily diabetes management regimen leads to developing appropriate pathways of care and minimizes risk for in-office emergencies.

## References

1. Christgau M, Palitzsch KD, Schmalz G, Kreiner U, Frenzel S. Healing response to non-surgical periodontal therapy in patients with diabetes mellitus: clinical, microbiological, and immunological results. *J Clin Periodontol* 1998; 25: 112–124.
2. Tervonen T, Knuuttila M, Pohjamo L, Nurkkala H. Immediate response to non-surgical periodontal treatment in subjects with diabetes mellitus. *J Clin Periodontol* 1991; 18: 65–68.
3. Tervonen T, Karjalainen K. Periodontal disease related to diabetic status. A pilot study of the response to periodontal therapy in type 1 diabetes. *J Clin Periodontol* 1997; 24: 505–510.
4. Westfelt E, Rylander H, Blohme G, Jonasson P, Lindhe J. The effect of periodontal therapy in diabetics. Results after 5 years. *J Clin Periodontol* 1996; 23: 92–100.
5. Costa FO, Miranda Cota LO, Pereira Lages EJ, Soares Dutra Oliveira AM, Dutra Oliveira PA, Cyrino RM, Medeiros Lorentz TC, Cortelli SC, Cortelli JR. *J Periodontol* 2012, Jul 6 (ePub ahead of print).
6. Mealey BL, Oates TW. Diabetes mellitus and periodontal diseases. *J Periodontol* 2006; 77: 1289–1303.
7. Lu H, Kraut D, Gerstenfeld LC, Graves DT. Diabetes interferes with bone formation by affecting the expression of transcription factors that regulate osteoblast differentiation. *Endocrinology* 2003; 144: 346–352.
8. Vestergaard P. Discrepancies in bone mineral density and fracture risk in patients with type 1 and type 2 diabetes—a meta-analysis. *Osteoporos Int* 2007; 18: 427–444.
9. Nevins ML, Karimbux NY, Weber HP, Giannobile WV, Fiorellini JP. Wound healing around endosseous implants in experimental diabetes. *Int J Oral Maxillofac Implants* 1998; 13: 620–629.
10. Fiorellini JP, Nevins ML, Norkin A, Weber HP, Karimbux NY. The effect of insulin therapy on osseointegration in a diabetic rat model. *Clin Oral Implants Res* 1999; 10: 362–368.
11. Moy PK, Medina D, Shetty V, Aghaloo TL. Dental implant failure rates and associated risk factors. *Int J Oral Maxillofac Implants* 2005; 20: 569–577.
12. Morris HF, Ochi S, Winkler S. Implant survival in patients with type 2 diabetes: placement to 36 months. *Ann Periodontol* 2000; 5: 157–165.

13. Alsaadi G, Quirynen M, Komárek A, van Steenberghe D. Impact of local and systemic factors on the incidence of oral implant failures, up to abutment connection. *J Clin Periodontol* 2007; 34: 610–617.
14. Alsaadi G, Quirynen M, Komárek A, van Steenberghe D. Impact of local and systemic factors on the incidence of late oral implant loss. *Clin Oral Implants Res* 2008; 19: 670–676.
15. Bornstein MM, Cionca N, Mombelli A. Systemic conditions and treatments as risks for implant therapy. *Int J Oral Maxillofac Implants* 2009; 24(suppl): 12–27.
16. Dowell S, Oates TW, Robinson M. Implant success in people with type 2 diabetes mellitus with varying glycemic control: A pilot study. *J Am Dent Assoc* 2007; 138: 355–361.
17. Tawil G, Younan R, Azar P, Sleilati G. Conventional and advanced implant treatment in the type II diabetic patient: surgical protocol and long-term clinical results. *Int J Oral Maxillofac Implants* 2008; 23: 744–752.
18. Turkyilmaz I. One-year clinical outcome of dental implants placed in patients with type 2 diabetes mellitus: A case series. *Implant Dent* 2010; 19: 323–329.
19. Khandelwal N, Oates TW, Vargas A, Alexander PP, Schoolfield JD, Alex McMahan C. Conventional SLA and chemically modified SLA implants in patients with poorly controlled type 2 diabetes mellitus—a randomized controlled trial. *Clin Oral Implants Res* 2013; 24: 13–19.
20. Centers for Disease Control and Prevention. National diabetes fact sheet, 2011. http://www.cdc.gov/diabetes/pubs/factsheet11.htm Accessed December 4, 2013.
21. Mealey BL, Ocampo GL. Diabetes mellitus and periodontal disease. *Periodontology 2000* 2007; 44: 127–153.
22. Lalla E, Cheng B, Lal S, Kaplan S, Softness B, Greenberg E, Goland RS, Lamster IB. Diabetes-related parameters and periodontal conditions in children. *J Clin Periodontol* 2007; 42: 345–349.
23. Taylor GW, Burt BA, Becker MP, et al. Non-insulin dependent diabetes mellitus and alveolar bone loss progression over 2 years. *J Periodontol* 1998: 69: 76–83.
24. American Diabetes Association. Standards of Medical Care in Diabetes—2013 (Position Statement). *Diabetes Care* 2013; 36(suppl): S11–S66.
25. Kunzel C, Lalla E, Lamster IB. Management of the patient who smokes and the diabetic patient in the dental office. *J Periodontol* 2006; 77: 331–340.
26. Mealey BL. Managing patients with diabetes: First, do no harm. *J Periodontol* 2007; 78: 2072–2076.
27. Virtue MA, Furne JK, Nuttall FQ, Levitt MD. Relationship between GHb concentration and erythrocyte survival determined from breath carbon monoxide concentration. *Diabetes Care* 2004: 27: 931–935.
28. Nathan DM, Kuenen J, Borg R, Zheng H, Schoenfeld D, Heine RJ. Translating the A1c assay into estimated average glucose values. *Diabetes Care* 2008; 31:1473–1478.
29. Teeuw WJ, Gerdes VE, Loos BG. Effect of periodontal treatment on glycemic control of diabetic patients: a systematic review and meta-analysis. *Diabetes Care* 2010; 33: 421–427.
30. Grossi SG, Skrepcinski FB, DeCaro T, Robertson DC, Ho AW, Dunford RG, Genco RJ. Treatment of periodontal disease in diabetics reduces glycated hemoglobin. *J Periodontol* 1997: 68: 713–719.
31. Darre L, Vergnes JN, Gourdy P, Sixou M. Efficacy of periodontal treatment on glycaemic control in diabetic patients: A meta-analysis of interventional studies. *Diabetes Metab* 2008; 34: 497–506.
32. Tervonen T, Lamminsalo S, Hiltunen L, Raunio T, Knuuttila M. Resolution of periodontal inflammation does not guarantee improved glycemic control in type 1 diabetic subjects. *J Clin Periodontol* 2009; 36: 51–57.

33. Calabrese N, D'Aiuto F, Calabrese A, Patel K, Calabrese G, Massi-Benedetti M. Effects of periodontal therapy on glucose management in people with diabetes mellitus. *Diabetes Metab* 2011; 37: 456–459.
34. Diabetes Control and Complications Trial Research Group. The effect of intensive treatment of diabetes on the development and progression of long-term complications in insulin-dependent diabetes mellitus. *N Engl J Med* 1993: 329: 977–986.
35. U.K. Prospective Diabetes Study (UKPDS) Group. Intensive blood-glucose control with sulphonylureas or insulin compared with conventional treatment and risk of complications in patients with type 2 diabetes (UKPDS 33). *Lancet* 1998: 352: 837–853.
36. Diabetes Control and Complications Trial Research Group. Hypoglycemia in the Diabetes Control and Complications Trial. *Diabetes* 1997; 46: 271–286.
37. Bakatselos SO. Hypoglycemia unawareness. *Diabetes Res Clin Pract* 2011; 93 (suppl 1): S92–S96.

# Chapter 6

# Periodontal disease as a complication of diabetes mellitus

*George W. Taylor, DMD, DrPH; Dana T. Graves, DDS, DMSc; and Ira B. Lamster, DDS, MMSc*

The focus of this chapter is on the adverse effects of diabetes on periodontal health. The two major areas of emphasis are (1) discussions of the types and strength of empirical evidence from large-scale epidemiological and smaller clinical studies that support the concept that diabetes has an adverse effect on periodontal health in humans, and (2) the biologic mechanisms by which diabetes is thought to contribute to poorer periodontal health (i.e., the tissue, cellular, and molecular dynamics and their interactions).

Both diabetes and periodontal diseases are globally common chronic lifestyle-related diseases [1]. The epidemiology of diabetes mellitus was presented in Chapter 2. A potentially important commonality that is increasingly becoming recognized is the association of obesity with periodontal disease as well as diabetes [2, 3]. This commonality highlights the rationale for considering periodontal disease as having an important lifestyle component in its pathogenesis [1].

## Periodontal diseases: overview

The periodontal diseases are a group of chronic, microbial-induced inflammatory disease that most commonly occurs in two major forms, gingivitis and chronic periodontitis. Both forms of periodontal disease have bacterial etiologies in which Gram-negative anaerobes predominate as major periodontal pathogens. Gingivitis is a biofilm or plaque-induced inflammation of the gingiva that is reversible but can progress to chronic periodontitis, if not treated, in susceptible individuals. Gingivitis resolves clinically after mechanical disruption of the biofilm, usually by effective, regular oral hygiene. Chronic periodontitis occurs in susceptible individuals with long-term supra- and sub-gingival plaque accumulation. The chronic presence of plaque results in enrichment and maturation of the biofilm leading to sustained inflammation (or constant wounding). Chronic periodontitis is characterized by irreversible loss of the supporting tooth structures, including the connective tissue fibers of the gingiva, periodontal ligament, and alveolar bone. This local, irreversible destruction of periodontal tissues, in severe cases, may lead to partial or complete tooth loss [4, 5].

*Diabetes Mellitus and Oral Health: An Interprofessional Approach*, First Edition. Edited by Ira B. Lamster.
© 2014 John Wiley & Sons, Inc. Published 2014 by John Wiley & Sons, Inc.

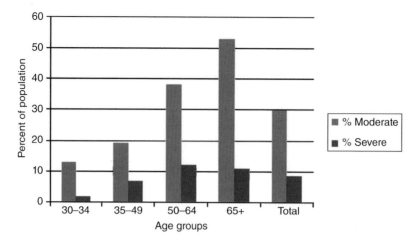

**Figure 6.1**   Prevalence of moderate or severe periodontitis in US adults: National Health and Nutrition Examination Survey 2009–2010 [7]. % Moderate: Moderate periodontitis is defined as 2 or more teeth with attachment loss greater than or equal to 4 mm, or 2 or more teeth with probing pocket depth greater than or equal to 5 mm at the interproximal sites. % Severe: Severe periodontitis is defined as 2 or more teeth with attachment loss greater than or equal to 6 mm, and 1 or more teeth with probing pocket depth greater than or equal to 5 mm at interproximal sites.

Like diabetes, periodontal diseases are common chronic diseases in the adult population in the United States. The prevalence of gingivitis is approximately 50% in all age groups [6]. In contrast, the prevalence of chronic periodontitis is associated with increasing age. Figure 6.1 presents the relative prevalence of moderate and severe periodontal disease (generally chronic adult periodontitis) in U.S. adults examined in the 2009–2010 National Health and Nutrition Examination Survey [7]. Figure 6.1 shows that there is a gradient for the prevalence of both moderate and severe periodontal disease as age increases. This age-related gradient is due, for the most part, to the accumulated exposure over time to other risk factors. On average, the overall prevalence of moderate and severe chronic periodontal disease is approximately 30% and 8.5%, respectively, in the United States.

## Evidence of adverse effects of diabetes mellitus on periodontal health

The evidence we will consider with regard to the adverse effects of diabetes on periodontal health comes from English language reports of studies conducted in numerous parts of the world.

As might be expected, reports in the literature provide answers to different kinds of questions, and vary in their ability to help us establish and understand causal associations between diabetes and periodontal diseases.

1 Studies of prevalence allow us to compare the proportion of individuals with periodontal disease between those with and without diabetes. Studies of prevalence also allow us to evaluate the association of degrees of glycemic control with the proportion of individuals who have periodontal disease among people with diabetes.

2 Studies of extent of periodontal disease are those assessing the number of teeth or sites affected, whereas studies of severity assess the amount of periodontal destruction in terms of severity of pocket depth, attachment loss, or alveolar bone loss.

3 Studies of incidence and progression of periodontal disease must follow people over time. Incidence is a measure of the rate of new cases of periodontal disease. Progression is a measure of worsening of periodontal status over time.

In terms of study designs' contributions to inferring causal relationships, cross-sectional studies are limited to studies of prevalence, extent, and severity. Because cross-sectional studies cannot establish temporal relationships, they are limited in providing evidence of causal relationships. In contrast, studies following individuals over time (i.e., prospective cohort or longitudinal studies) allow quantification of the risk of diabetes contributing to worsening periodontal health using any of the terms associated with the passage of time (i.e., incidence and progression) and can allow for inferences regarding causal relationships.

Several comprehensive narrative reviews [8–12] and three meta-analyses [13–15] have evaluated the body of literature for original research reports to assess the adverse effect of diabetes on periodontal health. The narrative reviews and the meta-analyses consistently conclude that diabetes adversely effects periodontal health in people with diabetes.

Tables 6.1 and 6.2 illustrate a way in which conclusions from reviews of the body of literature can be organized. These tables summarize the relative proportionate numbers of studies by study design (i.e., cohort and cross-sectional/descriptive) for each category of diabetes typically considered in reviews of the literature. These two tables are derived from the compilation of two comprehensive narrative reviews evaluating reports published between 1967 and 2007 [11, 12].

Table 6.1 summarizes the conclusions of studies reported in the literature that address the question of whether diabetes adversely affects periodontal health, comparing people with and without diabetes. The column headings indicate the type of diabetes included in the study and the row headings indicate the type of study design (i.e., cohort or cross-sectional/descriptive). In each category within Table 6.1, the numerator is the number of

Table 6.1 Effects of diabetes on periodontal health. Conclusions of the 89 studies that include a non-diabetes control group [16].

| Study design | Diabetes mellitus type | | | | | Total number of studies (number with effect/number of all studies) |
| | Type 1 | Type 2 | Type 1 or 2 | Gestational (GDM) | Type not reported | |
| --- | --- | --- | --- | --- | --- | --- |
| Cohort | 3/3 | 4/4 | 0/0 | 0/0 | 0/0 | 7/7 |
| Cross-sectional, descriptive | 22/23 | 20/23 | 15/18 | 3/3 | 11/15 | 72/83 |
| Total: | 25/26 | 24/27 | 15/18 | 3/3 | 11/15 | 79/89 |

The numerator represents the number of studies reporting diabetes having an adverse effect on periodontal health, the denominator the total number of studies in each group.

Table 6.2   Effects of diabetes on periodontal health. Conclusions of the 61 studies that include participants with both better and poorer glycemic control [16].

| Study design | Diabetes mellitus type | | | | Total number of studies (number with effect/number of all studies) |
| | Type 1 | Type 2 | Type 1 or 2 | Type not reported | |
| --- | --- | --- | --- | --- | --- |
| Cohort | 4/4 | 3/3 | 1/3 | 0/0 | 8/10 |
| Cross-sectional, descriptive | 11/18 | 15/17 | 7/11 | 1/5 | 34/51 |
| Total: | 15/22 | 18/20 | 8/14 | 1/5 | 42/61 |

The numerator represents the number of studies reporting poorer glycemic control having decreasing adverse effect on periodontal health, the denominator the total number of studies in each group.

studies confirming that diabetes adversely affects one or more of several measures of periodontal health (e.g., gingivitis, probing pocket depth, attachment loss, or radiographic bone loss). The denominator represents the total number of studies of that particular kind (e.g., cross-sectional studies with participants having type 2 diabetes). For example, all four of the reports from cohort studies that included people with type 2 diabetes concluded that periodontal health was worse in people who had diabetes than in those without diabetes. The information presented in Table 6.1 shows the vast majority of reports, specifically 79 of 89 studies, provided evidence that diabetes adversely affects periodontal health. The stronger evidence comes from the cohort studies with all seven reports supporting a conclusion that diabetes had an adverse effect on periodontal health. An updated review of the body of literature published from 1967 to 2011 found 101 of 115 reports concluding diabetes had an adverse effect on periodontal health (Table 6.3). In Table 6.3, proportions for the types of study designs, the types of diabetes included in the studies, and studies with positive results are relatively consistent with the earlier summary of published reports shown in Table 6.1.

Table 6.2 illustrates another way of organizing the literature to address the question of whether the degree of control of diabetes (i.e., glycemic control) is associated with poorer periodontal health. In this type of analysis the participants can be limited to people with diabetes who have better or poorer glycemic control. The degree to which diabetes is controlled or managed is usually assessed by measuring the amount of hemoglobin A1c (HbA1c) in the blood. HbA1c is an indicator of persisting hyperglycemia over the previous 60–90 days. For many people with diabetes the therapeutic target for good glycemic control is to achieve an HbA1c level that is 7% or less [17].

Table 6.2 summarizes the conclusions of studies that provided information comparing the effects of better or poorer glycemic control on periodontal health in people with diabetes. Similar to Table 6.1, the evidence was derived from both cohort and cross-sectional original research reports published between 1967 and 2007 [11, 12]. A large majority (two-thirds) of the studies in Table 6.2 concluded that people with poorer glycemic control had worse periodontal health than those with better glycemic control (42 of the 61 studies). Again, the stronger evidence comes from the set of cohort studies that followed

Table 6.3   Effects of diabetes on periodontal health. Conclusions of the 115 studies that include a non-diabetes control group for the period from 1967 to 2011.

| Study design | Diabetes mellitus type | | | | | Total number of studies (number with effect/number of all studies) |
|---|---|---|---|---|---|---|
| | Type 1 | Type 2 | Type 1 or 2 | Gestational (GDM) | Type not reported | |
| Cohort | 3/3 | 5/6 | 0/0 | 0/0 | 0/0 | 8/9 |
| Cross-sectional, descriptive | 26/28 | 35/38 | 15/18 | 3/3 | 14/19 | 93/106 |
| Total: | 29/31 | 40/44 | 15/18 | 3/3 | 14/19 | 101/115 |

The numerator represents the number of studies reporting diabetes having an adverse effect on periodontal health, the denominator the total number of studies in each group.

people over time, allowing for more definitive conclusions regarding a causal relationship. Eight of the 10 cohort studies supported the conclusion that poorer glycemic control leads to poorer periodontal health over time.

From the information provided in Tables 6.1 to 6.3 and persisting to the present, the preponderance of studies reporting on the adverse effects of diabetes are cross-sectional and involve convenience samples of patients, principally from hospitals and clinics. A smaller subset of longitudinal and population-based studies provides additional support for the association between diabetes and periodontal disease.

In extending our capacity to assess the body of evidence beyond comprehensive narrative reviews, meta-analyses provide the opportunity to combine the results of several studies and quantitatively summarize the results. Chavarry et al. (2009) published a systematic review and meta-analysis of the association of diabetes with poorer periodontal health and whether diabetes has an adverse impact on the response to periodontal treatment in 49 cross-sectional studies and eight cohort studies [13]. This meta-analysis found statistically significant greater mean clinical attachment loss and probing pocket depth in cross-sectional studies of people with type 2 diabetes compared to those without diabetes ($P=0.021$ and $P=0.046$ respectively). While not statistically significant and probably not clinically significant, the meta-analysis showed a tendency for people with type 1 diabetes in cross-sectional studies to have greater mean attachment loss than people without diabetes ($P=0.54$) and greater mean probing depths ($P=0.137$). The authors of this meta-analysis suggested that the lack of a statistically significant association of type 1 diabetes and poorer periodontal health could be explained by the low mean age of the participants with type 1 diabetes (between 11 and 15 years) and the concomitant observation that people in this age group do not frequently develop destructive periodontal disease. It should also be noted that this meta-analysis did not conduct analyses that distinguished between those with better and poorer controlled diabetes. This may have also limited their ability to find a significant difference in those with type 1 diabetes.

Although the meta-analysis by Chavarry et al. did not find a statistically significant impact of diabetes on periodontal health in those with type 1 diabetes, one rigorously conducted study of children and adolescents 6–18 years old who predominantly had type 1 diabetes found significantly poorer periodontal health in those with diabetes than the control group without diabetes [18–20]. In one report the investigators found statistically significant and clinically meaningful four-fold higher prevalence of teeth with clinical attachment loss in children with type 1 diabetes [20]. In another report the investigators considered the degree of glycemic control over a two-year period prior to the periodontal examination. In that report the investigators found statistically significant greater perio-dontal destruction in the participants with diabetes than the controls without diabetes, even when divided into two subgroups of 6- to 11-year-olds and 12- to 18-year olds [19]. In another analysis, HbA1c was significantly associated with the degree of periodontal destruction, suggesting the need to account for glycemic control in investigations of rela-tionships between diabetes and periodontal diseases in children and adolescents with type 1 diabetes [18].

Chavarry and colleagues' systematic review also investigated eight longitudinal studies; four assessed differences in the progression of periodontal disease between people with diabetes and those without and the effect of diabetes on the response to periodontal treatment. For the three longitudinal studies of participants with type 1 diabetes [21–23], one of the two studies of the progression of periodontal disease found the progression to be more pronounced in those with type 1 diabetes [21]. In the study that investigated diabetes effects on the response to periodontal therapy, there was no significant difference in improvements of periodontal outcomes between those with and without diabetes [23].

In Chavarry and colleagues' systematic review of the progression of periodontal dis-ease in type 2 diabetes, of the three studies included [24–26], two studies reported greater progression of periodontal disease [25, 26]. The study assessing the effect of diabetes on the response to periodontal treatment showed worsening of periodontal health at six months follow-up was greater in the participants with diabetes than in those who did not have diabetes [24]. In two studies investigating the response to periodontal treatment that included participants with either type 1 or type 2 diabetes, neither found differences in the changes to clinical periodontal outcomes after four months [27] and five years follow-up [28].

Additional evidence supporting diabetes having an adverse effect on periodontal health comes from studies of women with gestational diabetes mellitus (GDM). Gestational diabetes is defined as any degree of glucose intolerance, that is clearly not overt diabetes, with onset or first recognition during pregnancy [17]. Approximately 7% of all pregnan-cies are complicated by GDM [29]. For many women the impact of GDM goes beyond the end of the pregnancy. A systematic review and meta-analysis of 20 studies found women who had GDM to have at least a seven-fold greater risk for developing type 2 diabetes in the future than women who had a normoglycemic pregnancy [30]. Evidence is emerging that GDM contributes to poorer periodontal health during the pregnancy. Five studies published in English since 2006 have included pregnant women with and without GDM to evaluate the role of GDM as a risk indicator for periodontal disease [31–35]. The prevalence of periodontal disease ranged from 31% to 77% in women with GDM or a history of GDM and from 13% to 57% in women who had no history of GDM. Four of the five studies, conducted in Thailand (31) and the United States [33–35], concluded that

GDM was significantly associated with poorer periodontal health. These four studies estimated 2.6- to 9-fold greater odds of having periodontal disease for women with a history of GDM than women who had not had GDM. The other study, conducted in Brazil [32], did not find a significant difference in the prevalence of periodontal disease in women with and without GDM. This is an emerging body of evidence that will benefit from subsequent prospective studies to strengthen causal inferences.

The studies reviewed in this section provide an overview of the evidence supporting the conclusion that diabetes has an adverse effect on periodontal health in susceptible individuals. The studies included in the reviews were conducted in different settings and different countries, with different ethnic populations and age distributions, and with a variety of measures of periodontal disease status (i.e., gingival inflammation, pathologic probing pocket depth, loss of periodontal attachment, or radiographic evidence of alveolar bone loss). The studies used different parameters to assess periodontal disease occurrence (prevalence, incidence, extent, severity, or progression). Hence, this inevitable variation in methodology and study populations limits the possibility that the same biases or confounding factors apply in all the studies and provides support for concluding that diabetes is a risk factor for periodontal disease incidence, progression, and severity. In addition, there is substantial evidence to support a "dose-response" relationship (i.e., as glycemic control worsens, the adverse effects of diabetes on periodontal health become greater). Finally, there are no studies with superior design features to refute this conclusion.

## Biologic mechanisms contributing to the adverse effects of diabetes on periodontal health

This section reviews the biologic mechanisms that can explain the increased prevalence and severity of periodontal disease in people with diabetes. As with other complications of diabetes, biologic mechanisms important in diabetes-associated periodontitis are probably multi-factorial, arising from the altered cellular and molecular interactions due to the metabolic dysregulation that characterizes diabetes. The mechanisms to be considered in this section include altered subgingival microflora, altered host inflammatory response, advanced glycation end-product formation (AGEs) and their receptor (RAGE), uncoupling of bone resorption and bone formation, and several other mechanisms less frequently mentioned. Understanding the explanatory mechanisms leading to more frequent and more severe periodontal infection in diabetes involves synthesis of observations from these multiple perspectives. Sources providing major contributions to the content of this section on the biologic mechanisms include extensive reviews in journal articles [8, 11, 36] and book chapters [12, 16].

### *Altered subgingival microflora*

The question of whether diabetes contributes to a periodontal sulcular microflora that has a different composition and is more virulent due to elevated sulcular glucose levels has been studied since the 1980s. An extensive review of studies investigating the impact of diabetes on the periodontal microflora suggests neither diabetes nor the degree of glycemic control has an established, significant effect on the periodontal microflora [36]. The authors of that review recognize the limitations of the studies reviewed in this body of literature generally include inadequate control groups and restricted analysis of the dental plaque or biofilm species. The review's authors suggest that techniques of microbiomics and metagenomics could, in the future, provide a different perspective on the influence of diabetes on the oral microbiome. An example of application of such techniques is a report by Casarin and colleagues using 16S rRNA gene cloning and sequencing [37]. In that report investigators found significant dissimilarities in the subgingival biodiversity of participants who had severe generalized chronic periodontitis when comparing those with poorly controlled type 2 diabetes (n = 12) to those who did not have diabetes (n = 11).

### Altered host inflammatory response

Whereas the evidence for diabetes having an effect on the periodontal microbiome is inconclusive, evidence that diabetes contributes to an altered host response to the periodontal bacterial challenge is more compelling. A number of earlier investigations reported that diabetes contributes to impaired neutrophil function. The reports indicate that impaired chemotaxis [38–44], adherence [45, 46], phagocytosis, and bacteriocidal activity [47–49] could result in greater propensity for colonization and proliferation of periodontal pathogens in the dental plaque biofilm. Additional evidence also suggests that chronic hyperglycemia in diabetes contributes to defects in neutrophil function that mediate diabetes-related tissue damage to the periodontium by stimulating exaggerated production of inflammatory mediators and superoxide release by neutrophils, enhanced leukocyte rolling and attachment to the vascular endothelium in periodontal vessels, and impaired transendothelial migration [50, 51]. Neutrophils in patients with diabetes who have severe periodontitis have also been shown to have defective apoptosis, leading to longer retention of neutrophils in the periodontal tissue and prolonged and greater tissue destruction by continued release of matrix metalloproteinases (MMPs) and reactive oxygen species (ROS) [52]. Metabolic routes linked to leukocyte dysfunction include advanced protein glycosylation, the polyol pathway, oxygen free radical formation, and the nitric oxide-cyclic guanosine monophosphate pathway [53].

To further assess the effects of diabetes on altering the host's inflammatory response, a number of small-scale, mainly cross-sectional studies have investigated whether diabetes influences the cytokine and other mediator profiles (growth factors, prostanoids, and MMPs), quantitatively or qualitatively, of patients with periodontal disease. An extensive systematic review [36] notes this group of studies has investigated pro-inflammatory biomarkers from samples of human saliva, gingival crevicular fluid, and gingival tissues to provide additional evidence regarding the role of diabetes in increasing the inflammatory response in the periodontal tissues.

Human studies noted in the review [36] included investigations of mediator profiles in individuals with type 1 and type 2 diabetes. For type 1 diabetes the review found the number of human studies was very limited. A consistent finding was that individuals with both type 1 diabetes and periodontitis had higher levels of the pro-inflammatory cytokines prostaglandins E2 (PGE2) and interleukin-1 β (IL-1β). For type 2 diabetes the review found that the most consistent findings were higher levels of IL-1β and IL-6 in individuals with both diabetes and chronic periodontal disease than in individuals who had chronic periodontal disease but not diabetes. The review noted that evidence for elevated levels of tumor necrosis factor-$\alpha$ (TNF-$\alpha$) in oral fluids or gingival tissue in individuals with type 2 diabetes and chronic periodontitis was inconsistent. Other studies reviewed provided evidence of type 2 diabetes adversely influencing the receptor activator of nuclear factor $\kappa$B ligand (RANKL) to osteoprotegrin ratio (RANKL:OPG) in individuals with both type 2 diabetes and chronic periodontitis. Also considered in the review were studies investigating the effect of glycemic control on markers of inflammation in individuals with type 2 diabetes and chronic periodontal disease. Higher levels of salivary IL-6, IL-1$\beta$, and gingival crevicular fluid levels of RANKL:OPG were reported to be associated with poor glycemic control in individuals with type 2 diabetes and chronic periodontitis.

Additional insight into mechanisms of diabetes-enhanced periodontitis come from *in vitro* and animal studies that have demonstrated cause-and-effect relationships between specific cellular and molecular events, which cannot be performed easily in human studies [54]. Cell culture studies indicate that a substantial subset of individuals with type 1 diabetes have a monocytic hyperresponsive phenotype that predisposes them to an exaggerated response to Gram-negative bacterial infections [55–59]. Several important putative periodontal pathogens are Gram-negative anaerobes. Salvi and colleagues have reported enhanced peripheral blood monocytic response to LPS challenge, as evidenced by the previously mentioned elevated gingival crevicular fluid levels of PGE2, IL-1$\beta$, and TNF-$\alpha$ in individuals with type 1 diabetes and periodontal disease when compared to controls without diabetes [57, 58]. They reported that enhanced inflammatory mediator response is functionally consistent with the type and levels of mediators required to induce alveolar bone resorption and other periodontal connective tissue destruction. This evidence suggests that the enhanced PGE2, IL-1$\beta$, and TNF-$\alpha$ secretory responsiveness of peripheral blood monocytes in individuals with type 1 diabetes mellitus may contribute to the increased risk for severe periodontal disease. Neutrophils from individuals with diabetes have been reported to demonstrate increased production of superoxides, which enhance oxidative stress [60].

In an animal model, injection of *Porphyromonas gingivalis* (*P. gingivalis*), an established periodontal pathogen, into connective tissue was shown to stimulate more prolonged formation of an inflammatory infiltrate with higher levels of inflammatory cytokines [61]. This was linked to higher levels of TNF-$\alpha$ because a specific TNF-$\alpha$ inhibitor reversed the increased and prolonged inflammation in the diabetic mice stimulated by *P. gingivalis* [62]. In another animal model, type 2 diabetes was shown to significantly enhance periodontal inflammation induced by the onset of periodontal disease more so than matched healthy rats [63]. Diabetic rats had significantly more prolonged gingival inflammation as well as greater osteoclast numbers and bone loss.

A study of ligature-induced periodontitis in rats showed diabetes-enhanced inflammation in the periodontium leads to up-regulation of genes involved in the host response, apoptosis, and coagulation/homeostasis/complement and down-regulation of energy/metabolism-associated genes [64]. That study also showed that peroxisome proliferator-activated receptor-$\alpha$ (PPAR-$\alpha$), a contributor in the resolution of periodontitis through its anti-inflammatory properties, was up-regulated during the resolution of periodontal inflammation in the gingiva of the control rats and suppressed in the diabetic rats. Using gingival intravital microscopy, a study of diabetic and control mice found that the pro-inflammatory state induced by diabetes affects the gingival microcirculation to increase vascular permeability and activation of leukocytes and endothelial cells. This then leads to microvascular damage, which in turn may contribute to periodontal tissue damage in diabetes [65].

## Advanced glycation end-product formation

Other studies have provided additional insight into potential metabolic and genetic factors that could contribute to the increased risk and severity of periodontal tissue destruction in diabetes. Persistent hyperglycemia causes non-enzymatic glycation and oxidation of proteins and lipids and subsequent formation of advanced glycation end products (AGEs), which accumulate in the plasma and tissues [66–68]. AGEs are long-lived molecules formed by the irreversible binding of glucose to protein and lipids in the plasma and tissues during persistent hyperglycemia. Diabetes enhances formation of AGEs in the periodontium and increases expression of RAGE [69]. Hyperglycemia and resultant AGE formation are considered to be a major causal factor in the pathogenesis of diabetic complications [66, 70, 71]. RAGE is the principal signal transducer for the AGE ligand [72]. Expression of cell surface binding sites or receptors for AGE (i.e., RAGE) is increased in diabetes, and RAGE has been identified on the cell surfaces of several cell types exhibiting a heightened inflammatory response and involved with the pathogenesis of complications of diabetes. These cell types include mononuclear phagocytes, endothelial cells, fibroblasts, smooth muscle cells, lymphocytes, podocytes, and neurons [67, 73]. In subjects with diabetes who also have periodontitis, AGEs and increased oxidative stress have been demonstrated in gingival tissues [74] and periodontal ligament cells [69]. A recent extensive review by Lalla and Papapanou describing the role of AGEs and RAGE in the diabetes-periodontitis relationship [8] mentions that levels of AGEs in serum have been shown to be associated with the extent of periodontitis in adults with type 2 diabetes [75] and increased RAGE expression has been observed in the gingival tissues of people with diabetes and periodontal disease [76]. The review also mentions that *in vitro* studies have reported that AGEs are involved in suppressed collagen production by gingival and periodontal ligament fibroblasts [77, 78].

Also discussed in the review by Lalla and Papapanou is the role of AGEs and RAGE in periodontal tissue destruction and an exaggerated inflammatory response to the challenge of periodontal pathogens for people with diabetes [8]. A study using a murine model of oral infection with *P. gingivalis* reported increased alveolar bone loss in diabetic mice compared to nondiabetic controls. Increased expression of RAGE, AGEs, and tissue-destructive MMPs in the gingival tissues were observed in conjunction with the alveolar bone loss [79]. Another study discussed in the review reported that treatment of diabetic mice that had periodontal infection with soluble RAGE, the antagonist of the extracellular ligand-binding domain of RAGE, resulted in decreased levels of TNF-α, IL-6, and MMPs in gingival tissues. This treatment also suppressed alveolar bone loss in the diabetic mice [80]. Suppressed expression of RAGE and its ligands in the gingival tissues accompanied the beneficial effects of the RAGE antagonist. The review mentions there is also evidence that accumulation of AGEs and their interaction with RAGE may contribute to osteoclastogenesis via increased expression of receptor activator of RANKL and down-regulation of osteoprotegerin [81, 82].

In addition to its impact on periodontal tissue destruction, AGE-RAGE interaction has been shown to contribute to impaired wound repair. The review by Lalla and Papapanou describes three studies of excisional wounds in diabetic mice. In one study inhibition of RAGE signaling improved the rate of wound closure and repair and down-regulated MMP activity [83]. Another study using osteoblast cultures and craniotomy defects reported that RAGE and its interaction with carboxymethyllysine-albumin, an AGE ligand, contributed to delayed bone healing in the absence of infection [84]. Another study, also using osteo-blast cultures and craniotomy defects, reported that carboxymethyllysine-collagen had an apoptotic effect on osteoblasts that was mediated through RAGE. This study also reported mitogen-activated protein kinases, c-Jun N-terminal kinase, caspase 3, and caspase 8 had increased activity and were involved in this outcome [85].

### Uncoupling of bone resorption and bone formation

Another perspective on mechanisms proposed to contribute to greater bone loss in dia-betic animals is uncoupling of bone resorption and bone formation [63]. The process of coupling refers to the repair of resorbed bone by new bone formation [86]. Although bone repair occurs, not all resorbed bone is replaced by this reparative process. Thus, the amount of bone lost is equal to the amount of bone resorption minus the amount of repar-ative new bone formation. In another study of ligature-induced periodontitis in rats, the diabetic animals had significantly less coupling than the non-diabetic controls, so that there was less reparative bone formation following an episode of resorption, contributing to a net bone loss. The decreased numbers of bone-lining and periodontal ligament cells, due to higher levels of cell death (apoptosis), suggested an explanatory mechanism [63]. This interpretation is supported by studies in which a cause-effect relationship between diabetes-enhanced apoptosis and the ability to form bone after an episode of resorption has been inferred [87], in which inhibition of apoptosis with a caspase inhibitor signifi-cantly improved the amount of reparative bone formation in diabetic animals following bone resorption induced by *P. gingivalis*. Inflammation could also affect bone-lining cells by reducing proliferation or interfering with differentiation to osteoblasts [52]. A sche-matic of this process is shown in Figure 6.2.

TNF-α dysregulation has also been suggested as a mechanism because a TNF-α inhibi-tor significantly reduced cell death and improved bone formation [88]. Inhibition of TNF-α reduces prolonged cytokine expression, leukocyte infiltration, and bone resorption [89]. At the same time TNF-α inhibition reduces apoptosis and enhances proliferation of bone-lining cells and increases expression of fibroblast growth factor 2, transforming growth factor β-1, and bone morphogenetic proteins-2 and -6. This demonstrates that much of the detrimental effect of diabetes is due to enhanced and prolonged inflammation and the effect of this inflammation on bone resorption and limiting the normal reparative process (i.e., bone coupling) [89]. Interestingly, TNF-α inhibition significantly improved these parameters in diabetic animals, but not in non-diabetic control animals, suggesting that the level of TNF-α in the diabetic group is especially problematic.

A study of *A. actinomycetemcomitans*-induced periodontitis using type 2 diabetic rats found a greater degree of gingival epithelial and connective tissue cell death in the diabetic rats than in the controls through a caspase-3-dependent mechanism [90]. This may enhance

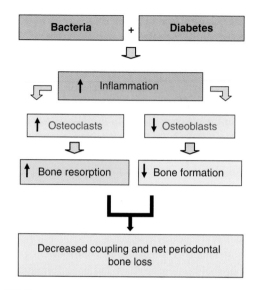

**Figure 6.2** Impact of diabetes on periodontal bone loss. Diabetes enhances the inflammatory response to oral bacteria. Increased inflammation could affect alveolar bone by increasing resorption as well as inhibiting bone formation resulting in uncoupling and greater net bone loss. One of the mechanisms of diminished bone formation is through reduced numbers of osteoblasts caused by the impact of inflammation on apoptosis, proliferation, or differentiation of bone-lining cells [16].

susceptibility to microulceration and interfere with repair following damage caused by inflammation. Additionally, this study found that the diabetic rats preferentially benefitted from antibiotic treatment after the *A. actinomycetemcomitans* inoculation, suggesting that the diabetic rats had more difficulty resisting infection [90]. Decreased bacterial killing may potentially enhance the growth of pathogens and increase the possibility that opportunistic bacteria cause periodontal tissue loss. An altered host response to bacteria can lead to greater or prolonged expression of cytokines that stimulate bone resorption and may limit bone repair.

## Other mechanisms

### *Lipid dysregulation and impaired wound healing*

Three reviews have discussed investigations that address another perspective on metabolic dysregulation in diabetes, focusing on the effects of hyperlipidemia on monocyte/macrophage function in wound signaling [91–93]. The monocyte/macrophage is considered the major mediator of the inflammatory phase in wound healing, having primary roles in wound signal transduction and in the initiation of the transition of healing from the inflammatory to the granulation phase. One hypothesized effect of hyperlipidemia occurs through fatty acid interaction with the monocyte cell membrane, causing impaired function of membrane-bound receptors and enzyme systems. This leads to impaired amplification and transduction of the wound signal. Another postulated pathway leading to impaired monocyte function in diabetes and wound signaling is via the non-enzymatic glycosylation of lipids and triglycerides in addition to proteins. These AGEs are thought to affect normal differentiation and maturation of specific monocyte phenotypes throughout the different stages of wound healing. The net result of both of these pathways is exacerbated host-mediated inflammatory responses and tissue destruction. In impairing monocyte function, diabetes-associated lipid dysregulation, leading to high levels of low-density lipoproteins and triglycerides, may be a major factor in the incidence and severity of periodontal disease.

## Other metabolic pathways

A number of metabolic pathways are affected by diabetes. In many cases they have been linked to hyperglycemia, although the potential contribution of hypoinsulinemia should also be considered. One of the changes that occurs is increased shunting through the polyol pathway that leads to enhanced aldose reductase activity and greater production of the sugars sorbitol and fructose. As a result there is increased formation of AGEs and enhanced formation of ROS and nitric oxide (NO). As previously mentioned, AGEs, ROS, and NO are pro-inflammatory. That this pathway is important in diabetes has been shown by the use of aldose reductase inhibitors. When aldose reductase is inhibited there is reduced protein kinase C (PKC) activation, less nuclear translocation of NF-κB, and reduced expression of markers of inflammation. Inhibiting aldose reductase also decreases the production of ROS [94, 95]. In addition, bacterial killing by neutrophils, which is reduced in individuals with diabetes, is improved by use of an aldose reductase inhibitor [96]. This may have implications for periodontal disease as diabetes reduces the capacity of neutrophils to kill periodontal pathogens such as *P. gingivalis* [97]. As indicated previously, oxidative stress is significantly increased by diabetes and is associated with both enhanced formation of ROS and decreased anti-oxidant capacity [52, 98]. One of the mechanisms through which this occurs is through overloading the electron transport chains in mitochondria, which leads to escape of electrons that react with oxygen producing superoxides. ROS cause cell damage and also stimulate the production of inflammatory cytokines. The importance of oxidative stress in diabetic conditions has been demonstrated by improvements of diabetic complications by treatment of diabetic animals with anti-oxidants [99]. In addition, diabetes causes increased nitrosative stress in the periodontium [100].

## Elevated activation of protein kinase C

Complications of diabetes have been linked to elevated activation of PKC. Diabetes increases glycolysis, which in turn causes increased levels of dihydroxyacetone phosphate that may be converted to diacylglycerol. PKC is activated by diacylglycerol and by an increased ratio of nicotinamide adenine dinucleotide (reduced form) to nicotinamide adenine dinucleotide associated with diabetes [101]. Increased PKC activity then stimulates formation of ROS and inflammation. PKC-α/PKC-β inhibitors reverse this increase. Hyperglycemia is also linked to increased formation of advanced glycation end products, which, as previously mentioned, are proinflammatory [80, 102].

## *Obesity*

As mentioned early in this chapter, obesity is an important factor in the pathogenesis of type 2 diabetes. It is important to consider the close relationship of type 2 diabetes mellitus and obesity (Chapter 2) when considering the impact of diabetes on periodontal health. This relationship may confound or modify the findings of the increased severity of periodontal disease in individuals with diabetes, because evidence is emerging for an association between obesity and periodontal disease [2, 103]. Obesity is an inflammatory state. Adipose tissue is now recognized as important in chronically activating the innate immune system and contributing to a chronic, low-grade, systemic inflammatory burden. Among the adverse effects of obesity-related chronic activation of systemic inflammation include development of insulin resistance, glucose intolerance, and increased risk for the development of type 2 diabetes [104]. The finding of poorer periodontal health in individuals with metabolic syndrome [105] and pre-diabetes [106], who are often overweight or obese, underscores the potential impact of obesity on glucose dysregulation, even before overt diabetes, and the subsequent potential impact on the occurrence and progression of periodontitis [107–109].

Animal studies have demonstrated that in addition to increased weight gain, increased bone loss was observed in rats fed a calorie-rich diet. This was seen both with the placement of silk ligatures to induce bone loss [110] and without ligature placement [111].

A number of systemic reviews have examined obesity as a risk factor for periodontitis. A review in 2010 [2] indicated that the relative risk was 1.35 (CI of 1.23 to 1.47) with stronger associations observed for younger as opposed to older adults, women vs. men, and non-smokers. A later review also found a significant association of periodontitis and obesity (OR = 1.81, CI = 1.42–2.30), periodontitis and being overweight (OR = 1.27, CI = 1.06 – 1.15), and periodontitis and being overweight or obese (OR = 2.13, CI = 1.40 – 3.26) [103]. In both reviews, a causal relationship could not be assessed because the vast majority of studies were cross-sectional. Two inflammatory mechanisms were proposed to explain this association:

1  Excess production of a range of inflammatory cytokines by adipocytes, macrophages, and other cells in adipose tissue.
2  An elevation in the concentration of c-reactive protein and other acute phase plasma proteins in obesity, and an increase in the number of circulating leukocytes.

To support this concept, elevated levels of TNF-α in gingival fluid have been reported in patients with obesity [112]. TNF-α and other inflammatory cytokines have been shown to reduce insulin sensitivity, contributing to development of type 2 diabetes mellitus.

Adipose tissue produces inflammatory cytokines, and excess adipose tissue can be an important contributor to the total systemic inflammatory burden. When a person is overweight or obese, macrophage recruitment into adipose tissue occurs [113], and there is increased production of important inflammatory mediators such as TNF-α [114].

The infiltration of macrophages into adipose tissue is considered a particularly important component of the inflammatory response associated with obesity. In an animal model, obesity was associated with increased macrophages influx into adipose tissue [113]. Two subclasses of macrophages are recognized: pro-inflammatory and anti-inflammatory [115].

In obesity, there is shift toward the pro-inflammatory type [116], with production of pro-inflammatory cytokines such as IL-6 [117]. Adipocytes also have inflammatory potential. In addition to production of interleukins and cytokines, adipocytes produce important adipokines such as leptin and adiponectin. Leptin can function as a pro-inflammatory cytokine and induce macrophage phagocytosis, influx of polymorphonuclear leukocytes, and oxygen radical production [118, 119]. Adiponectin has both pro-inflammatory and anti-inflammatory activities, and low levels of this adipokine have been reported in obesity, indicating a lack of suppression of production of both TNF-α and IL-6 [120].

## Summary

This chapter has provided a detailed description of the evidence supporting the long-held belief by dental clinicians and some medical care providers that diabetes has an adverse effect on periodontal health. Recognizing that the relationship between diabetes and periodontal disease is actually bi-directional [8, 12], this chapter focused on evidence for the direction of this relationship in which diabetes and poor control of diabetes can lead to greater periodontal disease in susceptible individuals. The evidence presented in this chapter from observational studies includes population-based studies that enhance generalizability and longitudinal studies that provide basis for causal inference. The evidence from *in vitro* and animal studies provides further evidence to support the adverse impact of diabetes on periodontal health as well as evidence for the biologic plausibility of this relationship by illuminating inter-related explanatory mechanisms.

## References

1. Petersen PE, Ogawa H. The global burden of periodontal disease: towards integration with chronic disease prevention and control. *Periodontol 2000* 2012; 60(1): 15–39.
2. Chaffee BW, Weston SJ. Association between chronic periodontal disease and obesity: a systematic review and meta-analysis. *J Periodontol* 2010; 81(12): 1708–24.
3. Genco RJ, Borgnakke WS. Risk factors for periodontal disease. *Periodontol 2000* 2013; 62(1): 59–94.
4. Genco RJ. Classification and clinical and radiographic features of periodontal disease. In: Genco RJ, Goldman HM, Cohen DW, eds. *Contemporary Periodontics*. St. Louis: Mosby; 1990. pp. 63–81.
5. Pihlstrom BL, Michalowicz BS, Johnson NW. Periodontal diseases. *Lancet* 2005; 366(9499): 1809–20.
6. Albandar JM, Kingman A. Gingival recession, gingival bleeding, and dental calculus in adults 30 years of age and older in the United States, 1988–1994. *J Periodontol* 1999; 70(1): 30–43.
7. Eke PI, Dye BA, Wei L, Thornton-Evans GO, Genco RJ, CDC Periodontal Disease Surveillance workgroup: James Beck GDRP. Prevalence of periodontitis in adults in the United States: 2009 and 2010. *J Dent Res* 2012; 91(10): 914–20.
8. Lalla E, Papapanou PN. Diabetes mellitus and periodontitis: a tale of two common interrelated diseases. *Nat Rev Endocrinol* 2011; 7(12): 738–48.

9. Lamster IB, Lalla E, Borgnakke WS, Taylor GW. The relationship between oral health and diabetes mellitus. *J Am Dent Assoc* 2008; 139 (Suppl):19S-24S. Epub 2008/11/01.

10. Mealey BL, Ocampo GL. Diabetes mellitus and periodontal disease. *Periodontol 2000* 2007; 44:127–53. Epub 2007/05/04.

11. Taylor GW, Borgnakke WS. Periodontal disease: associations with diabetes, glycemic control and complications. *Oral Dis* 2008; 14(3): 191–203. Epub 2008/03/14.

12. Taylor GW, Borgnakke WS. Treatment of established complications: periodontal disease. In: Herman WH, Kinmouth AL, Wareham NJ, Williams R, eds. *The Evidence Base in Diabetes Care*, 2nd edition. Chichester, The United Kingdom: John Wiley & Sons; 2010.

13. Chavarry NGM, Vettore MV, Sansone C, Sheiham A. The relationship between diabetes mellitus and destructive periodontal disease: a meta-analysis. *Oral Health Prev Dent* 2009; 7(2): 107–27.

14. Khader YS, Dauod AS, El-Qaderi SS, Alkafajei A, Batayha WQ. Periodontal status of diabetics compared with nondiabetics: a meta-analysis.[see comment in: Evid Based Dent. 2006;7(2):45; PMID: 16858380]. *J Diabetes Complications* 2006; 20(1): 59–68.

15. Papapanou PN. Periodontal diseases: epidemiology. *Ann Periodontol* 1996; 1(1): 1–36.

16. Taylor GW, Borgnakke WS, Graves DT. Association between Periodontal Diseases and Diabetes Mellitus. In: Genco RJ, Williams RC, eds. *Periodontal Disease and Overall Health: A Clinician's Guide*. Yardley, Pennsylvania: Professional Audience Communications, Inc.; 2010. p. 331.

17. American Diabetes Association. Standards of medical care in diabetes—2013. *Diabetes Care* 2013; 36 (Suppl 1): S11–66.

18. Lalla E, Cheng B, Lal S, Kaplan S, Softness B, Greenberg E, et al. Diabetes-related parameters and periodontal conditions in children. *J Periodontal Res* 2007; 42(4): 345–9.

19. Lalla E, Cheng B, Lal S, Kaplan S, Softness B, Greenberg E, et al. Diabetes mellitus promotes periodontal destruction in children. *J Clin Periodontol* 2007; 34(4): 294–8.

20. Lalla E, Cheng B, Lal S, Tucker S, Greenberg E, Goland R, et al. Periodontal changes in children and adolescents with diabetes: a case-control study. *Diabetes Care* 2006; 29(2): 295–9.

21. Firatli E. The relationship between clinical periodontal status and insulin-dependent diabetes mellitus. Results after 5 years. *J Periodontol* 1997; 68(2): 136–40.

22. Sbordone L, Ramaglia L, Barone A, Ciaglia RN, Tenore A, Iacono VJ. Periodontal status and selected cultivable anaerobic microflora of insulin-dependent juvenile diabetics. *J Periodontol* 1995; 66(6): 452–61.

23. Tervonen T, Karjalainen K. Periodontal disease related to diabetic status. A pilot study of the response to periodontal therapy in type 1 diabetes. *J Clin Periodontol* 1997; 24(7): 505–10.

24. Faria-Almeida R, Navarro A, Bascones A. Clinical and metabolic changes after conventional treatment of type 2 diabetic patients with chronic periodontitis. *J Periodontol* 2006; 77(4): 591–8.

25. Novaes Junior AB, Gutierrez FG, Novaes AB. Periodontal disease progression in type II non-insulin-dependent diabetes mellitus patients (NIDDM). Part I—Probing pocket depth and clinical attachment. *Braz Dent J* 1996; 7(2): 65–73.

26. Taylor GW, Burt BA, Becker MP, Genco RJ, Shlossman M, Knowler WC, et al. Non-insulin dependent diabetes mellitus and alveolar bone loss progression over 2 years. *J Periodontol* 1998a; 69(1): 76–83.

27. Christgau M, Palitzsch KD, Schmalz G, Kreiner U, Frenzel S. Healing response to non-surgical periodontal therapy in patients with diabetes mellitus: clinical, microbiological, and immunologic results. *J Clin Periodontol* 1998; 25(2): 112–24.

28. Westfelt E, Rylander H, Blohme G, Jonasson P, Lindhe J. The effect of periodontal therapy in diabetics. Results after 5 years. *J C Periodontol* 1996; 23(2): 92–100.

29. American Diabetes Association. Diagnosis and classification of diabetes mellitus. *Diabetes Care* 2013; 36 (Suppl 1): S67–S74.
30. Bellamy L, Casas J-P, Hingorani AD, Williams D. Type 2 diabetes mellitus after gestational diabetes: a systematic review and meta-analysis. *Lancet* 2009; 373(9677): 1773–9.
31. Chokwiriyachit A, Dasanayake AP, Suwannarong W, Hormdee D, Sumanonta G, Prasertchareonsuk W, et al. Periodontitis and gestational diabetes mellitus in non-smoking females. *J Periodontol* 2013; 84(7): 857–62.
32. Esteves Lima RP, Miranda Cota LO, Costa FO. Association between periodontitis and gestational diabetes mellitus: a case-control study. *J Periodontol* 2013; 84(9): 1257–65.
33. Novak KF, Taylor GW, Dawson DR, Ferguson JE, 2nd, Novak MJ. Periodontitis and gestational diabetes mellitus: exploring the link in NHANES III. *J Public Health Dent* 2006; 66(3): 163–8.
34. Xiong X, Buekens P, Vastardis S, Pridjian G. Periodontal disease and gestational diabetes mellitus. *Am J Obstet Gynecol* 2006; 195(4): 1086–9.
35. Xiong X, Elkind-Hirsch KE, Vastardis S, Delarosa RL, Pridjian G, Buekens P. Periodontal disease is associated with gestational diabetes mellitus: a case-control study. *J Periodontol* 2009; 80(11): 1742–9.
36. Taylor JJ, Preshaw PM, Lalla E. A review of the evidence for pathogenic mechanisms that may link periodontitis and diabetes. *J Periodontol* 2013; 84(4 Suppl): S113–S134.
37. Casarin RCV, Barbagallo A, Meulman T, Santos VR, Sallum EA, Nociti FH, et al. Subgingival biodiversity in subjects with uncontrolled type-2 diabetes and chronic periodontitis. *J Periodontal Res* 2013; 48(1): 30–6.
38. Brayton RG, Stokes PE, Schwartz MS, Louria DB. Effect of alcohol and various diseases on leukocyte mobilization, phagocytosis and intracellular bacterial killing. *N Engl J Med* 1970; 282(3): 123–8.
39. Golub LM, Nicoll GA, Iacono VJ, Ramamurthy NS. In vivo crevicular leukocyte response to a chemotactic challenge: inhibition by experimental diabetes. *Infect Immun* 1982; 37(3): 1013–20.
40. Hill HR, Sauls HS, Dettloff JL, Quie PG. Impaired leukotactic responsiveness in patients with juvenile diabetes mellitus. *Clin Immunol Immunopathol* 1974; 2(3): 395–403.
41. Manouchehr-Pour M, Spagnuolo PJ, Rodman HM, Bissada NF. Comparison of neutrophil chemotactic response in diabetic patients with mild and severe periodontal disease. *J Periodontol* 1981; 52(8): 410–5.
42. Miller ME, Baker L. Leukocyte functions in juvenile diabetes mellitus: humoral and cellular aspects. *J Pediatr* 1972; 81(5): 979–82.
43. Molenaar DM, Palumbo PJ, Wilson WR, Ritts RE, Jr. Leukocyte chemotaxis in diabetic patients and their nondiabetic first-degree relatives. *Diabetes* 1976; 25(2 Suppl): 880–3.
44. Mowat A, Baum J. Chemotaxis of polymorphonuclear leukocytes from patients with diabetes mellitus. *N Engl J Med* 1971; 284(12): 621–7.
45. Bagdade JD, Stewart M, Walters E. Impaired granulocyte adherence. A reversible defect in host defense in patients with poorly controlled diabetes. *Diabetes* 1978; 27(6): 677–81.
46. Bagdade JD, Walters E. Impaired granulocyte adherence in mildly diabetic patients: effects of tolazamide treatment. *Diabetes* 1980; 29(4): 309–11.
47. Bagdade JD, Nielson KL, Bulger RJ. Reversible abnormalities in phagocytic function in poorly controlled diabetic patients. *Am J Med Sci* 1972; 263(6): 451–6.
48. Bagdade JD, Root RK, Bulger RJ. Impaired leukocyte function in patients with poorly controlled diabetes. *Diabetes* 1974; 23(1): 9–15.
49. Walters MI, Lessler MA, Stevenson TD. Oxidative metabolism of leukocytes from nondiabetic and diabetic patients. *J Lab Clin Med* 1971; 78(1): 158–66.

50. Collison KS, Parhar RS, Saleh SS, Meyer BF, Kwaasi AA, Hammami MM, et al. RAGE-mediated neutrophil dysfunction is evoked by advanced glycation end products (AGEs). *J Leukoc Biol* 2002; 71(3): 433–44.

51. Gyurko R, Siqueira CC, Caldon N, Gao L, Kantarci A, Van Dyke TE. Chronic hyperglycemia predisposes to exaggerated inflammatory response and leukocyte dysfunction in Akita mice. *J Immunol* 2006; 177(10): 7250–6.

52. Graves DT, Liu R, Alikhani M, Al-Mashat H, Trackman PC. Diabetes-enhanced inflammation and apoptosis—impact on periodontal pathology. *J Dent Res* 2006; 85(1): 15–21.

53. Alba-Loureiro TC, Munhoz CD, Martins JO, Cerchiaro GA, Scavone C, Curi R, et al. Neutrophil function and metabolism in individuals with diabetes mellitus. *Braz J Med Biol Res* 2007; 40(8): 1037–44.

54. Graves DT, Fine D, Teng YT, Van Dyke TE, Hajishengallis G. The use of rodent models to investigate host-bacteria interactions related to periodontal diseases. *J Clin Periodontol* 2008; 35(2): 89–105. Epub 2008/01/18.

55. Pociot F, Molvig J, Wogensen L, Worsaae H, Dalboge H, Baek L, et al. A tumour necrosis factor beta gene polymorphism in relation to monokine secretion and insulin-dependent diabetes mellitus. *Scand J Immunol* 1991; 33: 37–49.

56. Pociot F, Wilson AG, Nerup J, Duff GW. No independent association between a tumor necrosis factor-a promotor region polymorphism and insulin-dependent diabetes mellitus. *Eur J Immunol* 1993; 23: 3043–9.

57. Salvi GE, Collins JG, Yalda B, Arnold RR, Lang NP, Offenbacher S. Monocytic TNFa secretion patterns in IDDM patients with periodontal diseases. *J Clin Periodontol* 1997a; 24: 8–16.

58. Salvi GE, Yalda B, Collins JG, Jones BH, Smith FW, Arnold RR, et al. Inflammatory mediator response as a potential risk marker for periodontal diseases in insulin-dependent diabetes mellitus patients. *J Periodontol* 1997b; 68(2): 127–35.

59. Santamaria P, Gehrz RC, Bryan MK, Barbosa JJ. Involvement of class II MHC molecules in the LPS-induction of IL-1/TNF secretions by human monocytes. Quantitative differences at the polymorphic level. *J Immunol* 1989; 143(3): 913–22.

60. Omori K, Ohira T, Uchida Y, Ayilavarapu S, Batista EL, Jr., Yagi M, et al. Priming of neutrophil oxidative burst in diabetes requires preassembly of the NADPH oxidase. *J Leukoc Biol* 2008; 84(1): 292–301. Epub 2008/04/09.

61. Graves DT, Naguib G, Lu H, Leone C, Hsue H, Krall E. Inflammation is more persistent in type 1 diabetic mice. *J Dent Res* 2005; 84(4): 324–8. Epub 2005/03/26.

62. Naguib G, Al-Mashat H, Desta T, Graves DT. Diabetes prolongs the inflammatory response to a bacterial stimulus through cytokine dysregulation. *J Invest Dermatol* 2004; 123(1): 87–92. Epub 2004/06/12.

63. Liu R, Bal HS, Desta T, Krothapalli N, Alyassi M, Luan Q, et al. Diabetes enhances periodontal bone loss through enhanced resorption and diminished bone formation. *J Dent Res* 2006a; 85(6): 510–4. Epub 2006/05/26.

64. Andriankaja OM, Galicia J, Dong G, Xiao W, Alawi F, Graves DT. Gene expression dynamics during diabetic periodontitis. *J Dent Res* 2012; 91(12): 1160–5. Epub 2012/10/30.

65. Sima C, Rhourida K, Van Dyke TE, Gyurko R. Type 1 diabetes predisposes to enhanced gingival leukocyte margination and macromolecule extravasation in vivo. *J Periodontal Res* 2010; 45(6): 748–56. Epub 2010/08/05.

66. Brownlee M. Lilly Lecture 1993. Glycation and diabetic complications. *Diabetes* 1994; 43(6): 836–41.

67. Ramasamy R, Vannucci SJ, Yan SSD, Herold K, Yan SF, Schmidt AM. Advanced glycation end products and RAGE: a common thread in aging, diabetes, neurodegeneration, and inflammation. *Glycobiology* 2005; 15(7): 16R–28R.

68. Schmidt AM, Hori O, Cao R, Yan SD, Brett J, Wautier JL, et al. RAGE: a novel cellular receptor for advanced glycation end products. *Diabetes* 1996b; 45(Suppl 3): S77–S80.
69. Chang PC, Chien LY, Chong LY, Kuo YP, Hsiao JK. Glycated matrix up-regulates inflammatory signaling similarly to Porphyromonas gingivalis lipopolysaccharide. *J Periodontal Res* 2013; 48(2): 184–93. Epub 2012/08/29.
70. Vlassara H. Recent progress on the biologic and clinical significance of advanced glycosylation end products. *J Lab Clin Med* 1994; 124(1): 19–30.
71. Yan SF, Ramasamy R, Schmidt AM. Receptor for AGE (RAGE) and its ligands—cast into leading roles in diabetes and the inflammatory response. *J Molec Med* 2009; 87(3): 235–47.
72. Schmidt AM, Yan SD, Yan SF, Stern DM. The biology of the receptor for advanced glycation end products and its ligands. *Biochim Biophys Acta* 2000; 1498(2–3): 99–111.
73. Brett J, Schmidt AM, Yan SD, Zou YS, Weidman E, Pinsky D, et al. Survey of the distribution of a newly characterized receptor for advanced glycation end products in tissues. *Am J Pathol* 1993; 143(6): 1699–712.
74. Schmidt AM, Weidman E, Lalla E, Yan SD, Hori O, Cao R, et al. Advanced glycation endproducts (AGEs) induce oxidant stress in the gingiva: a potential mechanism underlying accelerated periodontal disease associated with diabetes. *J Periodontal Res* 1996a; 31(7): 508–15.
75. Takeda M, Ojima M, Yoshioka H, Inaba H, Kogo M, Shizukuishi S, et al. Relationship of serum advanced glycation end products with deterioration of periodontitis in type 2 diabetes patients. *J Periodontol* 2006; 77(1): 15–20.
76. Katz J, Bhattacharyya I, Farkhondeh-Kish F, Perez FM, Caudle RM, Heft MW. Expression of the receptor of advanced glycation end products in gingival tissues of type 2 diabetes patients with chronic periodontal disease: a study utilizing immunohistochemistry and RT-PCR. *J Clin Periodontol* 2005; 32(1): 40–4.
77. Murillo J, Wang Y, Xu X, Klebe RJ, Chen Z, Zardeneta G, et al. Advanced glycation of type I collagen and fibronectin modifies periodontal cell behavior. *J Periodontol* 2008; 79(11): 2190–9.
78. Ren L, Fu Y, Deng Y, Qi L, Jin L. Advanced glycation end products inhibit the expression of collagens type I and III by human gingival fibroblasts. *J Periodontol* 2009; 80(7): 1166–73.
79. Lalla E, Lamster IB, Feit M, Huang L, Schmidt AM. A murine model of accelerated periodontal disease in diabetes. *J Periodontal Res* 1998b; 33(7): 387–99.
80. Lalla E, Lamster IB, Feit M, Huang L, Spessot A, Qu W, et al. Blockade of RAGE suppresses periodontitis-associated bone loss in diabetic mice. *J Clin Invest* 2000; 105(8): 1117–24.
81. Ding K-H, Wang Z-Z, Hamrick MW, Deng Z-B, Zhou L, Kang B, et al. Disordered osteoclast formation in RAGE-deficient mouse establishes an essential role for RAGE in diabetes related bone loss. *Biochem Biophys Res Comm* 2006; 340(4): 1091–7.
82. Yoshida T, Flegler A, Kozlov A, Stern PH. Direct inhibitory and indirect stimulatory effects of RAGE ligand S100 on sRANKL-induced osteoclastogenesis. *J Cell Biochem* 2009; 107(5): 917–25.
83. Goova MT, Li J, Kislinger T, Qu W, Lu Y, Bucciarelli LG, et al. Blockade of receptor for advanced glycation end-products restores effective wound healing in diabetic mice. [see comment]. *Am J Pathol* 2001; 159(2): 513–25.
84. Santana RB, Xu L, Chase HB, Amar S, Graves DT, Trackman PC. A role for advanced glycation end products in diminished bone healing in type 1 diabetes. *Diabetes* 2003; 52(6): 1502–10.
85. Alikhani M, Alikhani Z, Boyd C, MacLellan CM, Raptis M, Liu R, et al. Advanced glycation end products stimulate osteoblast apoptosis via the MAP kinase and cytosolic apoptotic pathways. *Bone* 2007; 40(2): 345–53.
86. Parfitt AM. The coupling of bone formation to bone resorption: a critical analysis of the concept and of its relevance to the pathogenesis of osteoporosis. *Metab Bone Dis Relat Res* 1982; 4(1): 1–6. Epub 1982/01/01.

87. Al-Mashat HA, Kandru S, Liu R, Behl Y, Desta T, Graves DT. Diabetes enhances mRNA levels of proapoptotic genes and caspase activity, which contribute to impaired healing. *Diabetes* 2006; 55(2): 487–95. Epub 2006/01/31.

88. Liu R, Bal HS, Desta T, Behl Y, Graves DT. Tumor necrosis factor-alpha mediates diabetes-enhanced apoptosis of matrix-producing cells and impairs diabetic healing. *Am J Pathol* 2006b; 168(3): 757–64. Epub 2006/03/02.

89. Pacios S, Kang J, Galicia J, Gluck K, Patel H, Ovaydi-Mandel A, et al. Diabetes aggravates periodontitis by limiting repair through enhanced inflammation. *FASEB J* 2012; 26(4): 1423–30. Epub 2011/12/20.

90. Kang J, de Brito Bezerra B, Pacios S, Andriankaja O, Li Y, Tsiagbe V, et al. Aggregatibacter actinomycetemcomitans infection enhances apoptosis in vivo through a caspase-3-dependent mechanism in experimental periodontitis. *Infect Immun* 2012; 80(6): 2247–56. Epub 2012/03/28.

91. Iacopino AM. Diabetic periodontitis: possible lipid-induced defect in tissue repair through alteration of macrophage phenotype and function. *Oral Dis* 1995; 1(4): 214–29.

92. Iacopino AM. Periodontitis and diabetes interrelationships: role of inflammation. *Ann Periodontol* 2001; 6(1): 125–37. Epub 2002/03/13.

93. Cutler CW, Iacopino AM. Periodontal disease: links with serum lipid/ triglyceride levels? Review and new data. *J Int Acad Periodontol* 2003; 5(2): 47–51. Epub 2003/05/23.

94. Ihm SH, Yoo HJ, Park SW, Park CJ. Effect of tolrestat, an aldose reductase inhibitor, on neutrophil respiratory burst activity in diabetic patients. *Metabolism* 1997; 46(6): 634–8.

95. Tebbs SE, Lumbwe CM, Tesfaye S, Gonzalez AM, Wilson RM. The influence of aldose reductase on the oxidative burst in diabetic neutrophils. *Diabetes Res Clin Pract* 1992; 15(2): 121–9.

96. Boland OM, Blackwell CC, Clarke BF, Ewing DJ. Effects of ponalrestat, an aldose reductase inhibitor, on neutrophil killing of *Escherichia coli* and autonomic function in patients with diabetes mellitus. *Diabetes* 1993; 42(2): 336–40.

97. Cutler CW, Eke P, Arnold RR, Van Dyke TE. Defective neutrophil function in an insulin-dependent diabetes mellitus patients. A case report. *J Periodontol* 1991; 62(6): 394–401.

98. Silva JA, Lorencini M, Reis JR, Carvalho HF, Cagnon VH, Stach-Machado DR. The influence of type I diabetes mellitus in periodontal disease induced changes of the gingival epithelium and connective tissue. *Tissue Cell* 2008; 40(4): 283–92. Epub 2008/04/29.

99. Stosic-Grujicic SD, Miljkovic DM, Cvetkovic ID, Maksimovic-Ivanic DD, Trajkovic V. Immunosuppressive and anti-inflammatory action of antioxidants in rat autoimmune diabetes. *J Autoimmun* 2004; 22(4):267–76.

100. Nishikawa T, Naruse K, Kobayashi Y, Miyajima S, Mizutani M, Kikuchi T, et al. Involvement of nitrosative stress in experimental periodontitis in diabetic rats. *J Clin Periodontol* 2012; 39(4): 342–9. Epub 2012/01/27.

101. Koya D, King GL. Protein kinase C activation and the development of diabetic complications. *Diabetes* 1998; 47(6): 859–66.

102. King GL. The role of inflammatory cytokines in diabetes and its complications. *J Periodontol* 2008; 79(8 Suppl): 1527–34.

103. Suvan J, D'Aiuto F, Moles DR, Petrie A, Donos N. Association between overweight/obesity and periodontitis in adults. A systematic review. *Obes Rev* 2011; 12(5): e381–404.

104. Tataranni PA, Ortega E. A burning question: does an adipokine-induced activation of the immune system mediate the effect of overnutrition on type 2 diabetes? *Diabetes* 2005; 54(4): 917–27. Epub 2005/03/29.

105. Nibali L, Tatarakis N, Needleman I, Tu Y-K, D'Aiuto F, Rizzo M, et al. Clinical review: Association between metabolic syndrome and periodontitis: a systematic review and meta-analysis. *J Clin Endocrinol Metab* 2013; 98(3): 913–20.

106. Choi Y-H, McKeown RE, Mayer-Davis EJ, Liese AD, Song K-B, Merchant AT. Association between periodontitis and impaired fasting glucose and diabetes. *Diabetes Care* 2011; 34(2): 381–6.

107. Gorman A, Kaye EK, Apovian C, Fung TT, Nunn M, Garcia RI. Overweight and obesity predict time to periodontal disease progression in men. *J Clin Periodontol* 2012; 39(2): 107–14.

108. Gorman A, Kaye EK, Nunn M, Garcia RI. Changes in body weight and adiposity predict periodontitis progression in men. *J Dent Res* 2012; 91(10): 921–6.

109. Jimenez M, Hu FB, Marino M, Li Y, Joshipura KJ. Prospective associations between measures of adiposity and periodontal disease. *Obesity* 2012; 20(8): 1718–25.

110. Cavagni J, Wagner TP, Gaio EJ, Rego RO, Torres IL, Rosing CK. Obesity may increase the occurrence of spontaneous periodontal disease in Wistar rats. *Arch Oral Biol* 2013; 58(8): 1034–9.

111. Verzeletti GN, Gaio EJ, Linhares DS, Rosing CK. Effect of obesity on alveolar bone loss in experimental periodontitis in Wistar rats. *J Appl Oral Sci* 2012; 20(2): 218–21.

112. Lundin M, Yucel-Lindberg T, Dahllof G, Marcus C, Modeer T. Correlation between TNF-alpha in gingival crevicular fluid and body mass index in obese subjects. *Acta Odontol Scand* 2004; 62(5): 273–7.

113. Weisberg SP, McCann D, Desai M, Rosenbaum M, Leibel RL, Ferrante AW, Jr. Obesity is associated with macrophage accumulation in adipose tissue. *The Journal of Clinical Investigation* 2003; 112(12): 1796–808.

114. Hotamisligil GS, Shargill NS, Spiegelman BM. Adipose expression of tumor necrosis factor-alpha: direct role in obesity-linked insulin resistance. *Science* 1993; 259(5091): 87–91.

115. Goerdt S, Politz O, Schledzewski K, Birk R, Gratchev A, Guillot P, et al. Alternative versus classical activation of macrophages. *Pathobiology* 1999; 67(5–6): 222–6.

116. Lumeng CN, Bodzin JL, Saltiel AR. Obesity induces a phenotypic switch in adipose tissue macrophage polarization. *J Clin Invest* 2007; 117(1): 175–84.

117. Lumeng CN, Deyoung SM, Bodzin JL, Saltiel AR. Increased inflammatory properties of adipose tissue macrophages recruited during diet-induced obesity. *Diabetes* 2007; 56(1): 16–23.

118. Caldefie-Chezet F, Poulin A, Vasson MP. Leptin regulates functional capacities of polymorphonuclear neutrophils. *Free Radic Res* 2003; 37(8): 809–14.

119. Loffreda S, Yang SQ, Lin HZ, Karp CL, Brengman ML, Wang DJ, et al. Leptin regulates proinflammatory immune responses. *FASEB J* 1998; 12(1): 57–65.

120. Fantuzzi G. Adiponectin and inflammation: consensus and controversy. *J Allergy Clin Immunol* 2008; 121(2): 326–30.

# Chapter 7

# The influence of periodontal disease on glycemic control in diabetes

*Dana Wolf, DMD, MS and Evanthia Lalla, DDS, MS*

Periodontitis is a chronic inflammatory condition that is initiated by bacteria and results in the destruction of the tissues that anchor and support the teeth in the oral cavity. As reviewed in Chapter 6, it is well established that individuals with diabetes mellitus are at high risk for periodontitis. Moreover, the current thinking about the relationship between these two disease entities is that it is bi-directional [1]. Not only does diabetes mellitus negatively impact periodontal status, but periodontitis also adversely affects glycemic control and other outcomes in diabetic patients. In this chapter, we summarize the evidence that explores the potential effects of periodontitis on the diabetic state, including glycemic control, development of complications, and incident diabetes, and briefly describe possible mechanisms that lend biologic plausibility to this aspect of the association between the two diseases.

## Longitudinal observational studies

A number of longitudinal observational studies have assessed whether periodontitis negatively affects glycemic outcomes in patients with diabetes. One of the first and most widely cited reports on glycemic control in particular was based on data collected from the Pima Indians of the Gila River Indian Community in Arizona [2]. The prevalence of type 2 diabetes mellitus is very high in this population. Taylor et al. used data collected from residents of this community for the National Institute of Diabetes, Digestive and Kidney Diseases (NIDDK) follow-up study and a related oral health study to test the hypothesis that severe periodontal disease confers risk for poor glycemic control. Subjects were dentate individuals aged 18–67 who had had a diagnosis of non-insulin-dependent diabetes and a glycosylated hemoglobin A1 (HbA1) less than 9% at baseline. Severe periodontitis at baseline was defined as either the presence of radiographic bone loss of 50% or more on one or more teeth, or a maximum of 6 mm of clinical attachment loss on one of six Ramfjord index teeth. Most subjects had one follow-up exam two years after baseline and 17 subjects had an additional follow-up exam at four years after baseline. The authors adjusted for multiple covariates and found that severe periodontitis at baseline

*Diabetes Mellitus and Oral Health: An Interprofessional Approach*, First Edition. Edited by Ira B. Lamster.
© 2014 John Wiley & Sons, Inc. Published 2014 by John Wiley & Sons, Inc.

was associated with increased risk for poor glycemic control (HbA1 greater than 9%) at follow-up.

Other investigations have focused on the relationship between periodontitis and diabetic complications. In one of the first such studies, Thorstensson et al. divided type 1 diabetic subjects into 39 pairs of those with severe periodontitis (cases) and those with gingivitis or mild periodontitis (controls) [3]. Cases and controls were matched for age, sex, and diabetes duration. Over the median follow-up time of six years, cases were found to have a significantly higher prevalence of proteinuria and cardiovascular complications including stroke, transient ischemic attack, angina, myocardial infarct, and intermittent claudication compared to controls.

Saremi et al. assessed how periodontal disease affected overall and cardiovascular disease (CVD) mortality in subjects of the Gila River Indian Community with type 2 diabetes [4]. Data from 628 subjects who were part of the NIDDK follow-up study and who had undergone at least one dental examination were analyzed. Over an average of 11 years of follow-up, 204 of the subjects died. Among individuals with severe periodontal disease, the death rate from ischemic heart disease was 2.3 times higher and the death rate from diabetic nephropathy was 8.5 times higher than among individuals with no, mild, or moderate periodontal disease after adjustment for age, sex, and duration of diabetes.

In the same population of Pima Indians with type 2 diabetes, Shultis et al. investigated the effect of periodontitis on the development of overt nephropathy (defined as macroalbuminuria) and end-stage renal disease (ESRD) [5]. Of the 529 subjects included, 20% had no or mild periodontitis at baseline, 38% had moderate periodontitis, 22% had severe periodontitis, and 20% were fully edentulous. Over the follow-up period of up to 22 years (median of 9.4 years), 193 subjects developed macroalbuminuria and 68 developed ESRD. After adjusting for various confounders, the incidence of these diabetic complications was higher in subjects who had severe periodontitis or who were edentulous at baseline. The authors concluded that severe periodontitis and edentulism predict the development of overt nephropathy and ESRD in patients with type 2 diabetes.

Li et al. assessed the association between tooth loss and subsequent mortality in subjects with type 2 diabetes [6]. Ten thousand eight hundred and fifty-eight subjects who were part of the large cohort study Action in Diabetes and Vascular Disease: Preterax and Diamicron Modified-Release Controlled Evaluation (ADVANCE) trial counted the number of teeth in their mouths and reported the number of days their gums had bled over the preceding year. After controlling for several potential confounders, it was found that both the presence of fewer teeth and complete edentulism were significantly associated with an increased risk of death from all causes, CVD and non-CVD, over a five-year period. It is important to note that although tooth loss can occur for different reasons, periodontal disease is a major cause of tooth loss in adults.

There have been two studies to date which have examined whether periodontitis is associated with the development of type 2 diabetes. Demmer et al. used data from the first National Health and Nutrition Examination Survey (NHANES I) and its Epidemiologic Follow-up Study (NHEFS) to test the hypothesis that baseline periodontal status could predict incident type 2 diabetes [7]. A total of 9,296 non-diabetic subjects who had completed a baseline dental examination and had at least one follow-up evaluation were included in the analysis. Dentate subjects were classified into categories of periodontal disease severity based on the Periodontal Index (a clinical index in which higher scores represent increased levels of disease). Over a follow-up period of $17\pm4$ years, 817 cases of incident diabetes were found. The adjusted odds ratios for incident diabetes in periodontal index categories 1 and 2 were not elevated, whereas those in categories 3, 4, and 5 were 2.26, 1.71, and 1.50, respectively. The authors speculated that the substantially elevated odds at intermediate periodontal index levels might have been a consequence of the fact that examiners assigned the lesser of two periodontal index values when periodontal findings were equivocal. The authors concluded that periodontal disease at baseline could predict incident type 2 diabetes. Limitations of this study were the use of an outdated clinical index to assess periodontal status and the unavailability of laboratory measures to exclude undiagnosed diabetes at baseline.

In contrast to the findings from the NHANES I data, a large prospective study out of Japan failed to demonstrate an association between periodontitis and incident diabetes [8]. Ide et al. analyzed 5,848 civil service officers aged 30–59 who were diabetes-free (verified with a negative fasting plasma glucose test result at baseline). Periodontal status was defined again with a rather imprecise method, using the Community Periodontal Index of Treatment Needs (CPITN), an index which examines only certain teeth in the mouth [9]. Based on a positive fasting plasma glucose test result, 287 new cases of diabetes were identified over a mean follow-up period of 6.5 years (range: 2–7 years). There was a statistically significantly increased risk of developing diabetes among those with moderate and severe periodontitis at baseline, but the association did not hold after adjustment for various confounders.

There are other reports in the literature on diabetes-free subjects which have examined the impact of periodontal disease on longitudinal changes in HbA1c [10] and the development of glucose intolerance [11], but enrolled subjects did not develop frank diabetes over the course of these trials.

## Treatment studies

Several intervention studies aimed at testing the hypothesis that periodontal therapy may result in improved glycemic control in patients with diabetes have been published since the 1990s. Unfortunately, many of the reports are based on uncontrolled studies with small sample sizes and short duration of post-treatment follow-up. The two most recent systematic reviews which analyzed data from available randomized controlled trials (RCT) and controlled clinical trials (CCT) were published in 2010 [12, 13]. Table 7.1 summarizes the studies included in the meta-analyses of these two reviews.

The first, by Teeuw et al. [13], sought publications that met the following inclusion criteria:

1  Were original intervention studies of diabetic subjects with periodontitis who received periodontal therapy
2  Included a control group of diabetic subjects with periodontitis who received no periodontal treatment (i.e., were either RCT or CCT)
3  Reported outcomes related to glycemic control
4  Had a duration of at least three months

**Table 7.1** Intervention studies testing the impact of periodontal therapy on glycemic control in diabetes included in the two most recent meta-analyses [12, 13].

| Publication | Study design | Intervention | Main outcome variables and results |
|---|---|---|---|
| Stewart et al. 2001 [18] | CCT; subjects with type 2 DM; T – n=36 C – n=36 F/u - 3 months | T: SRP, extraction of hopeless teeth C: None, dental status of controls unknown | **HbA1c** T: Δ −0.8 (P=0.0001) C: Δ −1.9 (P=0.02) Statistically significant difference in change between T and C |
| Kiran et al. 2005 [17]* | RCT, subjects with type 2 DM; T – n=22 C – n=22 F/u – 3 months | T: OHI, SRP C: None | **HbA1c** T: Δ −0.86; C: Δ +0.31 Statistically significant difference in change between T and C **FPG** T: Δ −3.96; C: Δ +1.22 Statistically significant difference in change between T and C |
| Promsudthi et al. 2005 [15] | CCT; subjects with type 2 DM; T – n=27 C – n=36 F/u – 3 months | T: OHI, SRP, systemic doxycycline C: None | **HbA1c** T: Δ −0.19; C: Δ +0.12 Non-statistically significant difference in change between T and C **FPG** T: Δ −3.63; C: Δ +0.2 Non-statistically significant difference in change between T and C |
| Jones et al. 2007 [16]* | RCT; DM type not reported T – n=82 C – n=83 F/u – 4 months | T: SRP, systemic, chlorhexidine gluconate rinses C: "usual dental care": participants did not alter dental care routine. Some used dental services, others did not. | **HbA1c** T: Δ −0.65 C: Δ −0.49 Non-statistically significant difference in change between T and C |
| Yun et al. 2007 [23] | RCT; subjects with type 2 DM; T – n=23 C – n=23 F/u – 16 weeks | T: SRP, systemic doxycycline C: systemic doxycycline | **HbA1c** T: Δ −0.77 C: Δ −0.58 Between group (T and C) analysis not reported |
| Katigiri et al. 2009 [14] | RCT; subjects with type 2 DM; T – n=32 C – n=17 F/u – 1, 3, 6 months | T: OHI, SRP, locally administered minocycline ointment C: OHI | **HbA1c** T: Statistically significant reduction at 1 month but not at 3 or 6 months C: No statistically significant change at any time point **FPG** No statistically significant change at any time point |

*Studies included in both meta-analyses.
CCT=controlled clinical trial; RCT=randomized control trial; DM=diabetes mellitus; T=treatment group; C=control group; F/u=follow-up; OHI=oral hygiene instruction; SRP=scaling and root planing; HbA1c= hemoglobin A1c; FPG=fasting plasma glucose.

The authors identified five studies that met the inclusion criteria [14–18], with a total of 382 patients with type 2 diabetes (199 in the intervention groups and 183 in the control groups). Sample sizes of the individual studies ranged from 44 to 165 subjects. The intervention groups received mechanical periodontal therapy (scaling and root planing) with [14–16] or without [17, 18] adjunctive local or systemic antibiotics.

All five studies identified assessed changes in HbA1c after periodontal therapy. Two of the five studies showed statistically significant improvement in glycemic control in cases (as measured by a decrease in HbA1c levels) compared to controls [17, 18]. The other three studies showed a non-statistically significant decrease in HbA1c in the treatment group [14–16]. Three of the five studies also reported changes in fasting plasma glucose (FPG) after therapy [14, 15, 17]. Two of the studies showed a non-statistically significant decrease in FPG after treatment [15, 17], while one showed a non-significant increase [14]. The data from the individual studies were pooled for two separate meta-analyses using either change in HbA1c (all five studies, 382 subjects) or FPG (3 studies, 145 subjects) as the main outcome variable. Mean changes in HbA1c in the treatment groups ranged from −1.90 to −0.14% while in the control groups they ranged from −0.40 to +0.31%. The weighted mean difference (WMD) in HbA1c between test and control before and after periodontal therapy was −0.40% (95% CI: −0.04 to −0.77%) indicating a statistically significant HbA1c reduction in the treatment group. Mean changes in FPG ranged from −3.63 to +19.00 mg/dl for the treatment groups versus −3.00 to +1.22 mg/dl for the controls. The WMD of mean FPG differences between test and control groups was a non-significant increase by 2.30 mg/dl (95% CI: -13.64 to +18.24 mg/dl).

The second systematic review was a Cochrane Collaboration review that included only RCTs with a follow-up period of at least 90 days [12]. Seven studies were identified that met the inclusion criteria [16, 17, 19–23]. Sample sizes of the individual studies ranged from 30 to 193 subjects. Five of the studies only recruited subjects with type 2 diabetes and the other two studies enrolled mostly subjects with type 2 diabetes, but also some subjects with type 1 diabetes [16, 19]. Test groups received mechanical periodontal therapy alone [17, 19] or with the addition of a systemic antibiotic [16, 20, 22, 23], and one study tested mechanical therapy with adjunctive use of an oral bisphosphonate [21]. The control groups in five of the included studies had some form of intervention ranging from mechanical therapy to systemic antibiotic administration [19–23]. Three of the identified studies [16, 17, 23], with a total of 244 subjects, were deemed similar enough to have their data pooled for the meta-analysis which revealed a statistically significant reduction in HbA1c of 0.40% (95% CI: of −0.78% to −0.01%) in the treatment group.

The treatment effect of 0.40% reduction in HbA1c observed in both meta-analyses described above is clinically relevant. Analysis of data from the United Kingdom Prospective Diabetes Study indicated an apparently linear 35% reduction in the risk of microvascular complications for every percentage point decrease in levels of HbA1c [24], and there is evidence that an average 0.2% reduction in HbA1c is associated with a 10% reduction in mortality [25].

While promising, the results of these studies should be interpreted with caution. There is a lack of robustness due to significant heterogeneity in the included studies. The strength of the data is also limited by both the small number of included studies and the small sample sizes of those individual studies. It is unclear how the use of adjunctive antibiotics influenced the observed effects, because systemic antibiotics can affect extra-oral sources of inflammation. Additionally, pretreatment levels of periodontal disease and glycemic control were dissimilar, possibly influencing treatment effects observed.

Since the publication of these two systematic reviews, a number of randomized controlled trials testing the effect of periodontal treatment on glycemic control have been published and are summarized in Table 7.2. Sun et al. [26] evaluated the effects of periodontal therapy on inflammatory cytokines, adiponectin, insulin resistance, and metabolic control in type 2 diabetes. One hundred and ninety subjects with baseline HbA1c ranging from 7.5–9.5% and chronic periodontitis were randomly distributed to either a treatment or no-treatment group. Periodontal therapy consisted of oral hygiene instruction, full mouth mechanical debridement, extraction of teeth with a hopeless prognosis, and surgical periodontal therapy when indicated. Patients in the treatment group were also given a three-day course of systemic antibiotic (tinidazole and ampicillin) before and after periodontal therapy. Periodontal parameters improved after therapy and there was a statistically significant difference ($p < 0.01$) in the mean change in HbA1c from baseline to three months between groups favoring the treatment group (treatment group $-0.50 \pm 0.18$; no-treatment $-0.14 \pm 0.12$). The authors concluded that periodontal therapy can improve glycemic control.

In a study by Koromantzos et al. [27], 60 subjects with type 2 diabetes (baseline HbA1c 7–10%) and moderate to severe periodontitis were allocated to either a periodontal treatment test group or a delayed treatment control group. Periodontal intervention consisted of oral hygiene instruction, full-mouth scaling and root planing, and extraction of periodontally hopeless teeth. Subjects in the control group received a supra-gingival tooth debridement (prophylaxis) initially and had sub-gingival scaling and root planing after the final follow-up visit. Subjects were followed up at one, three, and six months. There was a statistically significant difference in the change in HbA1c from baseline to six months between the treatment and control groups ($p < 0.01$). HbA1c was reduced by $0.72 \pm 0.93\%$ ($p < 0.01$) in the treatment group and by $0.13 \pm 0.46\%$ in the control group.

In contrast to the studies by Sun et al. and Koromantzos et al., Chen et al. [28] failed to find a difference in the change in HbA1c between type 2 diabetic subjects treated for periodontitis and untreated controls. One hundred thirty-four subjects were allocated to one of two treatment groups (subgingival scaling and root planing with and without repeat subgingival instrumentation at three months) and a control group with no treatment. The periodontitis "case" definition used was quite liberal and subjects only had mild periodontal disease at baseline. This and the fact that the study was underpowered may explain failure to find a statistically significant treatment effect.

Another small RCT conducted by investigators in Iran found a statistically significant reduction in HbA1c after periodontal treatment in subjects with type 2 diabetes (HbA1c greater than 7% at baseline) [29]. Forty subjects were assigned to either a treatment group or a delayed treatment group. The treatment group received mechanical debridement without the use of adjunctive antibiotics. At the three-month follow-up, subjects in the treatment group had a mean reduction in HbA1c of 0.74% (variance not reported, $p < 0.003$), while controls demonstrated a non-significant increase in mean HbA1c. The difference in the mean change in HbA1c between cases and controls was statistically significant ($p < 0.003$).

**Table 7.2** Randomized controlled trials testing the impact of periodontal therapy on glycemic control in diabetes since 2010.

| Publication | Study design | Intervention | Main outcome variables and results |
|---|---|---|---|
| Sun et al. 2011 [26] | Subjects with type 2 DM; T – n=82 C – n=75 F/u – 3 months | T: OHI, SRP, periodontal surgery, extraction of hopeless teeth when indicated C: OHI | **HbA1c** T: Δ −0.50 C: Δ −0.14 Statistically significant difference in change between T and C **FPG** T: Δ −1.17 C: Δ −0.44 Statistically significant difference in change between T and C |
| Koromantzos et al. 2011 [27] | Subjects with type 2 DM; T – n=30 C – n=30 F/u – 1, 3, 6 months | T: OHI, SRP, extraction of hopeless teeth when indicated C: OHI, supragingival scaling | **HbA1c** T: Δ −0.72 C: Δ −0.13 Statistically significant difference in change between T and C |
| Chen et al. 2012 [28] | Subjects with type 2 DM; T1 – n=42 T2 – n=43 C – n=41 F/u – 1.5, 3, 6 months | T1: SRP at 1 and 3 months T2: SRP at 1 month and supragingival scaling at 3 months C: none | **HbA1c** T1: Δ −0.22 T2: Δ −0.42 C: Δ −0.13 No statistically significant difference between groups **FPG** T1: Δ −0.73 T2: Δ −0.20 C: Δ +0.20 No statistically significant difference between groups |
| Moeintaghavi et al. 2012 [29] | Subjects with type 2 DM; T – n=22 C – n=18 F/u – 3 months | T: SRP C: None | **HbA1c** T: Δ −0.74 C: Δ +0.25 Statistically significant difference in change between T and C **FPG** T: Δ −17.5 C: Δ +9.78 No statistically significant difference between groups |
| Botero et al. 2013 [30] | Subjects with type 2 DM; T1 – n=33 T2 – n=37 C – n=35 F/u – 3, 6, 9 months | T1: SRP + Azithromycin T2: SRP + Placebo C: Supragingival scaling + Azithromycin | **HbA1c** T1: Δ −0.80 T2: Δ −0.30 C: No reduction No statistically significant difference between groups **FPG** T1: Δ −35.8 T2: Δ −19.2 C: No reduction No statistically significant difference between groups |

*(Continued)*

Table 7.2   (*Continued*)

| Publication | Study design | Intervention | Main outcome variables and results |
|---|---|---|---|
| de Oliveira Macedo et al. 2013 [31] | Subjects with type 2 DM; T – n=15 C – n=15 F/u – 3 months | T: SRP+antimicrobial photodynamic therapy C: SRP | **HbA1c** T: Δ –1.00 C: Δ –0.20 Statistically significant difference in change between T and C |

DM=diabetes mellitus; T=treatment group; C=control group; F/u=follow-up; OHI=oral hygiene instruction; SRP=scaling and root planing; HbA1c=hemoglobin A1c; FPG=fasting plasma glucose.

In a three-arm RCT, Botero et al. assessed changes in HbA1c after periodontal therapy and a systemic antibiotic (azithromycin) [30]. Both type 1 and type 2 diabetic subjects (n=105) were included in the study and were allocated into one of three groups: (1) subgingival mechanical debridement plus azithromycin 500 mg/day for three days, (2) subgingival mechanical debridement plus placebo for three days, or (3) supragingival prophylaxis plus azithromycin 500 mg/day for three days. Patients were followed up at three, six, and nine months. At nine months there was a reduction in HbA1c in both groups that received subgingival scaling; however, the reduction was only statistically significant for the group that received subgingival scaling plus the antibiotic (change: -0.8%, variance not reported; $p<0.05$). Between-group comparisons were not statistically significant. No reduction in HbA1c was seen in the group that received antibiotics plus supragingival prophylaxis.

Finally, de Oliveira Macedo et al. [31] tested the use of antimicrobial photodynamic therapy (aPDT) as an adjunct to scaling and root planing in 30 subjects with type 2 diabetes and chronic periodontitis. Although the use of aPDT did not show any additional benefit beyond scaling and root planing with respect to periodontal clinical parameters, it was associated with a significant reduction in HbA1c ($p<0.01$). There was a non-significant reduction in HbA1c in the control group and no test-control difference.

## Underlying mechanisms

It is well established that inflammation is critically involved in the pathogenesis of diabetes and contributes to enhanced insulin resistance and poor glycemic control [32–35].

Mounting evidence (reviewed in [36–38]) is demonstrating that periodontal infections increase levels of inflammatory cells and mediators systemically, that they promote insulin resistance, and that periodontal treatment in non-diabetic individuals has the potential to reduce systemic inflammation.

In the setting of diabetes, emerging evidence suggests that periodontal infections may indeed promote systemic inflammation and adversely affect glycemia and insulin sensitivity (Figure 7.1). In animal studies of ligature-induced alveolar bone loss in Zucker pre-diabetic and diabetic fatty rats, periodontitis was associated with deterioration of glucose metabolism and accelerated onset of severe insulin resistance [39, 40]. In a more recent animal study, oral infection with a major periodontal pathogen in diabetic Tallyho/JngJ mice or C57BL/6 J mice with streptozotocin-induced diabetes led to increased levels of tumor necrosis factor (TNF)-α in serum [41]. A study in adults with type 2 diabetes previously reported a dose-response relationship between severity of periodontitis and plasma levels of TNF-α [42], a cytokine known to promote insulin resistance [43, 44]. In a recent study in adults with type 2 diabetes, periodontitis was associated with increased levels of markers of oxidative stress in plasma and decreased β-cell function (by HOMA-β, the homoeostasis model assessment which allows the derivation of β-cell secretory function) [45].

The first pilot study to suggest a systemic anti-inflammatory effect of periodontal therapy in patients with type 2 diabetes reported a suppression in serum levels of TNF-α following debridement and local antimicrobial treatment, which positively correlated with an improvement in HbA1c levels [46]. In another pilot study of subjects with type 1 diabetes, a positive effect of scaling and root planing on TNF-α secretion by peripheral

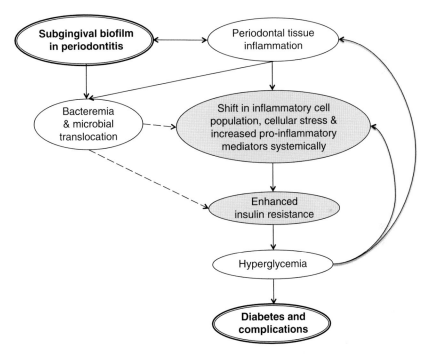

**Figure 7.1** Model of mechanistic pathways that may explain the impact of periodontitis on diabetes. The subgingival biofilm in periodontitis leads to periodontal tissue inflammation locally (which further helps pathogenic bacteria to thrive), but also systemically. Indeed, studies have demonstrated both a shift in the circulating inflammatory cells (that also become more pro-inflammatory) in patients with periodontitis, and enhanced cytokine levels in the serum/plasma. It is well established that systemic inflammation, in turn, enhances insulin resistance and hyperglycemia (which further promotes inflammation), contributing to poor glycemic control and the development of complications in diabetes. In addition, subgingival microbiota have been shown to gain entry to the systemic circulation through the highly vascular ulcerated epithelial interface of the periodontal pocket and may even have a direct effect in promoting systemic inflammation and insulin resistance. Such a direct effect is biologically plausible, but has been studied considerably less thus far (dashed arrows).

blood-derived macrophages and on serum levels of C-reactive protein and E-selectin was demonstrated [47]. A number of studies since have corroborated the notion that periodontal therapy in diabetic subjects can reduce circulating pro-inflammatory mediators, such as TNF-α, C-reactive protein, IL-6, and fibrinogen, and also increase adiponectin levels [14, 26, 28, 48–51]. These effects may ultimately result in improved insulin sensitivity, and contribute to improved glycemic control and overall health outcomes in affected individuals.

Oral/periodontal bacteria and bacterial products have been shown to disseminate systemically [52]. Indeed, transient bacteremias are common and frequent regardless of periodontal status, but their incidence and intensity positively correlate with the extent and severity of periodontitis [53–56]. Whether bacteria that gain access to the systemic circulation have any impact on mediating insulin resistance directly, beyond their indirect effect through the inflammatory response, has barely been assessed [57, 58] and warrants further investigation (Figure 7.1).

As the clinical and epidemiologic evidence mounts for an adverse effect of periodontitis on diabetes outcomes, there is an increased need for more mechanistic studies to explain this direction of the association between the two conditions. Dissecting the underlying mechanisms is indeed critical in (a) improving the design of relevant treatment strategies to achieve glycemic goals and/or limit other diabetes complications, and (b) identifying patient populations that may most benefit from periodontal therapy in this context.

## Concluding remarks

There has been significant progress in understanding the link between periodontitis and diabetes. Nonetheless, larger scale, well-designed studies are needed to further elucidate the role of periodontal infections on glycemic outcomes in diabetes. For example, as previously mentioned, treatment studies to date have had small sample sizes and were extremely variable in design. Because most of the observational and intervention studies published primarily enrolled subjects with type 2 diabetes, the findings cannot necessarily be generalized to individuals with type 1 diabetes.

In summary, the available evidence from clinical studies suggests (1) that severe periodontitis at baseline is associated with poor glycemic control and diabetic complications at follow-up, and (2) that periodontal treatment may be associated with an improvement in glycemic control. Emerging mechanistic studies support the notion that periodontal infections can negatively impact glycemic status in individuals with diabetes through the resultant increase in systemic inflammation.

## References

1. Lalla E, Papapanou PN. Diabetes mellitus and periodontitis: a tale of two common interrelated diseases. *Nat Rev Endocrinol* 2011; 7(12): 738–48.
2. Taylor GW, Burt BA, Becker MP, Genco RJ, Shlossman M, Knowler WC, et al. Severe periodontitis and risk for poor glycemic control in patients with non-insulin-dependent diabetes mellitus. *J Periodontol* 1996; 67(10 Suppl): 1085–93.

3. Thorstensson H, Kuylenstierna J, Hugoson A. Medical status and complications in relation to periodontal disease experience in insulin-dependent diabetics. *J Clin Periodontol* 1996; 23: 194–202.
4. Saremi A, Nelson RG, Tulloch-Reid M, Hanson RL, Sievers ML, Taylor GW, et al. Periodontal disease and mortality in type 2 diabetes. *Diabetes Care* 2005; 28(1): 27–32.
5. Shultis WA, Weil EJ, Looker HC, Curtis JM, Shlossman M, Genco RJ, et al. Effect of periodontitis on overt nephropathy and end-stage renal disease in type 2 diabetes. *Diabetes Care* 2007; 30(2): 306–11.
6. Li Q, Chalmers J, Czernichow S, Neal B, Taylor BA, Zoungas S, et al. Oral disease and subsequent cardiovascular disease in people with type 2 diabetes: a prospective cohort study based on the Action in Diabetes and Vascular Disease: Preterax and Diamicron Modified-Release Controlled Evaluation (ADVANCE) trial. *Diabetologia* 2010; 53(11): 2320–7.
7. Demmer RT, Jacobs DR, Jr., Desvarieux M. Periodontal disease and incident type 2 diabetes: results from the First National Health and Nutrition Examination Survey and its epidemiologic follow-up study. *Diabetes Care* 2008; 31(7): 1373–9.
8. Ide R, Hoshuyama T, Wilson D, Takahashi K, Higashi T. Periodontal disease and incident diabetes: a seven-year study. *J Dent Res* 2011; 90(1): 41–6.
9. Ainamo J, Barmes D, Beagrie G, Cutress T, Martin J, Sardo-Infirri J. Development of the World Health Organization (WHO) community periodontal index of treatment needs (CPITN). *Int Dent J* 1982; 32(3): 281–91.
10. Morita I, Inagaki K, Nakamura F, Noguchi T, Matsubara T, Yoshii S, et al. Relationship between periodontal status and levels of glycated hemoglobin. *J Dent Res* 2012; 91(2): 161–6.
11. Saito T, Shimazaki Y, Kiyohara Y, Kato I, Kubo M, Iida M, et al. The Severity of periodontal disease is associated with the development of glucose intolerance in non-diabetics: The Hisayama Study. *J Dent Res* 2004; 83(6): 485–90.
12. Simpson TC, Needleman I, Wild SH, Moles DR, Mills EJ. Treatment of periodontal disease for glycaemic control in people with diabetes. *Cochrane Database Syst Rev* 2010; 12(5).
13. Teeuw WJ, Gerdes VE, Loos BG. Effect of periodontal treatment on glycemic control of diabetic patients: a systematic review and meta-analysis. *Diabetes Care* 2010; 33(2): 421–7.
14. Katagiri S, Nitta H, Nagasawa T, Uchimura I, Izumiyama H, Inagaki K, et al. Multi-center intervention study on glycohemoglobin (HbA1c) and serum, high-sensitivity CRP (hs-CRP) after local anti-infectious periodontal treatment in type 2 diabetic patients with periodontal disease. *Diabetes Res Clin Pract* 2009; 83(3): 308–15.
15. Promsudthi A, Pimapansri S, Deerochanawong C, Kanchanavasita W. The effect of periodontal therapy on uncontrolled type 2 diabetes mellitus in older subjects. *Oral Dis* 2005; 11(5): 293–8.
16. Jones JA, Miller DR, Wehler CJ, Rich SE, Krall-Kaye EA, McCoy LC, et al. Does periodontal care improve glycemic control? The Department of Veterans Affairs Dental Diabetes Study. *J Clin Periodontol* 2007; 34(1): 46–52.
17. Kiran M, Arpak N, Unsal E, Erdogan MF. The effect of improved periodontal health on metabolic control in type 2 diabetes mellitus. *J Clin Periodontol* 2005; 32(3): 266–72.
18. Stewart JE, Wager KA, Friedlander AH, Zadeh HH. The effect of periodontal treatment on glycemic control in patients with type 2 diabetes mellitus. *J Clin Periodontol* 2001; 28(4): 306–10.
19. Al-Mubarak S, Ciancio S, Aljada A, Mohanty P, Mohanty P, Ross C, et al. Comparative evaluation of adjunctive oral irrigation in diabetics. *J Clin Periodontol* 2002; 29(4): 295–300.
20. Grossi SG, Skrepcinski FB, DeCaro T, Robertson DC, Ho AW, Dunford RG, et al. Treatment of periodontal disease in diabetics reduces glycated hemoglobin. *J Periodontol* 1997; 68(8): 713–9.
21. Rocha M, Nava LE, de la Torre CV, Sánchez-Marín F, Garay-Sevilla ME, Malacara JM. Clinical and radiological improvement of periodontal disease in patients with type 2 diabetes mellitus treated with alendronate: A randomized, placebo-controlled trial. *J Periodontol* 2001; 72(2): 204–9.

22. Rodrigues DC, Taba MJ, Novaes AB, Souza SL, Grisi MF. Effect of non-surgical periodontal therapy on glycemic control in patients with type 2 diabetes mellitus. *J Periodontol* 2003; 74(9): 1361–7.

23. Yun F, Firkova EI, Jun-Qi L, Xun H. Effect of non-surgical periodontal therapy on patients with type 2 diabetes mellitus. *Folia Med (Plovdiv)* 2007; 49(1–2): 32–6.

24. Stratton IM, Adler AI, Neil HAW, Matthews DR, Manley SE, Cull CA, et al. Association of glycaemia with macrovascular and microvascular complications of type 2 diabetes (UKPDS 35): prospective observational study. *BMJ* 2000; 321(7258): 405–12.

25. Khaw K-T, Wareham N, Bingham S, Luben R, Welch A, Day N. Association of hemoglobin A1c with cardiovascular disease and mortality in adults: The European Prospective Investigation into Cancer in Norfolk. *Ann Intern Med* 2004; 141(6): 413–20.

26. Sun W-L, Chen L-L, Zhang S-Z, Wu Y-M, Ren Y-Z, Qin G-M. Inflammatory cytokines, adiponectin, insulin resistance and metabolic control after periodontal intervention in patients with type 2 diabetes and chronic periodontitis. *Intern Med* 2011; 50(15): 1569–74.

27. Koromantzos PA, Makrilakis K, Dereka X, Katsilambros N, Vrotsos IA, Madianos PN. A randomized, controlled trial on the effect of non-surgical periodontal therapy in patients with type 2 diabetes. Part I: effect on periodontal status and glycaemic control. *J Clin Periodontol* 2011; 38(2): 142–7.

28. Chen L, Luo G, Xuan D, Wei B, Liu F, Li J, et al. Effects of non-surgical periodontal treatment on clinical response, serum inflammatory parameters, and metabolic control in patients with type 2 diabetes: a randomized study. *J Periodontol* 2012; 83(4): 435–43.

29. Moeintaghavi A, Arab HR, Bozorgnia Y, Kianoush K, Alizadeh M. Non-surgical periodontal therapy affects metabolic control in diabetics: a randomized controlled clinical trial. *Aust Dent J* 2012; 57(1): 31–7.

30. Botero JE, Yepes FL, Ochoa SP, Hincapie JP, Roldan N, Ospina CA, Castrillon CA, Becerra MA. Effects of periodontal non-surgical therapy plus azithromycin on glycemic control in patients with diabetes: a randomized clinical trial. *J Periodontal Res* 2013; Epub Feb 27th 2013.

31. de Oliveira Macedo G, Novaes A, Jr., Souza SS, Taba M, Jr., Palioto D, Grisi MM. Additional effects of aPDT on nonsurgical periodontal treatment with doxycycline in type II diabetes: a randomized, controlled clinical trial. *Lasers Med Sci* 2013; 1–6.

32. Pradhan AD, Manson JE, Rifai N, Buring JE, Ridker PM. C-reactive protein, interleukin 6, and risk of developing type 2 diabetes mellitus. *JAMA* 2001; 286(3): 327–34.

33. Donath MY, Shoelson SE. Type 2 diabetes as an inflammatory disease. *Nat Rev Immunol* 2011; 11(2): 98–107.

34. King GL. The role of inflammatory cytokines in diabetes and its complications. *J Periodontol* 2008; 79(8 Suppl): 1527–34.

35. Shoelson SE, Lee J, Goldfine AB. Inflammation and insulin resistance. *J Clin Invest* 2006; 116(7): 1793–801.

36. Loos BG. Systemic markers of inflammation in periodontitis. *J Periodontol* 2005; 76(11 Suppl): 2106–15.

37. Paraskevas S, Huizinga JD, Loos BG. A systematic review and meta-analyses on C-reactive protein in relation to periodontitis. *J Clin Periodontol* 2008; 35(4): 277–90.

38. Kebschull M, Demmer RT, Papapanou PN. "Gum bug, leave my heart alone!"—epidemiologic and mechanistic evidence linking periodontal infections and atherosclerosis. *J Dent Res* 2010; 89(9): 879–902.

39. Pontes Andersen CC, Flyvbjerg A, Buschard K, Holmstrup P. Periodontitis is associated with aggravation of prediabetes in Zucker fatty rats. *J Periodontol* 2007; 78(3): 559–65.

40. Watanabe K, Petro BJ, Shlimon AE, Unterman TG. Effect of periodontitis on insulin resistance and the onset of type 2 diabetes mellitus in Zucker diabetic fatty rats. *J Periodontol* 2008; 79(7): 1208–16.

41. Li H, Yang H, Ding Y, Aprecio R, Zhang W, Wang Q, et al. Experimental periodontitis induced by Porphyromonas gingivalis does not alter the onset or severity of diabetes in mice. *J Periodontal Res* 2013: Epub 2013/01/16.

42. Engebretson S, Chertog R, Nichols A, Hey-Hadavi J, Celenti R, Grbic J. Plasma levels of tumour necrosis factor-alpha in patients with chronic periodontitis and type 2 diabetes. *J Clin Periodontol* 2007; 34(1): 18–24.

43. Gupta A, Ten S, Anhalt H. Serum levels of soluble tumor necrosis factor-alpha receptor 2 are linked to insulin resistance and glucose intolerance in children. *J Pediatr Endocrinol Metab* 2005; 18(1): 75–82.

44. Pickup JC. Inflammation and activated innate immunity in the pathogenesis of type 2 diabetes. *Diabetes Care* 2004; 27(3): 813–23.

45. Allen EM, Matthews JB, O'Halloran DJ, Griffiths HR, Chapple IL. Oxidative and inflammatory status in Type 2 diabetes patients with periodontitis. *J Clin Periodontol* 2011; 38(10): 894–901.

46. Iwamoto Y, Nishimura F, Nakagawa M, Sugimoto H, Shikata K, Makino H, et al. The effect of antimicrobial periodontal treatment on circulating tumor necrosis factor-alpha and glycated hemoglobin level in patients with type 2 diabetes. *J Periodontol* 2001; 72(6): 774–8.

47. Lalla E, Kaplan S, Yang J, Roth GA, Papapanou PN, Greenberg S. Effects of periodontal therapy on serum C-reactive protein, sE-selectin, and tumor necrosis factor-alpha secretion by peripheral blood-derived macrophages in diabetes. A pilot study. *J Periodontal Res* 2007; 42(3): 274–82.

48. Correa FO, Goncalves D, Figueredo CM, Bastos AS, Gustafsson A, Orrico SR. Effect of periodontal treatment on metabolic control, systemic inflammation and cytokines in patients with type 2 diabetes. *J Clin Periodontol* 2010; 37(1): 53–8.

49. Matsumoto S, Ogawa H, Soda S, Hirayama S, Amarasena N, Aizawa Y, et al. Effect of antimicrobial periodontal treatment and maintenance on serum adiponectin in type 2 diabetes mellitus. *J Clin Periodontol* 2009; 36(2): 142–8.

50. O'Connell PA, Taba M, Nomizo A, Foss Freitas MC, Suaid FA, Uyemura SA, et al. Effects of periodontal therapy on glycemic control and inflammatory markers. *J Periodontol* 2008; 79(5): 774–83.

51. Sun WL, Chen LL, Zhang SZ, Ren YZ, Qin GM. Changes of adiponectin and inflammatory cytokines after periodontal intervention in type 2 diabetes patients with periodontitis. *Arch Oral Biol* 2010; 55(12): 970–4.

52. Iwai T. Periodontal bacteremia and various vascular diseases. *J Periodontal Res* 2009; 44(6): 689–94.

53. Crasta K, Daly CG, Mitchell D, Curtis B, Stewart D, Heitz-Mayfield LJ. Bacteraemia due to dental flossing. *J Clin Periodontol* 2009; 36(4): 323–32.

54. Forner L, Larsen T, Kilian M, Holmstrup P. Incidence of bacteremia after chewing, tooth brushing and scaling in individuals with periodontal inflammation. *J Clin Periodontol* 2006; 33(6): 401–7.

55. Kinane DF, Riggio MP, Walker KF, MacKenzie D, Shearer B. Bacteraemia following periodontal procedures. *J Clin Periodontol* 2005; 32(7): 708–13.

56. Lockhart PB, Brennan MT, Sasser HC, Fox PC, Paster BJ, Bahrani-Mougeot FK. Bacteremia associated with toothbrushing and dental extraction. *Circulation* 2008; 117(24): 3118–25.

57. Makiura N, Ojima M, Kou Y, Furuta N, Okahashi N, Shizukuishi S, et al. Relationship of Porphyromonas gingivalis with glycemic level in patients with type 2 diabetes following periodontal treatment. *Oral Microbiol Immunol* 2008; 23(4): 348–51.

58. Nishihara R, Sugano N, Takano M, Shimada T, Tanaka H, Oka S, et al. The effect of Porphyromonas gingivalis infection on cytokine levels in type 2 diabetic mice. *J Periodontal Res* 2009; 44(3): 305–10.

# Chapter 8

# Non-periodontal oral complications of diabetes mellitus

*Ira B. Lamster, DDS, MMSc*

## Introduction

Periodontal disease is the most important oral complication of diabetes mellitus. Not only is the severity of periodontal disease greater in patients with diabetes (Chapter 6), but periodontal disease can adversely affect metabolic control in patients with the disease (Chapter 7). However, a number of other oral lesions and disorders have been shown to occur in patients with diabetes. The prevalence of diabetes, and this spectrum of oral pathology, suggests that diabetes mellitus is the most important systemic disease encountered in patients presenting to the dental office.

## Dental caries

Dental caries is the result of acid demineralization of the teeth. Four components are required for dental caries to develop: a susceptible host (the tooth surface), specific bacteria that colonize the host (*Streptococcus mutans*, *Lactobacillus* species), a substrate available for metabolism (fermentable carbohydrates in the diet), and time. The metabolism of carbohydrates by bacteria yields lactic acid as a byproduct. Lactic acid acts on the tooth surface to cause demineralization. Time is important because the frequency of acid exposure is related to demineralization of the tooth surface.

Dental caries can be broadly defined as coronal caries and root caries. Coronal caries affects the crown portion of the teeth, which is covered by enamel, and is the part of the tooth generally visible in the oral cavity. Enamel is inert. Below the enamel is the dentin, which contains cell process from odontoblasts that line the pulp chamber. Dentin has the capacity to repair.

Root caries affects the roots of teeth, which in the completely healthy state are not exposed to the oral cavity. A root surface is exposed when the coronal aspect of the gingiva (and the underlying bone) is lost as a result of trauma (such as toothbrush abrasion), anatomical factors (if the teeth are positioned towards the buccal, away from the central portion of the alveolar bone), and periodontal disease (gingival recession occurs when periodontitis

*Diabetes Mellitus and Oral Health: An Interprofessional Approach*, First Edition. Edited by Ira B. Lamster.
© 2014 John Wiley & Sons, Inc. Published 2014 by John Wiley & Sons, Inc.

is present). As a result of the inflammatory process that characterizes periodontitis, both mineralized and non-mineralized supporting tissues for the dentation are lost, and the tooth appears longer in the mouth. The root surface is covered with a thin layer of mineralized tissue known as cementum. Cementum is more susceptible than enamel to the effects of lactic acid.

Coronal dental caries is an extremely common disorder of childhood, and affects both the primary and permanent dentitions. Root caries is a lesion seen in adults.

The effect of diabetes mellitus on the prevalence of dental caries has been widely studied. This assessment is complicated by the overlapping effects of lifestyle and metabolic management, as well as other complications of diabetes on oral health. For dental caries, potential influences include diet, salivary flow, the effect of medications, availability of susceptible tooth surfaces, the frequency with which people with diabetes engage in self-care, and access to professional dental services.

Three animal models of oral disease in diabetes have suggested a relationship of dental caries and diabetes mellitus. At about 10 months of age, male WBN/KobSIc rats develop spontaneous diabetes mellitus secondary to pancreatitis. Caries, alveolar bone loss, and peri-apical bone loss were assessed radiographically and histologically in male diabetic WBN/KobSIc animals and unaffected female controls [1]. The caries scores were significantly higher for the male diabetic rats. The difference was most pronounced in the maxilla. Alveolar bone loss and periapical periodontitis (indicative of pulpal necrosis that resulted from extensive caries) were also evident in the male animals.

The WBN/KobSIc rats develop dental caries even in the absence of a cariogenic diet or inoculation with cariogenic bacteria, so this is a model that clearly favors the development of tooth demineralization. While the authors conclude that the hyperglycemia is the cause of the increased dental disease, they did not investigate or suggest specific reasons to account for this increased susceptibility.

In another animal study, a murine model was used to assess the relationship of hyperglycemia and dental caries [2]. The Akita −/− murine model is similar to type 1 diabetes mellitus. The animals demonstrate reduced insulin production, retinopathy, neuropathy, and early death. Dental caries and salivary flow had not previously been studied in these animals. Controls were nondiabetic mice from the same strain. Tooth morphology and biochemistry, caries development, salivary flow, and histology of the salivary glands were assessed over a nine-week period. The animals with diabetes demonstrated altered tooth morphology and hypomineralization. Subsequently pulpal abscesses developed, leading to necrosis of the pulp and apical bone loss (periapical periodontitis). When challenged with the drug pilocarpine, the non-diabetic animals produced copious amounts of saliva while the diabetic animals produced virtually none. Gross morphology of the salivary glands did not reveal differences for the diabetic animals, but histologic analysis suggested that diabetes led to reduced granule secretion, implying a neuropathy.

Another murine model was used to study the relationship of diabetes mellitus to dental caries in type 2 diabetes mellitus [3]. The db/db mouse model is characterized by obesity and early evidence of elevated insulin levels in blood. This model has been used to evaluate both nephropathy and neuropathy as complications of diabetes. The db/+ mice served as controls, because these animals do not manifest diabetes mellitus.

Both extent and severity of dental caries were pronounced in the db/db mice. At one year, dental caries was present in 85% of animals with diabetes, but only 22% of controls. In this model dental caries was associated with gingival inflammation, as well as pulpal involvement and apical periodontitis.

The literature examining the occurrence of coronal caries in patients with diabetes mellitus contains conflicting reports of increased caries compared to age-matched controls, as well as no differences or even decreased caries in affected individuals.

A number of studies have found an increased caries incidence in patients with type 1 diabetes mellitus [4–9]. These studies generally focus on children and adolescents, and two of the studies examined salivary flow as part of the analysis. Reduced flow, and lower salivary pH, has been reported in patients with diabetes [4]. Another study did not observe differences in salivary flow or buffering capacity [9]. Higher caries rates have also been reported in patients with type 2 diabetes mellitus [10–16]. Type 2 diabetes is primarily a disease of adults, and that was reflected in the age of the patients. Differences were observed primarily for root caries, and less so for coronal caries. Two of the studies examined salivary flow and chemistry [10, 11], and both suggested reduced production of saliva, lower concentrations of calcium and phosphate ions, and lower salivary pH.

In contrast, an approximately equal number of studies of both children and adults with type 1 and adults with type 2 diabetes mellitus failed to find differences in caries when compared with controls [17–25].

What is clear is that the studies differ in terms of populations and methodology. Furthermore, there are a number of important confounders that ideally should be considered when examining the prevalence and incidence of dental caries in patients with diabetes mellitus [26]. These can be considered as primary and secondary. Primary confounders include the patient's metabolic status, the use of xerogenic medications, and presence of periodontal disease (primarily in adults, which is associated with gingival recession and greater exposure of susceptible root surfaces).

A number of studies have examined the relationship of dental caries to metabolic control of diabetes mellitus. Children or adults with diabetes and poor metabolic control were compared to children or adults who are diabetic and demonstrate good control. While a limited number of studies report no effect of metabolic control on the caries rate [23, 27, 28], a greater number of studies report an increased caries rate in poorly controlled vs. well-controlled patients [29–34].

In summary, unlike the situation for periodontitis, caries is not a recognized complication of diabetes mellitus. Some children with type 1 and type 2 diabetes can be expected to demonstrate a high caries rate, especially if the diet is high in cariogenic food. For adults, it appears that the prevalence of root caries is higher in patients with diabetes versus age-related controls (Figure 8.1). This may relate to exposure of root surfaces secondary to periodontal disease and loss of periodontal tissues. The caries prevalence also may be linked to reduced salivary flow or altered salivary chemistry, which in turn may be secondary to neuropathy affecting the salivary glands. The situation is further complicated by the fact that patients with diabetes mellitus do not access oral health care services as frequently as individuals without diabetes mellitus, and studies suggest that patients with diabetes mellitus are not knowledgeable about the oral complications of the disease (see below).

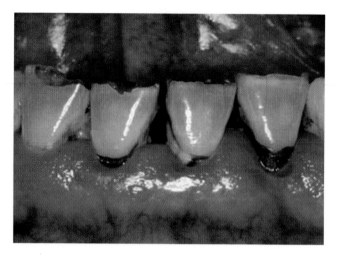

**Figure 8.1**   Root caries in a patient with diabetes mellitus. Xerostomia is also present. Courtesy of Dr. Angus Walls.

The caries risk for patients with diabetes should be assessed and managed on an individual basis. Personalized recommendations for oral hygiene and self-care, diet, and the appropriate schedule of professional visits should be provided.

## Xerostomia

Saliva is an exocrine secretion, and has a number of important functions in the oral cavity. Mixing with the bolus of food, saliva contains amylase, which begins the digestion of starch in food. Saliva also has an important role in maintenance of homeostasis in the oral cavity. This fluid contains antimicrobial substances, and has a buffering capacity that neutralizes acid produced by cariogenic bacteria. The lubricating function is also important; individuals with hyposalivation often complain of discomfort, an inability to eat, and a lack of enjoyment from eating.

Saliva is produced by three sets of major salivary glands: the parotids (the largest, located laterally and below the ear and lateral to the ramus of the mandible), the submandibular (located below the mandible and tongue), and the sublingual (located below and to the sides of the tongue and anterior to the submandibular glands). The parotid glands empty into the oral cavity through Stenson's ducts located in the cheek, at about the line where the teeth occlude. The submandibular glands empty into the oral cavity at Warton's ducts, located on the ridge of tissue at the anterior of the floor of the mouth. Saliva from the sublingual glands enters the oral cavity through a diffuse ductal system. There are also hundreds of minor salivary glands distributed throughout the mouth, in the submucosa, and found primarily on the soft palate, interior of the lips and vestibules, and buccal surfaces. In a normal adult, approximately 700 ml of saliva are produced in a 24-hour period.

Salivary hypofunction and the complaint of xerostomia have been repeatedly demonstrated in patients with diabetes mellitus. This finding has been reported in patients of all ages. Adolescents with type 1 diabetes were shown to have reduced salivary flow, and mouth dryness was a more common complaint on a quality of life questionnaire. Quality of life for these adolescents with diabetes was also related to their dental caries experience [35]. Similar findings were reported in a cohort of diabetic patients with a mean age of 33 years [36]. Both subjective and objective assessments indicated that patients with type 1 diabetes mellitus were affected by mouth dryness more frequently than controls (15.8% vs. 10.3%, p=0.047) and were also shown to have reduced salivary flow rate at rest (0.22±0.014 mL/minute vs. 0.28±0.016 mL/minute, p=0.005) and when saliva was stimulated (0.89±0.047 mL/minute vs. 1.02±0.054 mL/minute, p=0.071). Differences were even more pronounced when stratified by very low resting and stimulated flow rates (< 0.10 mL/minute). Both the use of medications that have reduced salivary flow as a side effect, and a higher fasting plasma glucose level, were associated with reduced flow in patients with diabetes. Of interest, they found that of the medical complications of diabetes, only peripheral neuropathy was associated with reduced salivary flow. Similar findings were reported by other investigators [37]. Xerostomia was present in nearly twice as many individuals with diabetes (62%) as compared to people without diabetes (36%; p=0.001). When salivary flow was measured, reduced flow was seen in 46% of patients vs. 28% of controls. Another study is noteworthy because potentially confounding variables were considered [38]. Patients using medications that were potentially xerogenic were excluded, and lacrimal fluid and other measures of exocrine function, indicating dryness on other mucosal surfaces, were assessed. Here 43% of the patients with diabetes complained of xerostomia, and more than 80% of those individuals were women. Patients with a complaint of xerostomia also reported ocular and vaginal dryness. Xerostomia was associated with a reduced resting salivary flow rate, but no differences were seen between patients and controls for the stimulated flow rate. The reduced flow was inversely related to the level of HbA1c, but was not related to function of the autonomic nervous system.

Continuing along the life course, salivary flow has been examined in older patients [39]. All individuals were at least 60 years of age, independent, and lived in the community. Of the 315 individuals who were examined, 52 reported that they had diabetes mellitus. The occurrence of dry mouth and reduced salivary flow was high. For the later, the percentage approached 50% in both unstimulated and stimulated conditions. It is important to note that while the majority of reports observed that xerostomia is a complication of diabetes mellitus, this finding is not universal [40].

A reduction in salivary flow adversely affects quality of life. Adolescents with complaints of a dry mouth and observed hyposalivation had lower scores on the Oral Health Impact Profile assessment scale compared to adolescents with type 1 diabetes but without xerostomia/hyposalivation [41].

While reduced salivary flow and complaints of oral dryness are seen in patients with diabetes mellitus, the relationship of this finding to other important measures of diabetic status is not clear. Compared to people without diabetes, lower salivary flow rates have been reported for individuals with both well-controlled and poorly controlled diabetes mellitus. The reduction in saliva flow was not related to metabolic control as assessed by glycosylated hemoglobin or fasting plasma glucose [42]. In contrast, other studies [43, 44] found a relationship between salivary flow and glycemic control. Patients with poorly controlled diabetes mellitus demonstrated lower stimulated parotid salivary flow than patients with well-controlled diabetes. Interestingly, there was no correlation of reduced salivary flow with patient complaints of mouth dryness. Therefore, both qualitative and quantitative assessment of salivary flow may be warranted when there is concern about xerostomia in patients with diabetes.

In an interesting study that sheds light on the relationship of diabetes mellitus and xerostomia, children and adolescents with newly diagnosed type 1 diabetes were evaluated [45]. Examining salivary flow upon initial diagnosis and the two weeks after initiation of treatment with insulin, increased stimulated salivary flow was seen with establishment of better glycemic control ($5.4 \pm 3.3$ ml/5 minutes vs. $7.3 \pm 2.6$ ml/5 minutes; $p < 0.01$). These data argue that xerostomia associated with diabetes is directly linked to serum levels of glucose and not to peripheral neuropathy, a late-occurring complication of diabetes mellitus.

The presence of diabetes changes the chemistry of saliva. The most common alteration is an increase in the concentration of glucose. In some studies that increase has been linked to the concentration of glucose in blood [46], and in other studies no association was observed [42, 45]. The elevated levels of glucose in saliva have been associated with an increase in some constituents of the oral microflora (*Candida* spp), but not others (*Streptococcus mutans*, lactobacilli; [45, 47]).

Other alterations in salivary chemistry have been examined in patients with diabetes. Elevated levels of total protein and urea in saliva were observed in patients with the disease [46]. Furthermore, increased concentrations of antimicrobial constituents in saliva (i.e., lactoferrin, myeloperoxidase, and secretory IgA), have been reported when diabetes is present [45]. In both cases, the increase in concentration of constituents may actually reflect the decreased production of fluid.

Inflammatory mediators in saliva from patients with diabetes have also been examined. This analysis is potentially important considering the pro-inflammatory nature of diabetes mellitus, and the increased prevalence of periodontitis in patients with diabetes (Chapter 6). Periodontitis is associated with production of increased gingival crevicular fluid (GCF), which has the characteristics of an inflammatory exudate when periodontitis is present. GCF enters the oral cavity via the gingival crevice, and constituents of GCF are routinely detected in saliva. Matrix metalloproteinase (MMP) levels has been evaluated in saliva from patients with diabetes and controls. Diabetes patients demonstrated both poor metabolic control (mean HbA1c of 8.7%) and increased periodontal disease [48]. The concentration of MMP-8 was elevated in saliva from patients with diabetes who also demonstrated periodontal disease. MMP-8 is derived from polymorphonuclear leukocytes (PMN), which are important cells in the acute inflammatory response in the gingiva. Furthermore, a study examining protease levels in serum, urine, and saliva from patients with diabetes observed higher levels of MMP-2 (which degrades type IV collagen) and MMP-9 (which degrades the extracellular matrix) in serum from patients with diabetes [49]. They also reported higher levels of MMP-9 in saliva from patients with diabetes mellitus who also demonstrated microvascular complications (nephropathy, retinopathy). Other reports have noted that as compared to controls, patients with diabetes mellitus have lower salivary levels of the antimicrobial glycoside hydrolase lysozyme [50], as well as lower levels of epidermal growth factor [51], suggesting a reduced mucosal healing capacity in the oral cavity.

## *Candida* infection

One of the most often mentioned oral complications of diabetes mellitus is *Candida* infection. *Candida* is a genus of yeast, and *Candida albicans* is the most common species that exists as a commensal organism in the oral cavity and gastrointestinal track. In the unperturbed individual, *Candida* does not cause disease. However, *Candida albicans* infection is observed with immunosuppression, or when homeostasis has been altered. *C. albicans* infections are seen in patients with HIV/AIDS, when malignancy is present and patients receive cancer chemotherapy, and in patients with poorly controlled diabetes mellitus. *Candida* infection can also occur in patients who receive an extended course of treatment with antibiotics or corticosteroids.

Not unexpectedly, oral *Candida* infection, and the clinical manifestations of this infection, are influenced by many variables. It has been proposed that in diabetes mellitus, elevated levels of glucose in blood and the tissue promote growth of *Candida* [52]. Elevated levels of glucose in blood have been examined as a risk factor for oral candidiasis. Evaluating patients with type 2 diabetes, a positive relationship was seen between the concentration of glucose in saliva and the presence of *Candida* in the oral cavity [53]. Confirming other work, the concentration of glucose in saliva from patients with diabetes was higher than that of controls. The number of *Candida* colony forming units correlated with the glucose concentration in unstimulated and stimulated saliva, as well as in the serum glucose concentration in patients with diabetes.

Furthermore, the reduced phagocytosis and killing capacity of PMN observed in people with diabetes has also been proposed to explain *Candida* overgrowth [54]. A study of PMN function in patients with diabetes mellitus revealed reduced cell function (phagocytosis, oxygen radical production, and intracellular killing of *Candida*) when diabetes and *Candida* infection were both present. Of interest, following treatment of the fungal infection, the reduced PMN function improved, but not to the level of the normal/control cells. The authors suggest that with any case of unexplained oral infection (fungal or odontogenic), clinicians should consider assessing the blood glucose level to rule-out diabetes mellitus [55].

The saliva of patients with diabetes has an elevated concentration of glucose. The constant bathing of the mucosal surfaces in saliva may account for the higher prevalence of *Candida* in the oral cavity of individuals with diabetes. This bathing does not occur in the esophagus, and consequently a lower prevalence of esophageal vs. oral candidiasis is seen in patients with diabetes [56].

There is an increased carriage rate of oral *Candida* in patients with diabetes who were treated with insulin [57]. Using a rinse technique, *Candida* was detected in 77% of patients. The species most frequently identified was *C. albicans*. Clinically, erythematous candidiasis was the most common form of candidiasis, but 40% of those with microbiologically detected candidiasis did not display a clinical lesion. The significant risk factor for an increased carriage rate was cigarette smoking, and the presence of a denture approached significance.

Confirmatory findings in patients with insulin-dependent diabetes mellitus have been reported [58]. Patients with diabetes were five times more likely to demonstrate clinical signs of candidiasis than were controls (15.1% vs. 3%). These manifestations included angular cheilitis, median rhomboid glossitis, and denture stomatitis. Taking a cytological smear, pseudohyphae (indicative of yeast infection) were found nearly four times as often in patients with diabetes vs. controls (23% vs. 5.7%), and when detected, higher pseudohyphae counts were seen for patients with diabetes. Risk factors for pseudohyphae in the cytological smear included cigarette smoking (OR = 2.4), the presence of a denture (OR = 2.3), and poor glycemic control as indicated by an elevated level of HbA1c (OR = 1.9). Other variables were not significant risk factors, including the use of potentially xerogenic medications.

Nevertheless, while certain risk factors for *Candida* infection and *Candida* overgrowth in the oral cavity have been identified, not all studies have been able to confirm these findings [59, 60].

The species of *Candida* that is most frequently isolated from the oral cavity in healthy individuals and patients with diabetes mellitus is *Candida albicans*. However, other species of *Candida* can be detected in the oral cavity. The species of *Candida* in the oral cavity of patients with type 1 diabetes, type 2 diabetes, and controls has been examined [61]. Using salivary samples, *Candida albicans* was the most frequently detected species in all groups, but additional species detected in patients with both type 1 and type 2 diabetes mellitus were *C. stellatoidea*, *C. lipolytica*, *C. parapsilosis*, *C. krusei*, *C. tropicalis*, and *C. glabrata*. *C. kefyr* was detected in one control patient. The susceptibility of the isolates to different antifungal medications was also examined. All isolates were susceptible to flucytosine and amphotericin B, but a limited number of isolates from type 2 diabetes mellitus were resistant to ketoconazole.

The different species of oral *Candida* present in patients with diabetes has been examined with different levels of metabolic control [62]. As in other studies, *C. albicans* was the most prevalent species in both patients with poorly controlled diabetes (53% positive) and well controlled diabetes (33%). Other species detected in the poorly controlled patients were *C. glabrata* (20%), *C. tropicalis* (6%), and *C. parapsilosis* (6%). The non-albicans species detected in the well-controlled patients was *C. glabrata* (13%). *C. tropicalis* and *C. parapsilosis* were not present in this group.

There has been interest in the presence of *C. dubliniensis* in the oral cavity of patients with diabetes. *C. dubliniensis* is a species of *Candida* identified in the oral cavity of immunosuppressed patients with human immunodeficiency virus [63]. It is believed that the natural habitat for this organism is the oral cavity. There is evidence for the presence of *C. dubliniensis* in patients with diabetes mellitus [57, 64], but another study failed to identify this species in the oral cavity of patients with diabetes [62].

One important risk factor for clinical *Candida* infection in patients with diabetes mellitus is the presence of a removable denture. This is observed on the oral mucosal surfaces of patients with complete dentures and removable partial dentures. The *Candida* infection tends to occur on the mucosal surface below the acrylic portion of the denture, and both tissue inflammation and the carriage rate of *Candida* infection in those patients has been examined [65]. The prevalence of denture stomatitis was greater in patients with type 2 diabetes vs. healthy controls. While the percentage of individuals with diabetes who were colonized by *Candida* was higher than that of the normal controls, this difference was not significant. However, the concentration of *Candida* infection was greater in the individuals with diabetes. Furthermore, *C. albicans* showed greater adherence to palatal epithelial cells from patients with diabetes compared to controls. The increased adherence of *Candida albicans* to buccal epithelial cells from patients with diabetes had previously been demonstrated [66].

Colonization of the underside of maxillary dentures by *C. albicans* in edentulous patients is increased when diabetes is present. This increased density correlated with higher serum glucose levels and the duration of denture use [67].

A study of denture stomatitis in patients with type 2 diabetes mellitus revealed an increased prevalence of stomatitis in patients with diabetes vs. healthy edentulous individuals (57% vs. 30%; $p=0.002$) [68]. Accompanying the denture stomatitis was a more than two-fold increase in clinical complaints, primarily of a burning sensation. Oral dryness, glossitis, and angular cheilitis were also much more commonly observed in patients with diabetes. The subjective and objective symptoms of denture stomatitis were associated with higher serum levels of HbA1c (Figure 8.2). This study also suggested that a number of mucosal symptoms occurred concurrently in patients with diabetes and diffuse inflammation. These include burning mouth syndrome and oral dryness, and to a lesser degree traumatic ulcers, angular cheilitis, and glossitis (Figure 8.3).

The clinical appearance of *Candida* infection in the mouth can vary markedly. The lesions include acute pseudomembranous candidiasis, acute atrophic candidiasis, median rhomboid glossitis, chronic atrophic candidiasis (denture stomatitis), chronic hypertrophic candidiasis, and angular cheilitis.

Acute pseudomembranous candidiasis is characterized by erythematous (red) areas with milky white to light yellow "curds" (Figures 8.4 and 8.5). The "curds" are aggregations of

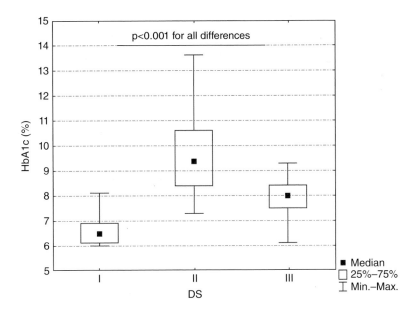

**Figure 8.2**   Mean HbA1c and type of mucosal inflammation. Mean HbA1c values (and 25th and 75th percentiles) for edentulous patients with type 2 diabetes mellitus and different types of mucosal inflammation (DS I=localized simple inflammation, DS II=diffuse inflammation, DS III=localized hyperemic inflammation) [68].

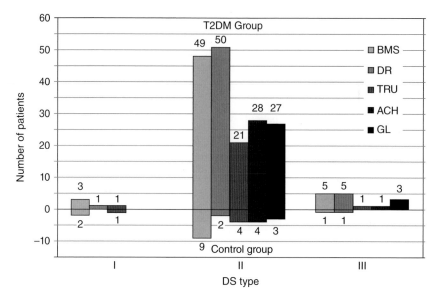

**Figure 8.3**   The number of complete denture patients with different oral symptoms. When diabetes mellitus was present, symptoms were markedly increased (BMS=burning mouth syndrome, DR=oral dryness, TRU=traumatic ulcer, ACH=angular cheilitis, GL=glossitis) [68].

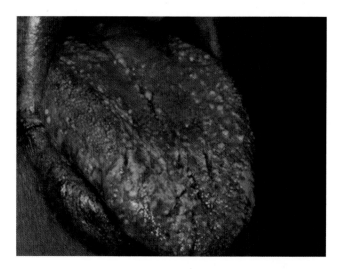

**Figure 8.4**   Acute pseudomembranous candidiasis of the tongue. Courtesy of Dr. David Zegarelli.

fungal organisms. Acute atrophic candidiasis is characterized by an erythematous mucosa but without the aggregations of fungal organisms. Acute pseudomembranous candidiasis may transform into acute atrophic candidiasis as the fungal infection resolves with treatment (Figure 8.6). In both acute pseudomembranous candidiasis and acute atrophic candidiasis, the dorsal surface of the tongue may appear red and atrophic (referred to as "bald" and also known as median rhomboid glossitis). This is due to the temporary loss of

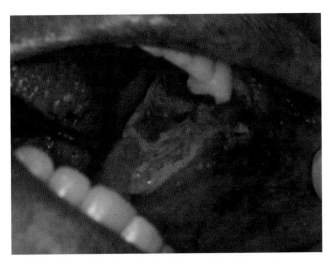

**Figure 8.5**   Acute pseudomembranous candidiasis of the buccal mucosa. Courtesy of Dr. David Zegarelli.

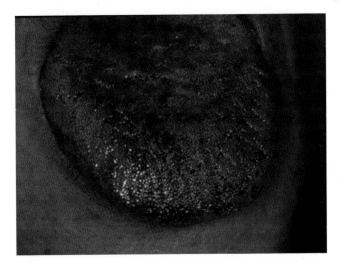

**Figure 8.6**   Acute atrophic candidiasis of the tongue. Courtesy of Dr. David Zegarelli.

the filiform papillae (Figure 8.7). Chronic atrophic candidiasis appears as a red mucosal surface beneath a removable partial or complete denture. The erythema follows the outline of the prosthesis (Figures 8.8 and 8.9), and has also been referred to as "denture stomatitis." Chronic hypertrophic candidiasis is a lesion that reflects a chronic *Candida* infection. The persistent infection causes a mucosal response characterized by hyperplasia and hyperkeratosis. Here the white patch is adherent and cannot be removed (leukoplakia; Figures 8.10 and 8.11). This is often a difficult clinical diagnosis. Angular cheilitis is seen at the corner of the lips. Because these lesions demonstrate *Candida* when a smear is examined or when a culture is taken, they are considered a form of *Candida* infection

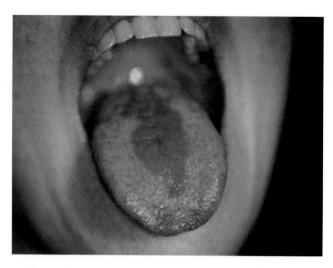

Figure 8.7    Median rhomboid glossitis. Courtesy of Dr. David Zegarelli.

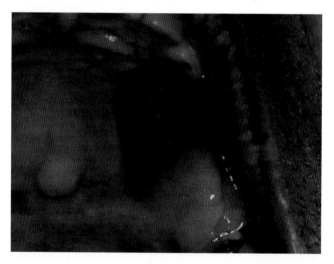

Figure 8.8    Chronic atrophic candidiasis (denture stomatitis) of the hard palate. Courtesy of Dr. David Zegarelli.

(Figure 8.12). It is important to emphasize that more than one type of clinical lesion can be seen in a patient. The most common complaint of patients with an intraoral *Candida* infection is a burning sensation, or report of a very sensitive mouth.

## Burning mouth syndrome

Burning mouth syndrome (BMS) is a complaint reported by patients with diabetes mellitus, but is not unique to patients with diabetes. Furthermore, as a symptom, there appear to be a number of underlying causes for BMS.

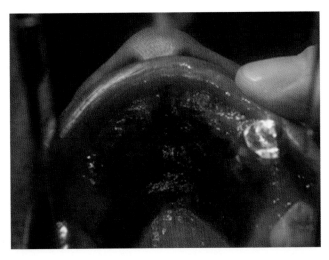

Figure 8.9   Chronic atrophic candidiasis (denture stomatitis) of the hard palate. Courtesy of Dr. David Zegarelli.

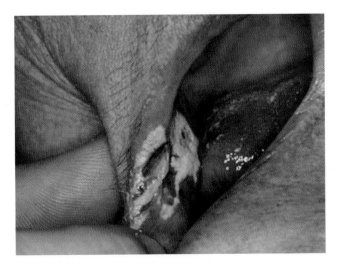

Figure 8.10   Chronic hypertrophic candidiasis of the buccal mucosa. Courtesy of Dr. David Zegarelli.

There is often no clear cause for BMS. Patients complain of burning or irritation of the mouth, often primarily involving the tongue. Taste disturbances can accompany a complaint of burning mouth, as can a subjective or objective complaint of mouth dryness.

A review of BMS concluded that the disorder is defined as a chronic condition characterized by a sensation of burning of the oral mucosa and/or tongue that occurs spontaneously, can be intense, and is not accompanied by any obvious clinical lesion that would account for the symptoms. The prevalence ranges from 0.7%–4.6% with postmenopausal women most often affected. Both idiopathic forms (referred to as primary BMS) and secondary BMS are recognized. The secondary forms are associated with an

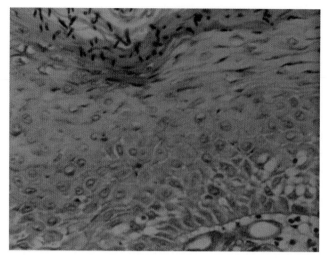

Figure 8.11 Histology of chronic hypertrophic candidiasis. Epithelium is thickened, and pseudohyphae are seen in the cornified layer. Courtesy of David Zegarelli.

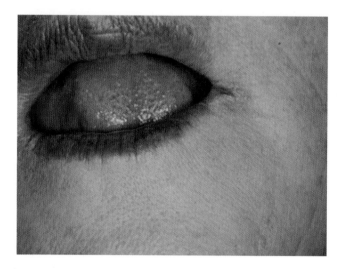

Figure 8.12 Angular cheilitis. Courtesy of David Zegarelli.

identifiable cause. Delays often occur in both the diagnosis and referral for appropriate treatment [69].

BMS is found in association with a number of disorders, including menopause, diabetes mellitus, *Candida* infection, mental illness including depression, Sjörgrens's syndrome, and contact sensitivity to a product or component of a product that is used in the mouth, mainly toothpastes [70].

BMS in patients with diabetes has been examined as a manifestation of neuropathy. A study of tactile sensory function in patients with BMS suggested that affected individuals could be grouped into different categories based on electrophysiologic findings, with particular attention to the blink reflex and the presence of trigeminal neuropathy. This study excluded patients with mucosal lesions or signs of *Candida* infection [71]. Four categories were defined (with some overlap): subclinical neuropathy of the trigeminal system (19% of patients), enhanced excitability of the blink reflex, which is indicative of hypofunction (21% of patients), thin fiber dysfunction, which also is indicative of hypofunction (76% of patients), and normal function (10% of patients). It was concluded that BMS has a neuropathic basis. This study did not include patients with diabetes mellitus. It is likely, however, that because neuropathy is one of the classical clinical complications of diabetes, this finding may be relevant for patients with diabetes. The prevalence of BMS has been evaluated in patients with type 1 diabetes [72]. All participants responded to questions related to abnormal sensations in their mouth. Eliminating those individuals with disorders that could account specifically for BMS (i.e., *Candida* infection, denture stomatitis), there were 12 of 371 (3.2%) patients and five of 233 (2.1%) controls with BMS. For those patients with diabetes, there were significant associations of symptoms with being female (p=0.042) and the presence of diabetic neuropathy (p=0.024).

The conclusions were that in the absence of an identifiable cause, BMS occurred in patients with diabetes at a slightly higher prevalence than individuals without diabetes. This study illustrates the challenge of defining BMS in the context of diabetes mellitus; there are a number of causes of this subjective symptom, and other oral disorders seen in patients with diabetes (such as *Candida* infection) are associated with symptoms of a burning mouth.

The relationship of oral complaints reported by patients with diabetes and neuropathy affecting these individuals has been of particular interest. Forty-five older patients with long-standing diabetes mellitus were assessed for neuropathy using neurophysiologic testing [73]. The prevalence of neuropathy was high in the patients with diabetes; peripheral neuropathy was identified in 42% of patients and none of the controls, whereas autonomic parasympathetic neuropathy was present in 54% of patients and 31% of controls. As for the oral disorders that were identified, more than half (56%) of the patients with diabetes demonstrated dry mouth, and nearly one in five (18%) reported a burning tongue (glossodynia). Temporomandibular joint dysfunction was also higher in patients than controls (27% vs. 16%). Analysis revealed that the presence of neuropathy was correlated with increased tooth loss, but not with dry mouth or glossodynia. Therefore, neuropathy was present but could not be related directly to either xerostomia or BMS.

It is worth noting that isolated case reports illustrate that BMS can be an important oral manifestation of diabetes, with implications for patient management. A 54-year old woman with type 2 diabetes was seen in a dental clinic with a chief complain of BMS. Upon review, her diabetes was poorly controlled (HbA1c of 14.1%). With improved metabolic management, the BMS improved during the following two years [74].

A review of BMS concluded that the relationship between BMS and diabetes mellitus is unresolved. The authors stated that because patients with diabetes are prone to oral infections, a diagnosis of BMS and BMS symptoms may be due more to oral candidiasis than to neuropathy [75]. Investigations into the BMS-candidiasis relationship suggest a cause and effect at least for some patients. One study evaluated 72 patients with BMS [76]. Eliminating patients who used steroid-containing inhalers for treatment of asthma, 52% demonstrated increased colonization with *Candida*; this infection was greater for patients with diabetes, and the symptoms of BMS resolved with treatment of the fungal infection. The authors proposed that the burning symptoms were the result of stimulation of the capsaicin receptors of the oral mucosa by metabolites derived from *Candida*.

In contrast, in a study of patients with BMS who had not previously been diagnosed with diabetes mellitus, only two individuals were found to have diabetes, and in the absence of diabetes no relationship between BMS and *Candida* was observed [77].

Another group that has been studied for the occurrence of BMS is patients with chronic kidney disease who are about to begin dialysis or require dialysis. End-stage renal disease is an important clinical complication of diabetes mellitus [78]. Patients with diabetes and those without diabetes were evaluated. No differences were seen in the percentage of patients in each group who reported oral discomfort. The frequency of oral problems in both groups was, however, quite high (e.g., xerostomia reported in 42% of patients with diabetes and 48% of patients without diabetes). BMS was observed in 6% and 5.7% of diabetic nephropathy and non-diabetic nephropathy patients, respectively. While no difference between groups was observed, it is important to note that these patients are severely compromised, taking multiple medications and suffering from a variety of co-morbidities. It would be difficult to discern specific risk factors that would account for BMS in these patients.

Similarly, a study of patients with and without diabetes mellitus who were receiving peritoneal dialysis revealed that patients with diabetes had lower salivary flow; lower salivary pH; and a higher frequency of dry mouth, oral ulcerations, and BMS [79]. Again, a complex patient population was being studied.

In conclusion, evidence suggests that BMS occurs as an oral complication of diabetes mellitus. The prevalence of this complication is low, certainly compared to other oral manifestations of diabetes. Furthermore, interpretation of the literature is complicated by the following points:

1 The definition of BMS is often not specific, and is inconsistent. Strictly defined, this definition includes the absence of other findings that could account for symptoms (i.e., *Candida* infection).
2 The complexity of the patients affected by BMS represents a challenge. These patients often use multiple medications, and the prevalence of BMS is higher in women who are experiencing or have experienced menopause.
3 The possible association of BMS and neuropathy is important because this may be the first or an early manifestation of diabetic neuropathy. To define this relationship, a comprehensive study design is needed, including a clear method of diagnosing neuropathy and a strict definition of BMS. Treatment studies might also prove useful. Assessment of the effect of medications that are used in the treatment of diabetic neuropathy can provide insight as to the underlying cause of BMS. These include antidepressants, antiepileptic drugs, and topical agents such as capsaicin [80].

## Parotid sialosis/benign parotid hypertrophy

Another interesting but infrequent and often overlooked complication of diabetes mellitus is parotid sialosis, also known as benign parotid hypertrophy. This is an asymptomatic, bilateral enlargement of the parotid glands. The result is a change in the appearance of

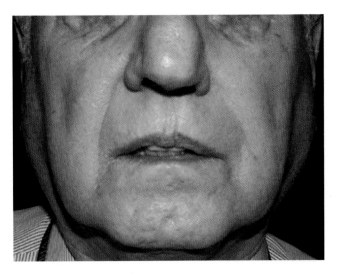

**Figure 8.13**   A patient with diabetes mellitus and bilateral parotid sialosis [84].

affected individuals. The midface can appear broader, as the parotid glands located at about the angle of the mandible enlarge and become prominent (Figure 8.13).

An early report of parotid sialosis in patients with diabetes mellitus stated that the prevalence ranges from 10% to 80% [81]. Sixteen patients with parotid sialosis were evaluated (14 with diabetes mellitus and two with glucose tolerance tests that were borderline abnormal). For five of the 16, the enlargement occurred before a diagnosis of dysglycemia was made.

An assessment of 200 patients with diabetes mellitus found that nearly one-quarter (24%) had bilateral parotid enlargement [82]. The author stated that most of the affected patients were unaware of this condition because it is asymptomatic.

A more recent report of 35 patients with sialosis, specifically defined as a diffuse and persistent enlargement without an inflammatory or neoplastic cause, indicated that the most common underlying disorders were diabetes mellitus and alcoholism [83].

A case report of a patient with long-standing diabetes mellitus who developed parotid sialosis may reveal information about the etiology of parotid sialosis [84]. The enlargement of the glands was attributed to a disorder of protein syntheses and secretion, perhaps related to autonomic sympathetic neuropathy. Based on an aspiration biopsy, there was an increase in the number of zymogen granules in the acinar cell cytoplasm, engorging the cells. The number of cells was not increased, but the cells were larger in size. They proposed that parotid sialosis may occur before other traditional clinical manifestations of diabetic neuropathy because the nerve fibers of the autonomic system are small, and are affected early in the development of diabetic neuropathy [84].

The two main causes of parotid sialosis are diabetes mellitus and chronic alcoholism. Parotid biopsy specimens were examined from patients with diabetes mellitus, alcoholic cirrhosis, and normal controls [85]. The parotid tissue from patients with diabetes mellitus vs. the tissue from the alcoholics was characterized by an increase in lipid in the cytoplasm of the acinar cells, as well as adipose deposition in the gland stroma. A subsequent study

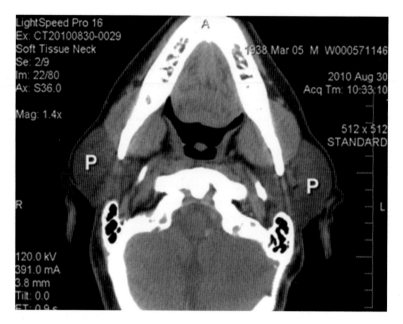

**Figure 8.14**   Computed axial tomogram of the patient in Figure 8.13. The parotid glands (P) are enlarged and uniformly dense [84].

by this same group [86] demonstrated that as compared to patients with diabetes, there was less adipose tissue in the glands from patients with chronic alcoholism. The authors also observed an association between sialosis and xerostomia.

Therefore, there is some confusion regarding the pathologic processes responsible for the enlargement of the parotid glands in individuals with diabetes. It has been proposed that in diabetes, gland enlargement begins as an increase in the size of the acinar cells, and the glands appear dense on an axial computed tomographic (CT) scan (Figure 8.14). In other cases, this enlargement either begins with fat infiltration or progresses to fat infiltration which may be a manifestation of altered lipid metabolism. If there is fat infiltration, the parotid glands will appear less dense on a CT scan [87].

The occurrence of parotid sialosis in diabetes mellitus is not thoroughly defined. The paucity of reports in the literature suggests that this complication of diabetes is not assessed when oral manifestations of diabetes are studied, or is overlooked. The absence of pain or discomfort with this enlargement could also lead to under-reporting. However, as the population ages and the prevalence of diabetes mellitus increases, this complication may be seen more often in the future. Of particular importance is the association of parotid sialosis, diabetic neuropathy, and reduced production of saliva.

## Other mucosal lesions

The occurrence of non-*Candida* mucosal lesions in patients with diabetes has been a theme in the literature for many years. Specifically, the literature regarding oral lichen planus as a complication of diabetes is conflicting. A number of studies have found an association [88–90], whereas others have not [91–93]. The focus on lichen planus is due in part to the potential for malignant transformation [94].

This relationship has also been examined from the opposite perspective. Patients with lichen planus who do not have a diagnosis of diabetes mellitus have been evaluated for their level of glycemic control. More than a quarter of patients with oral lichen planus were found to have diabetes mellitus [95]. It was suggested that screening for diabetes was warranted when lichen planus was identified. The relationship of non-oral and oral lichen planus to diabetes mellitus has also been examined (80% of the patients had oral lesions). Twenty-seven percent of patients with lichen planus were classified as having diabetes mellitus vs. only 3% in the control group [96]. Half of the patients with lichen planus and diabetes were first identified as having diabetes based on this analysis. Another 20% of the patients with lichen planus had altered glucose metabolism but not diabetes mellitus. Therefore, nearly 50% of patients with lichen planus had a disturbance of glucose metabolism. Examining the type of oral lichen planus, both erythematous and leukoplakic forms were observed [97]. In addition, two patients were identified with oral squamous cell carcinoma. Smoking (p=0.019) was found to be associated with dysplastic tissue changes, and alcohol use approached significance as a risk factor (p=0.085).

In contrast, a large study of patients with oral lichen planus in China (N=674) could not identify a relationship between lichen planus and diabetes mellitus [98]. It did observe malignant transformation in four patients. These individuals had been diagnosed with atrophic or erosive forms of the disorder.

Analyzing the relationship of oral lichen planus to diabetes mellitus is complicated by the development of oral lichenoid lesions as a side effect of medications used to treat diabetes and associated conditions such as hypertension. A case report described a patient with a lichenoid drug reaction who was taking both an oral hypoglycemic and oral anti-hypertensive medication [99]. The biopsy suggested lichen planus and the patient was treated with a topical steroid paste, and after changing the medications, the lesions disappeared. This case suggested that the lichen planus was related to drug usage for diabetes mellitus (and hypertension), and was not directly related to diabetes.

Compared to periodontitis or root caries, oral lichen planus is a less common complication of diabetes. However, evidence indicates that a small percentage of patients with oral lichen planus are at risk for malignant transformation to oral squamous cell carcinoma. For this reason, and the possibility that oral lichen planus can be a harbinger of undiagnosed diabetes mellitus, vigilance is required on the part of dental professionals.

Other studies have examined other oral mucosal lesions in patients with diabetes mellitus. Many of these studies actually reported lesions that are manifestations of *Candida* infection [100] or variations of normal anatomy [101].

## Diabetes mellitus and dental implants

Patients with diabetes mellitus demonstrate greater severity of periodontal disease and increased tooth loss compared to individuals without diabetes (Chapter 6). Consequently, these patients require tooth replacement to maintain a fully functional dentition that allows for proper mastication. In this regard, osseointegrated implants offer important clinical advantages. For the fully edentulous patient, the use of implant-retained restorations allows greater comfort and chewing efficiency than traditional complete dentures. For the partially edentulous patient, options are available that do not require modification of adjacent teeth, and can restore posterior occlusion, when in the past only a removable prosthesis would have provided a solution.

### Animal models

A number of animal models have been used to study dental implant healing in the context of diabetes mellitus. Models reflective of both type 1 and type 2 disease have been employed.

A streptozotocin-induced diabetes model in the rat has been used to examine osseointegration. Streptozotocin destroys the β cells of the pancreas and therefore mimics type 1 diabetes. Implants were placed in the femoral bone two weeks after animals were made diabetic and into control animals. Sacrifice was either four or eight weeks later. While the quantity of bone around the implants was similar for both groups, reduced bone-to-implant contact was seen for the diabetic animals at both time points [102]. To assess the effect of insulin replacement, in a subsequent study three groups of animals were established: unmodified controls, diabetic animals (established with injection of streptozotocin), and diabetic animals treated with insulin. Insulin therapy was able to increase bone-to-implant contact, but not to the level of the control animals [103].

A similar model was used to further examine the importance of insulin replacement on the outcome of implant therapy [104]. Three groups were established (normal animals, alloxan-induced diabetic animals, and alloxan-induced diabetic animals treated with insulin). Implants were placed into the tibia of all animals, and the outcome was assessed over 21 days. As compared to the non-diabetic animals, rats with induced diabetes demonstrated 50% less bone formation about the implants. The bone about the implants in the insulin-treated animals was equivalent to that observed in the non-diabetic animals. Of interest, the tissue about the implants in the diabetic animals was characterized as cartilaginous, suggesting that bone repair was delayed.

Another study examined implant healing in rats with induced diabetes, but the implants were placed into extracted molar tooth sockets [105]. After extraction of the maxillary molars, implants were immediately inserted. There was reduced bone deposition at 20 days following implant replacement in the animals with diabetes, which did not improve at 40 days. The authors suggested that immediate implant placement following extraction is not indicated in patients with poorly-controlled diabetes.

Another animal study modified the experimental conditions by examining the effect of diabetes on implant outcomes when diabetes developed after implant placement and implant integration had been achieved [106]. The implants were placed in the femur, and integration was allowed to progress for 28 days. Diabetes was then induced in all animals, and half received insulin replacement. Outcomes were assessed monthly for four months. A reduction in the bone-to-implant contact was observed for the untreated diabetic animals as compared to those animals that received insulin. This difference was significant for the three later observation periods. While integration was maintained, a decrease in bone-to-implant contact was observed for the untreated diabetic animals. These data suggest that development of diabetes after successful implant placement may still place those implants at risk for complications.

Another approach to assessing implant outcomes in a type 1 diabetes model in rats involved use of subtraction radiography to determine bone density about the implants [107]. Using an induced diabetes model, healing of implants in the tibia was followed by digital subtraction radiography. Differences were assessed by gray scale, comparing bone density at the time of implant surgery and at sacrifice. There was a significant ($p < 0.05$) reduction in bone density in the diabetic animals, as compared to non-diabetic animals and diabetic animals treated with insulin.

The majority of animal studies that have examined the effect of diabetes mellitus on implant healing have used a type 1 model in which the β cells of the pancreas are destroyed and there is no insulin production. A limited number of animal studies have explored implant healing in type 2 disease.

A rat model was used to evaluate implant osseointegration under conditions that mimic adult-onset diabetes. Genetically modified animals display characteristics of type 2 disease, including hyperglycemia occurring later in life and obesity [108]. Titanium implants were inserted into the femur of test and control animals. Differences were observed at four and eight weeks. For the implants placed in the test animals, bone volume in the cortical area was less than the controls, whereas no differences were observed in the marrow. They also assessed the percent of bone-to-implant contact, and observed a marked reduction at four weeks for the implants placed in the animals with diabetes. A less pronounced but still significant difference remained at eight weeks. There was a histologic difference between test and control animals, with the bone about the test animals characterized as fragmentary, with more deposition of non-mineralized tissue.

Another study compared implant outcomes in type 2 diabetes using a gerbil model (*Psammomys obesus*), in which diabetes is nutritionally induced [109]. Titanium implants were placed into the tibia of both test and control animals, and integration was evaluated over eight weeks. At two weeks, they noted a modest reduction in mature bone for the animals with diabetes, but this difference was not observed at later time points. No differences were observed for osseointegration or for volume of trabecular bone at any time point. This study illustrates possible differences that will be observed with different animal models, but also suggests differences between implant outcomes in patients with type 2 vs. type 1 diabetes mellitus.

Subsequent animal studies examined different modifications to the implant protocol that could improve the outcome in diabetic animals. The local delivery of insulin was observed to improve the percent of bone-to-implant contact in a type 2 diabetes model [110]. Furthermore, the effect of local delivery of insulin-like growth factor ($I_LGF$) resulted in a higher percent of bone-to-implant contact for diabetic animals vs. diabetic animals not receiving this growth factor [111]. Another biological adjunct that has been studied in the rat diabetes model is basic fibroblast growth factor (bFGF). bFGF stimulates growth of blood vessels. It is membrane bound and activated upon membrane perturbation. Using a rat model that initiated diabetes with a high-fat, high-calorie diet and low dose of streptozotocin, the bone-to-implant contact was equivalent for the control and bFGF-treated animals, but less for diabetic animals not receiving bFGF [112].

However, not all adjunctive biological therapies have proven to enhance bone-to-implant contact in animal models of diabetes. Parathyroid hormone (PTH), a regulator of blood levels of calcium, had been shown to increase bone deposition about dental implants. Systemic administration of PTH enhanced bone-to-implant contact in the non-diabetic animals, but failed to have that effect when diabetes was present [113].

In summary, the evidence from animal models suggests that the presence of diabetes adversely affects the integration of dental implants. This is particularly true for type 1 diabetes in the absence of treatment to improve glycemic control. With the addition of insulin, integration, as measured by bone-to-implant contact, improves to a level equivalent to or nearly equivalent to that seen in non-diabetic animals. Similar findings have been reported for implant integration in models of type 2 diabetes mellitus.

### Clinical studies

In contrast to animal studies examining dental implant outcomes as modified by diabetes mellitus, conclusions regarding the effect of diabetes mellitus on dental implants are not as clear. Large prospective studies have not been performed, and the available literature does not provide adequate information regarding the impact of different diabetes-associated variables (i.e., type 1 vs. type 2 disease, level of metabolic control, duration of diabetes) on implant outcomes. Nevertheless, some conclusions can be drawn from the study of dental implants in patients with diabetes.

Early studies examined the effect of diabetes mellitus on implant outcomes over various periods of time, but generally with limited follow-up. Diabetes mellitus was not identified as a contraindication to dental implant placement, and success rates were 90% and greater [114–116]. These studies did not, however, consider important variables that could influence clinical outcomes, including type of disease, metabolic control and duration of diabetes.

Subsequently, more defined studies of dental implant outcomes in patients with type 2 diabetes mellitus have been reported. A study of diabetes patients who received mandibular implants for an implant-retained overdenture and were followed for five years demonstrated a success rate of 90% [117]. The only diabetes-associated variable that was a predictor of implant failure was the duration of diabetes ($p<0.025$). This study did not include a non-diabetic control group, but the relatively high success rate over five years supports the application of implant-retained overdentures in patients with diabetes.

A retrospective chart review of patients with diabetes who were treated with dental implants revealed an overall success rate of 85.6% [118]. All patients were metabolically controlled, and no differences were seen for the maxilla vs. the mandible, or for implants placed in anterior vs. posterior locations. The failure rate was highest in the first year after prosthetic restoration. The authors concluded that the implant failure rate was higher than what is seen when diabetes is not present, but this therapy still offered a viable clinical option.

A larger study evaluated 663 patients and 2,887 implants over a three- year period. A total of 255 implants were placed in patients with type 2 diabetes. The data demonstrated a higher failure rate for implants placed in patients with diabetes vs. those patients without diabetes ($p=0.02$), and this difference remained significant when clustering of failed implants (within a patient) was considered (p=0.046). A more in-depth analysis indicated that the use of preoperative antibiotics improved implant survival by 4.5% for patients without diabetes and 10.5% for patients with type 2 diabetes [119].

Other studies have demonstrated that at least over the short-term, patients with diabetes could be successfully treated with dental implants. The success rate for implants in patients with diabetes and normal or near-normal serum glucose levels was 94.1% at one year [120]. A study of risk factors for implant complications considered local factors such as bone density and the reason why teeth were lost; systemic factors such as smoking; and the presence of systemic disease including hypertension, type 1 and type 2 diabetes, thyroid disease, and osteoporosis [121]. Three hundred and ninety-nine patients and 1,263 implants were followed, and the success rate was 97.8%. Diabetes mellitus was not identified as a risk factor for implant failure, whereas poor bone quality, heavy smoking, and chemotherapy were risk factors for failure. In another study of implant outcomes in patients with well-controlled type 2 diabetes mellitus, the success rates were 97.3% at one year and 94.4% at five years [122].

In contrast, other retrospective analyses have identified diabetes mellitus as a risk factor for implant failure or implant complications. A long-term (21-year) assessment of implant outcomes calculated the relative risk (RR) of failure for different modifiers. Significant risk factors included older age (60 to 79 years, compared to less than 40 years of age; RR=2.24), smoking (RR=1.56), post-menopausal women requiring estrogen replacement (RR=2.55), having received radiation to the head and neck (RR=2.73), and diabetes (RR=2.75). The implant failure rate was 8.2% for the maxilla and 4.9% for the mandible. The authors suggested that these risk factors are not contraindications to implant placement, but are to be considered when a treatment plan is developed and discussed with patients [123].

These earlier studies reported implant failure associated with an identified diagnosis of diabetes. As such, these findings did not identify earlier implant complications (peri-implant mucositis and peri-implantitis vs. implant failure), nor do they offer specific guidelines regarding the level of glycemic control that may increase risk for implant complications.

Assessing risk factors for adverse implant outcomes, both peri-implant mucositis and peri-implantitis were considered in 212 dentate patients who were treated with implants. Peri-implant mucositis occurred in 64.6% of patients, and peri-implantitis in 8.9% of patients. Both periodontitis and diabetes mellitus were associated with peri-implantitis [124].

Medical complications of diabetes mellitus are related to metabolic control and duration of the disease (Chapter 3). Consideration of glycosylated hemoglobin is a particularly important quantitative measure that has been examined in relation to implant complications. There is some evidence that poor glycemic control is associated with adverse outcomes, but the effect is not large.

A small study followed 35 patients (50 implants) until the point of restoration. HbA1c levels ranged from 4.5% to 13.8%. Only three complications occurred, in patients with an HbA1c that ranged from 7.4% to 8.3% [125]. Another study followed 45 patients with type 2 diabetes for up to 12 years [126]. Implant success was high (97.2% for the patients with type 2 diabetes and 98.8% for the control patients). No differences were seen in complications when metabolically well-controlled patients (HbA1c less than 7%) and less-well-controlled patients (HbA1c from 7% to 9%) were compared. Nevertheless, multivariate regression revealed that HbA1c was the only independent risk factor for implant failure (p=0.04). A smaller study followed 10 patients (23 implants) with well-controlled or moderately well-controlled diabetes for one year [127]. No implant complications were reported.

Surrogate markers for implant outcomes have also been studied [128]. Resonance frequency was used to compare implant stability after placement. Ten non-diabetic patients (12 implants) and 20 patients with type 2 diabetes (30 implants) were evaluated over the initial four months of healing. For the patients with diabetes, HbA1c raged from 4.7% to 12.6%. Implant stability decreased after placement for both diabetes patients and healthy controls, and the decrease was most pronounced for patients with diabetes with a level of HbA1c of 8.1% or greater. These data suggest impaired initial implant healing in patients with diabetes who do not display good metabolic control. It is important to emphasize that microvascular complications of diabetes mellitus are increased when the level of HbA1c is elevated, and the goal of diabetes treatment should be an HbA1c no more than 2% above the normal range ( = 8.5%; [129, 130]).

A recent comprehensive review of the relationship of clinical implant therapy outcomes to diabetes mellitus, with a focus on the importance of glycemic control, concluded that diabetes mellitus is not a contraindication to implant therapy, and the glycemic control was not associated with implant failure [131]. However, this review only was able to consider three clinical studies that met inclusion criteria: longitudinal assessment of at least 10 patients, with defined information about glycemic control [125–127].

Interpretation of the published clinical data on implant outcomes in patients with diabetes is limited by a lack of information about inclusion criteria and important variables associated with diabetes such as level of metabolic control (i.e., HbA1c) and duration of diabetes. At this time, however, certain conclusions can be drawn:

1 Healing of bone is impaired in diabetes mellitus. This is particularly true for patients with type 1 diabetes mellitus. The risk of fracture is also increased in patients with diabetes [132]. Consequently, concern is warranted when treating patients with osseointegrated implants. Possible modifications to treatment should include longer periods of initial healing [131].

2 Animal studies clearly indicate that implant healing (bone-to-implant contact) is adversely affected when metabolic control is poor.

3 Implant therapy is not contraindicated in patients with well-controlled and moderately well-controlled diabetes mellitus [133]. There are distinct advantages to the use of dental implants in partially edentulous or completely edentulous patients with diabetes, including improved masticatory function.

4 There is evidence that patients with diabetes can be successfully treated with dental implants if the level of HbA1c is below 8% [128, 134]. The prophylactic use of antibiotics may be warranted in patients with diabetes mellitus who receive dental implants [134].

5 It is essential that dental clinicians who plan to treat diabetic patients with implants fully understand the nature of their patient's disease (type 1 vs. type 2, duration of diabetes, degree of metabolic control and how the diabetes is managed). Dental and

medical providers should work collaboratively to optimize the patient's metabolic control prior to and after implant surgery. Implant placement is rarely emergent and all aspects of the patient's status should be optimized, including glycemic control, smoking cessation, treatment of existing periodontal disease, and evidence of ideal oral hygiene [135].

## Access to dental services

The preceding sections have documented that patients with diabetes mellitus bear a heavier oral disease burden than patients without diabetes.

To address this disparity, consideration must be given to the oral health preventative behavior, and utilization of dental services, by patients with diabetes. In terms of prevention, smoking (now or ever), tooth brushing (frequency), and use of a fluoridated toothpaste was comparable for patients and controls [136]. However, patients with diabetes were not fully aware of the oral complications of their disease, and a lower percentage of these patients believed that they had very good or good oral health (55.4%) as compared to controls (68.2%).

The frequency of dental visits by patients with diabetes has been assessed using the Behavioral Risk Factor Surveillance System. Data are available for more than 100,000 individuals, and more than 4,600 individuals were identified as having diabetes mellitus. Individuals who were dentate and had a diagnosis of diabetes did not see a dentist as often as those who were dentate but were not diabetic (65.8% vs. 73.1%, p=0.0001). Differences were more pronounced for Hispanic and African-American individuals with diabetes [137]. In a subsequent study [138] using the National Health Interview Survey from 2003, a difference in access to dental care was seen for women with diabetes, who had fewer visits to a dentist than women without diabetes. This difference was not seen for men. Furthermore, of the four recorded visits to diabetes-related health professionals (primary care, foot examination, dilated eye examination, dental visits), patients with diabetes were least likely to have visited a dentist. These same investigators determined that patients with diabetes and periodontitis were not more likely to have dental visits compared to patients with diabetes but without periodontitis [139]. These studies suggest that the importance of regular dental care is not being emphasized to patients with diabetes. Using different databases, other reports have confirmed that a lower percentage of patients with diabetes have an annual dental visit when compared patients who do not have diabetes [140].

A number of surveys of patients with diabetes suggest that as a group, these individuals are not fully aware of the importance of regular dental care as part of complete management of diabetes. Individuals with type 1 diabetes did not visit the dentist as regularly and reported more emergency visits than individuals without diabetes, and also did not demonstrate compliance with general diabetes-associated behaviors such as appropriate dietary management [141]. Patients with diabetes were also shown to be less aware of oral complications of diabetes (periodontal disease; 33%) as compared to their awareness of cardiovascular disease (84%), nephropathy (94%), retinopathy (98%), and circulatory abnormalities (99%; [142]). The findings regarding a lack of patient awareness of periodontal complications of diabetes have been confirmed in another study [143]. Less than 50% of patients were knowledge about periodontal complications of diabetes, or that periodontal disease may adversely affect glycemic control.

Studies also suggest that patients with diabetes who are careful about their oral health are also effective at controlling their blood glucose levels [144]. Furthermore, analysis of insurance utilization data has suggested that dental care visits are associated with improved health outcomes in patients with type 2 diabetes [145]. The outcomes were visits to the emergency room (odds ratio=0.61, 95% confidence internal 0.40–0.92) and reduced number of hospital admissions (odds ratio=0.61, 95% confidence internal 0.39–0.95).

Collectively, these reports indicate that patients with diabetes mellitus do not access dental services as frequently as individuals without diabetes. The reasons for this have not been thoroughly explored, but may relate to the time spent visiting other health professionals, as well as the effort required to personally manage their disease. Another reason is the absence of appropriate emphasis by medical professionals about the importance of regular dental examinations and care as part of disease management. The ideal time to mention this is when the patient is first diagnosed. Medical professionals should also examine the oral cavity for signs of tissue inflammation (periodontium and mucosa), as well as the presence of candidiasis and mouth dryness. Conversely, dental professionals must be thoroughly familiar with the subjective and objective signs and symptoms of the oral complications of diabetes mellitus, and when necessary refer patients to medical providers who they feel have undiagnosed or poorly managed diabetes mellitus. Patients may be seen in the dental office with an oral complaint directly related to undiagnosed diabetes, or a change in the patient's oral status may be reflective of poor metabolic management. Referral to a medical provider will both improve the patient's health as well as the outcome of dental treatment.

# References

1. Kodama Y, Matsuura M, Sano T, Nakahara Y, Ozaki K, Narama I, Matsuura T. Diabetes enhances dental caries and apical periodontitis in caries-susceptible WBN/KobSIc rats. *Comp Med*. 2011 Feb; 61(1):53–9.
2. Yeh CK, Harris SE, Mohan S, Horn D, Fajardo R, Chun YH, et al. Hyperglycemia and xerostomia are key determinants of tooth decay in type 1 diabetic mice. *Lab Invest*. 2012 June; 92(6):868–82.
3. Sano T, Matsuura T, Ozaki K, Narama I. Dental caries and caries-related periodontitis in type 2 diabetic mice. *Vet Pathol*. 2011 Mar; 48(2):506–12.
4. Rai K, Hegde AM, Kamath A, Shetty S. Dental caries and salivary alterations in type 1 diabetes. *J Clin Pediatr Dent*. 2011 Winter; 36(2):181–4.
5. Miralles L, Silvestre FJ, Hernández-Mijares A, Bautista D, Llambes F, Grau D. Dental caries in type 1 diabetics: influence of systemic factors of the disease upon the development of dental caries. *Med Oral Patol Oral Cir Bucal*. 2006 May 1; 11(3):E256–60.
6. Alavi AA, Amirhakimi E, Karami B. The prevalence of dental caries in 5- to 18-year-old insulin-dependent diabetics of Fars Province, southern Iran. *Arch Iran Med*. 2006 Jul; 9(3):254–60.

7. Miko S, Ambrus SJ, Sahafian S, Dinya E, Tamas G, Albrecht MG. Dental caries and adolescents with type 1 diabetes. *Br Dent J*. 2010 Mar 27; 208(6):E12.

8. Jones RB, McCallum RM, Kay EJ, Kirkin V, McDonald P. Oral health and oral health behaviour in a population of diabetic outpatient clinic attenders. *Community Dent Oral Epidemiol*. 1992 Aug; 20(4):204–7.

9. Edblad E, Lundin SA, Sjödin B, Aman J. Caries and salivary status in young adults with type 1 diabetes. *Swed Dent J*. 2001; 25(2):53–60.

10. Jawed M, Shahid SM, Qader SA, Azhar A. Dental caries in diabetes mellitus: role of salivary flow rate and minerals. *J Diabetes Complications*. 2011 May-Jun; 25(3):183–6.

11. Jawed M, Khan RN, Shahid SM, Azhar A. Protective effects of salivary factors in dental caries in diabetic patients of Pakistan. *Exp Diabetes Res*. 2012; 2012:947304.

12. Hintao J, Teanpaisan R, Chongsuvivatwong V, Dahlen G, Rattarasarn C. Root surface and coronal caries in adults with type 2 diabetes mellitus. *Community Dent Oral Epidemiol*. 2007 Aug; 35(4):302–9.

13. Hintao J, Teanpaisan R, Chongsuvivatwong V, Rattarasarn C, Dahlen G. The microbiological profiles of saliva, supragingival and subgingival plaque and dental caries in adults with and without type 2 diabetes mellitus. *Oral Microbiol Immunol*. 2007 Jun; 22(3):175–81.

14. Sandberg GE, Sundberg HE, Fjellstrom CA, Wikblad KF. Type 2 diabetes and oral health: a comparison between diabetic and non-diabetic subjects. *Diabetes Res Clin Pract*. 2000 Sep; 50(1):27–34.

15. Lin BP, Taylor GW, Allen DJ, Ship JA. Dental caries in older adults with diabetes mellitus. *Spec Care Dentist*. 1999 Jan-Feb; 19(1):8–14.

16. Jones RB, McCallum RM, Kay EJ, Kirkin V, McDonald P. Oral health and oral health behavior in a population of diabetic outpatient clinic attenders. *Community Dent Oral Epidemiol*. 1992 Aug; 20(4):204–7.

17. Tagelsir A, Cauwels R, van Aken S, Vanobbergen J, Martens LC. Dental caries and dental care level (restorative index) in children with diabetes mellitus type 1. *Int J Paediatr Dent*. 2011 Jan; 21(1):13–22.

18. Patiño Marín N, Loyola Rodríguez JP, Medina Solis CE, Pontigo Loyola AP, Reyes Macías JF, Ortega Rosado JC, et al. Caries, periodontal disease and tooth loss in patients with diabetes mellitus types 1 and 2. *Acta Odontol Latinoam*. 2008; 21(2):127–33.

19. Siudikiene J, Machiulskiene V, Nyvad B, Tenovuo J, Nedzelskiene I. Dental caries increments and related factors in children with type 1 diabetes mellitus. *Caries Res*. 2008; 42(5):354–62.

20. Moore PA, Weyant RJ, Etzel KR, Guggenheimer J, Mongelluzzo MB, Myers DE, Rossie K, et al. Type 1 diabetes mellitus and oral health: assessment of coronal and root caries. *Community Dent Oral Epidemiol*. 2001 Jun: 29(3):183:94.

21. Siudikiene J, Machiulskiene V, Nyvad B, Tenovuo J, Nedzelskiene I. Dental caries and salivary status in children with type 1 diabetes mellitus, related to the metabolic control of the disease. *Eur J Oral Sci*. 2006 Feb; 114(1):8–14.

22. Swanljung O, Meurman JH, Torkko H, Sandholm L, Kaprio E, Mäenpää J. Caries and saliva in 12- to 18-year-old diabetics and controls. *Scand J Dent Res*. 1992 Dec; 100(6)3:310–3.

23. Collin HL, Uusitupa M, Niskanen L, Koivisto AM, Markkanen H, Meurman JH. Caries in patients with non-insulin-dependent diabetes mellitus. *Oral Surg Oral Med Oral Pathol Oral Radiol Endod*. 1998 Jun; 85(6):680-5.

24. Tavares M, Depaola P, Soparkar P, Joshipura K. The prevalence of root caries in a diabetic population. *J Dent Res*. 1991 Jun; 70(6):979–83.

25. Cherry-Peppers G, Ship JA. Oral health in patients with type II diabetes and impaired glucose tolerance. *Diabetes Care*. 1993 Apr; 16(4):638–41.

26. Garton BJ, Ford PJ. Root caries and diabetes: risk assessing to improve oral and systemic health outcomes. *Aust Dent J.* 2012 Jun; 57(2):114–22.

27. Saes Busato IM, Bittencourt MS, Machado MA, Grégio AM, Azevedo-Alanis LR. Association between metabolic control and oral health in adolescents with type 1 diabetes mellitus. *Oral Surg Oral Med Oral Pathol Oral Radiol Endod.* 2010 Mar; 109(3):e51–6

28. Syrjälä AM, Niskanen MC, Ylöstalo P, Knuuttila ML. Metabolic control as a modifier of the association between salivary factors and dental caries among diabetic patients. *Caries Res.* 2003 Mar-Apr; 37(2):142–7.

29. Bakhshandeh S, Murtomaa H, Vehkalahti MM, Mofid R, Suomalainen K. Dental findings in diabetic adults. *Caries Res.* 2008; 42(1):14–8.

30. Twetman S, Johansson I, Birkhed D, Nederfors T. Caries incidence in young type 1 diabetes mellitus patients in relation to metabolic control and caries-associated risk factors. *Caries Res.* 2002 Jan-Feb; 36(1):31–5.

31. Gómez-Díaz RA, Ramírez-Soriano E, Tanus Hajj J, Bautista Cruz E, Jiménez Galicia C, Villasis-Keever MA, et al. Association between carotid intima-media thickness, buccodental status, and glycemic control in pediatric type 1 diabetes. *Pediatr Diabetes.* 2012 Nov; 13(7):552–8.

32. Siudikiene J, Maciulskiene V, Nedzelskiene I. Dietary and oral hygiene habits in children with type 1 diabetes mellitus related to dental caries. *Stomatologija.* 2005; 7(2):58–62.

33. Karjalainen KM, Knuuttila ML, Käär ML. Relationship between caries and level of metabolic balance in children and adolescents with insulin-dependent diabetes mellitus. *Caries Res.* 1997; 31(1):13–18.

34. Twetman S, Nederfors T, Stahl B, Aronson S. Two-year longitudinal observations of salivary status and dental caries in children with insulin-dependent diabetes mellitus. *Pediatr Dent.* 1992 May-Jun; 14(3):184–8.

35. Busato IM, Ignácio SA, Brancher JA, Moysés ST, Azevedo-Alanis LR. Impact of clinical status and salivary conditions on xerostomia and oral health-related quality of life of adolescents with type 1 diabetes mellitus. *Community Dent Oral Epidemiol.* 2012 Feb; 40(1):62–9.

36. Moore PA, Guggenheimer J, Etzel KR, Weyant RJ, Orchard T. Type 1 diabetes mellitus, xerostomia, and salivary flow rates. *Oral Surg Oral Med Oral Pathol Oral Radiol Endod.* 2001 Sep; 92(3):281–91.

37. Khovidhunkit SO, Suwantuntula T, Thaweboon S, Mitrirattanakul S, Chomkhakhai U, Khovidhunkit W. Xerostomia, hyposalivation, and oral microbiota in type 2 diabetic patients: a preliminary study. *J Med Assoc Thai.* 2009 Sep; 92(9):1220–8.

38. Sreebny LM, Yu A, Green A, Valdini A. Xerostomia in diabetes mellitus. *Diabetes Care.* 1992 Jul; 15(7):900–4.

39. Borges BC, Fulco GM, Souza AJ, de Lima KC. Xerostomia and hyposalivation: a preliminary report of their prevalence and associated factors in Brazilian elderly diabetic patients. *Oral Health Prev Dent.* 2010; 8(2):153–8.

40. Vasconcelos BC, Novaes M, Sandrini FA, Maranhão Filho AW, Coimbra LS. Prevalence of oral mucosa lesions in diabetic patients: a preliminary study. *Braz J Otorhinolaryngol.* 2008 May-Jun; 74(3):423–8.

41. Busato IM, Ignácio SA, Brancher JA, Grégio AM, Machado MA, Azevedo-Alanis LR. Impact of xerostomia on the quality of life of adolescents with type 1 diabetes mellitus. *Oral Surg Oral Med Oral Pathol Oral Radiol Endod.* 2009 Sep; 108(3):376–82.

42. Bernardi MJ, Reis A, Loguercio AD, Kehrig R, Leite MF, Nicolau J. Study of the buffering capacity, pH and salivary flow rate in type 2 well-controlled and poorly controlled diabetic patients. *Oral Health Prev Dent.* 2007; 5(1):73–8.

43. Chávez EM, Taylor GW, Borrell LN, Ship JA. Salivary function and glycemic control in older persons with diabetes. *Oral Surg Oral Med Oral Pathol Oral Radiol Endod*. 2000 Mar; 89(3):305–11.

44. Chávez EM, Borrell LN, Taylor GW, Ship JA. A longitudinal analysis of salivary flow in control subjects and older adults with type 2 diabetes. *Oral Surg Oral Med Oral Pathol Oral Radiol Endod*. 2001 Feb; 91(2):166–73.

45. Karjalainen KM, Knuuttila ML, Käär ML. Salivary factors in children and adolescents with insulin-dependent diabetes mellitus. *Pediatr Dent*. 1996 Jul-Aug; 18(4):306–11.

46. Carda C, Mosquera-Lloreda N, Salom L, Gomez de Ferraris ME, Peydró A. Structural and functional salivary disorders in type 2 diabetic patients. *Med Oral Patol Oral Cir Bucal*. 2006 Jul 1; 11(4):E309–14.

47. Karjalainen KM, Knuuttila ML, Käär ML. Relationship between caries and level of metabolic balance in children and adolescents with insulin-dependent diabetes mellitus. *Caries Res*. 1997; 31(1):13–18.

48. Collin HL, Sorsa T, Meurman JH, Niskanen L, Salo T, Rönkä H, et al. Salivary matrix metalloproteinase (MMP-8) levels and gelatinase (MMP-9) activities in patients with type 2 diabetes mellitus. *J Periodontal Res*. 2000 Oct; 35(5):259–65.

49. Caseiro A, Ferreira R, Quintaneiro C, Pereira A, Marinheiro R, Vitorino R, et al. Protease profiling of different biofluids in type 1 diabetes mellitus. *Clin Biochem*. 2012 Dec; 45(18):1613–9.

50. Pinducciu G, Micheletti L, Piras V, Songini C, Serra C, Pompei R, et al. Periodontal disease, oral microbial flora and salivary antibacterial factors in diabetes mellitus type 1 patients. *Eur J Epidemiol*. 1996 Dec; 12(6):631–6.

51. Oxford GE, Tayari L, Barfoot MD, Peck AB, Tanaka Y, Humphreys-Beher MG. Salivary EGF levels reduced in diabetic patients. *J Diabetes Complications*. 2000 May-Jun; 14(3):140–5.

52. Odds FC. *Candida* infections: an overview. *Crit Rev Microbiol*. 1987; 15(1):1–5.

53. Sashikumar R, Kannan R. Salivary glucose levels and oral candida carriage in type II diabetics. *Oral Surg Oral Med Oral Pathol Oral Radiol Endod*. 2010 May; 109(5):706–11.

54. Wilson RM, Reeves WG. Neutrophil phagocytosis and killing in insulin-dependent diabetes. *Clin Exp Immunol*. 1986 Feb; 63(2):478–84.

55. Ueta E, Osaki T, Yoneda K, Yamamoto T. Prevalence of diabetes mellitus in odontogenic infections and oral candidiasis: an analysis of neutrophil suppression. *J Oral Pathol Med*. 1993 Apr; 22(4):168–74.

56. Weerasuriya N, Snape J. Oesophageal candidiasis in elderly patients: risk factors, prevention and management. *Drugs Aging*. 2008; 25(2):119–30.

57. Willis AM, Coutler WA, Fulton CR, Hayes JR, Bell PM, Lamey PJ. Oral candida carriage and infection in insulin-treated diabetic patients. *Diabet Med*. 1999 Aug; 16(8):675–9.

58. Guggenheimer J, Moore PA, Rossie K, Myers D, Mongelluzzo MB, Block HM, et al. Insulin-dependent diabetes mellitus and oral soft tissue pathologies: II. Prevalence and characteristics of Candida and Candidal lesions. *Oral Surg Oral Med Oral Pathol Oral Radiol Endod*. 2000 May; 89(5):570–6.

59. Belazi M, Velegraki A, Fleva A, Gidarakou I, Papanaum L, Baka D, et al. Candidal overgrowth in diabetic patients: potential predisposing factors. *Mycoses*. 2005 May; 48(3):192–6.

60. Kumar BV, Padshetty NS, Bai KY, Rao MS. Prevalence of Candida in the oral cavity of diabetic subjects. *J Assoc Physicians India*. 2005 Jul; 53:599–602.

61. Bremenkamp RM, Caris AR, Jorge AO, Back-Brito GN, Mota AJ, Balducci I, et al. Prevalence and antifungal resistance profile of Candida spp. oral isolates from patients with type 1 and 2 diabetes mellitus. *Arch Oral Biol*. 2011 Jun; 56(6):549–55.

62. Melton JJ, Redding SW, Kirkpatrick WR, Reasner CA, Ocampo GL, Venkatesh A, et al. Recovery of Candida dubliniensis and other Candida species from the oral cavity of subjects with periodontitis who had well-controlled and poorly controlled type 2 diabetes: a pilot study. *Spec Care Dentist*. 2010 Nov-Dec; 30(6):230–4.

63. Schorling SR, Kortinga HC, Froschb M, Mühlschlegel FA. The role of *Candida dubliniensis* in oral candidiasis in human immunodeficiency virus-infected individuals. *Crit Rev Microbiol*. 2000 Jan; 26(1):59–68.

64. Tekeli A, Dolapci I, Emral R, Cesur S. Candida carriage and Candida dubliniensis in oropharyngeal samples of type-1 diabetes mellitus patients. *Mycoses*. 2004 Aug; 47(7):315–8.

65. Dorocka-Bobkowska B, Budtz-Jörgensen E, Wloch S. Non-insulin-dependent diabetes mellitus as a risk factor for denture stomatitis. *J Oral Pathol Med*. 1996 Sep; 25(8):411–5.

66. Darwazeh AM, Lamey PJ, Samaranayake LP, MacFarlane TW, Fisher BM, Macrury SM, et al. The relationship between colonisation, secretor status and *in-vitro* adhesion of Candida albicans to buccal epithelial cells from diabetics. *J Med Microbiol*. 1990 Sep; 33(1):43–9.

67. Lotfi-Kamran MH, Jafari AA, Falah-Tafti A, Tavakoli E, Falahzadeh MH. Candida colonization on the denture of diabetic and non-diabetic patients. *Dent Res J (Isfahan)*. 2009 Spring; 6(1):23–7.

68. Dorocka-Bobkowska B, Zozulinska-Ziolkiewicz D, Wierusz-Wysocka B, Hedzelek W, Szumala-Kakol A, Budtz-Jörgensen E. Candida-associated denture stomatitis in type 2 diabetes mellitus. *Diabetes Res Clin Pract*. 2010 Oct; 90(1):81–6.

69. Maltsman-Tseikhin A, Moricca P, Niv D. Burning mouth syndrome: will better understanding yield better management? *Pain Pract*. 2007 Jun; 7(2):151–62.

70. DeLattre VF. Factors contributing to adverse soft tissue reactions due to the use of tartar control toothpastes: report of a case and literature review. *J Periodontol*. 1999 Jul; 70(7):803–7.

71. Forssell H, Jääskeläinen S, Tenovuo O, Hinkka S. Sensory dysfunction in burning mouth syndrome. *Pain*. 2002 Sep; 99(1–2):41–7.

72. Moore PA, Guggenheimer J, Orchard T. Burning mouth syndrome and peripheral neuropathy in patients with type 1 diabetes mellitus. *J Diabetes Complications*. 2007 Nov-Dec; 21(6):397–402.

73. Collin HL, Niskanen L, Uusitupa M, Töyry, Collin P, Koivisto AM, et al. Oral symptoms and signs in elderly patients with type 2 diabetes. A focus on diabetic neuropathy. *Oral Surg Oral Med Oral Pathol Oral Radiol Endod*. 2000 Sep; 90(3):299–305.

74. Carrington J, Getter L, Brown RS. Diabetic neuropathy masquerading as glossodynia. *J Am Dent Assoc*. 2001 Nov; 132(11):1549–51.

75. Scala A, Checchi L, Montevecchi M, Marini I, Giamberardino MA. Update on burning mouth syndrome: overview and patient management. *Crit Rev Oral Biol Med*. 2003; 14(4):275–91.

76. Vitkov L, Weitgasser R, Hannig M, Fuchs K, Krautgartner WD. Candida-induced stomatopyrosis and its relation to diabetes mellitus. *J Oral Pathol Med*. 2003 Jan; 32(1):46–50.

77. Cavalcanti DR, Birman EG, Migliari DA, da Silveira FR. Burning mouth syndrome: clinical profile of Brazilian patients and oral carriage of Candida species. *Braz Dent J*. 2007; 18(4):341–5.

78. Vesterinen M, Ruokonen H, Furuholm J, Honkanen E, Meurman JH. *Clinical questionnaire study of oral health care and symptoms in diabetic vs. non-diabetic predialysis chronic kidney disease patients. Clin Oral Investig*. 2012 Apr; 16(2):559–63.

79. Eltas A, Tozoğlu U, Keleş M, Canakci V. Assessment of oral health in peritoneal dialysis patients with and without diabetes mellitus. *Perit Dial Int*. 2012 Jan-Feb; 32(1):81–5.

80. Vinik A. The approach to the management of the patient with neuropathic pain. *J Clin Endocrinol Metab*. 2010 Nov; 95(11):4802–11.

81. Davidson D, Leibel BS, Berris B. Asymptomatic parotid gland enlargement in diabetes mellitus. *Ann Intern Med.* 1969 Jan; 70(1):31–8.

82. Russotto SB. Asymptomatic parotid gland enlargement in diabetes mellitus. *Oral Surg Oral Med Oral Pathol.* 1981 Dec; 52(6):594–8.

83. Scully C, Bagán JV, Eveson JW, Barnard N, Turner FM. Sialosis: 35 cases of persistent parotid swelling from two countries. *Br J Oral Maxillofac Surg.* 2008 Sep; 46(6):468–72.

84. Mandel L, Khelemsky R. Asymptomatic bilateral facial swelling. *J Am Dent Assoc.* 2012 Nov; 143(11):1205–08.

85. Carda C, Carranza M, Arriaga A, Díaz A, Peydró A, Gomez de Ferraris ME. Structural differences between alcoholic and diabetic parotid sialosis. *Med Oral Patol Oral Cir Bucal.* 2005 Aug-Oct; 10(4):309–14.

86. Merlo C, Bohl L, Carda C, Gómez de Ferraris ME, Carranza M. Parotid sialosis: morphometrical analysis of the glandular parenchyme and stroma among diabetic and alcoholic patients. *J Oral Pathol Med.* 2010 Jan; 39(1):10–5.

87. Mandel L, Patel S. Sialadenosis associated with diabetes mellitus: a case report. *J Oral Maxillofac Surg.* 2002 Jun; 60(6):696–8.

88. Ahmed I, Nasreen S, Jehangir U, Wahid Z. Frequency of oral lichen planus in patients with noninsulin dependent diabetes mellitus. *J Pak Assoc Dermatol.* 2012; 22:30–4.

89. Albrecht M, Bánóczy J, Dinya E, Tamás G Jr. Occurrence of oral leukoplakia and lichen planus in diabetes mellitus. *J Oral Pathol Med.* 1992 Sep; 21(8):364–6.

90. Petrou-Amerikanou C, Markopoulos AK, Belazi M, Karamitsos D, Papanayotou P. Prevalence of oral lichen planus in diabetes mellitus according to the type of diabetes. *Oral Dis.* 1998 Mar; 4(1):37–40.

91. Van Dis ML, Parks ET. Prevalence of oral lichen planus in patients with diabetes mellitus. *Oral Surg Oral Med Oral Pathol Oral Radiol Endod.* 1995 Jun; 79(6):696–700.

92. Borghelli RF, Pettinari IL, Chuchurru JA, Stirparo MA. Oral lichen planus in patients with diabetes. An epidemiologic study. *Oral Surg Oral Med Oral Pathol.* 1993 Apr; 75(4):498–500.

93. Guggenheimer J, Moore PA, Rossie K, Myers D, Mongelluzzo MB, Block HM, et al. Insulin-dependent mellitus and oral soft tissue pathologies. I. Prevalence and characteristics of non-candidal lesions. *Oral Surg Oral Med Oral Pathol Oral Radiol Endod.* 2000; 89:563–9.

94. Lozada-Nur F, Miranda C. Oral lichen planus: epidemiology, clinical characteristics, and associated diseases. *Semin Cutan Med Surg.* 1997 Dec; 16(4):273–7.

95. Romero MA, Seoane J, Varela-Centelles P, Diz-Dios P, Garcia-Pola MJ. Prevalence of diabetes mellitus amongst oral lichen planus patients. Clinical and pathological characteristics. *Med Oral.* 2002 Mar-Apr; 7(2)121-9.

96. Seyhan M, Ozcan H, Sahin I, Bayram, Karincaoğlu Y. High prevalence of glucose metabolism disturbance in patients with lichen planus. *Diabetes Res Clin Pract.* 2007 Aug; 77(2):198–202.

97. Torrente-Castells E, Figueiredo R, Berini-Aytés L, Gay-Escoda C. Clinical features of oral lichen planus. A retrospective study of 65 cases. *Med Oral Patol Oral Cir Bucal.* 2010 Sep 1; 15(5):e685–90.

98. Xue JL, Fan MW, Wang SZ, Chen XM, Li Y, Wang L. A clinical study of 674 patients with oral lichen planus in China. *J Oral Pathol Med.* 2005 Sep; 34(8):467–72.

99. Kaomongkolgit R. Oral lichenoid drug reaction associated with antihypertensive and hypoglycemic drugs. *J Drugs Dermatol.* 2010 Jan; 9(1):73–5.

100. Saini R, Al-Maweri SA, Saini D, Ismail NM, Ismail AR. Oral mucosal lesions in non oral habit diabetic patients and association of diabetes mellitus with oral precancerous lesions. *Diabetes Res Clin Pract.* 2010 Sep; 89(3):320–6.

101. Vasconcelos BC, Novaes M, Sandrini FA, Maranhão Filho AW, Coimbra LS. Prevalence of oral mucosa lesions in diabetic patients: a preliminary study. *Braz J Otorhinolaryngol.* 2008 May-Jun; 74(3):423–8.
102. Nevins ML, Karimbux NY, Weber HP, Giannobile WV, Fiorellini JP. Wound healing around endosseous implants in experimental diabetes. *Int J Oral Maxillofac Implants.* 1998 Sept-Oct; 13(5):620–9.
103. Fiorellini JP, Nevins ML, Norkin A, Weber HP, Karimbux NY. The effect of insulin therapy on osseointegration in a diabetic rat model. *Clin Oral Implants Res.* 1999 Oct; 10(5):362–8.
104. Siqueira JT, Cavalher-Machado SC, Arana-Chavez VE, Sannomiya P. Bone formation around titanium implants in the rat tibia: role of insulin. *Implant Dent.* 2003; 12(3):242–51.
105. Shyng YC, Devlin H, Ou KL. Bone formation around immediately placed oral implants in diabetic rats. *Int J Prosthodont.* 2006 Sep-Oct; 19(5):513–4.
106. Kwon PT, Rahman SS, Kim DM, Kopman JA, Karimbux NY, Fiorellini JP. Maintenance of osseointegration utilizing insulin therapy in a diabetic lab rat model. *J Periodontol.* 2005 Apr; 76(4):621–6.
107. de Morais JA, Trindade-Suedam IK, Pepato MT, Marcantonio E Jr., Wenzel A, et al. Effect of diabetes mellitus and insulin therapy on bone density around osseointegrated dental implants: a digital subtraction radiography study in rats. *Clin Oral Implants Res.* 2009 Aug; 20(8):796–801.
108. Hasegawa H, Ozawa S, Hashimoto K, Takeichi T, Ogawa T. Type 2 diabetes impairs implant osseointegration capacity in rats. *Int J Oral Maxillofac Implants.* 2008 Mar-Apr; 23(2):237–46.
109. Casap N, Nimri S, Ziv E, Sela J, Samuni Y. Type 2 diabetes has minimal effect on osseointegration of titanium implants in Psammomys obesus. *Clin Oral Implants Res.* 2008 May; 19(5):458–64.
110. Wang B, Song Y, Wang F, Li D, Zhang H, Ma A, et al. Effects of local infiltration of insulin around titanium implants in diabetic rats. *Br J Oral Maxillofac Surg.* 2011 Apr; 49(3):225–9.
111. Wang F, Song YL, Li CX, Li DH, Zhang HP, et al. Sustained release of insulin-like growth factor-1 from poly(lactide-co-glycolide) microspheres improves osseointegration of dental implants in type 2 diabetic rats. *Eur J Pharmacol.* 2010 Aug; 640(1–3):226–32.
112. Zou GK, Song YL, Zhou W, Yu M, Liang LH, Sun DC et al. Effects of local delivery of bFGF from PLGA microspheres on osseointegration around implants in diabetic rats. *Oral Surg Oral Med Oral Pathol Oral Radiol.* 2012 Sep; 114(3):284–9.
113. Kuchler U, Spilka T, Baron K, Tangl S, Watzek G, Gruber R. Intermittent parathyroid hormone fails to stimulate osseointegration in diabetic rats. *Clin Oral Implants Res.* 2011 May; 22(5):518–23.
114. Smith RA, Berger R, Dodson TB. Risk factors associated with dental implants in healthy and medically compromised patients. *Int J Oral Maxillofac Implants.* 1992 Fall; 7(3):367–72.
115. Shernoff AF, Colwell JA, Bingham SF. Implants for type II diabetic patients: interim report. VA Implants in Diabetes Study Group. *Implant Dent.* 1994 Fall; 3(3):183–5.
116. Balshi TJ, Wolfinger GJ. Dental implants in the diabetic patient: a retrospective study. *Implant Dent.* 1999; 8(4):355–9.
117. Olson JW, Shernoff AF, Tarlow JL, Colwell JA, Sheetz JP, et al. Dental endosseous implant assessments in a type 2 diabetic population: a prospective study. *Int J Maxillofac Implants.* 2000 Nov-Dec; 15(6):811–8.
118. Fiorellini JP, Chen PK, Nevins M, Nevins ML. A retrospective study of dental implants in diabetic patients. *Int J Periodontics Restorative Dent.* 2000 Aug; 20(4):366–73.
119. Morris HF, Ochi S, Winkler S. Implant survival in patients with type 2 diabetes: placement to 36 months. *Ann Periodontol.* 2000 Dec; 5(1):157–65.

120. Farzad P, Andersson L, Nyberg J. Dental implant treatment in diabetic patients. *Implant Dent.* 2002; 11(3):262–7.
121. van Steenberghe D, Jacobs R, Desnyder M, Maffei G, Quirynen M. The relative impact of local and endogenous patient-related factors on implant failure up to the abutment stage. *Clin Oral Implants Res.* 2002 Dec; 13(6):617–22.
122. Peled M, Ardekian L, Tagger-Green N, Gutmacher Z, Machtei EE. Dental implants in patients with type 2 diabetes mellitus: a clinical study. *Implant Dent.* 2003; 12(2):116–22.
123. Moy PK, Medina D, Shetty V, Aghaloo TL. Dental implant failure rates and associated risk factors. *Int J Oral Maxillofac Implants.* 2005 Jul-Aug; 20(4):569–77.
124. Ferreira SD, Silva GL, Cortelli JR, Costa JE, Costa FO. Prevalence and risk variables for peri-implant disease in Brazilian subjects. *J Clin Periodontol.* 2006 Dec; 33(12):929–35.
125. Dowell S, Oates TW, Robinson M. Implant success in people with type 2 diabetes mellitus with varying glycemic control: a pilot study. *J Am Dent Assoc.* 2007 Mar; 138(3):355–61.
126. Tawil G, Younan R, Azar P, Sleilati G. Conventional and advanced implant treatment in the type II diabetic patient: surgical protocol and long-term clinical results. *Int J Oral Maxillofac Implants.* 2008 Jul-Aug; 23(4):744–52.
127. Turkyilmaz I. One-year clinical outcome of dental implants placed in patients with type 2 diabetes mellitus: a case series. *Implant Dent.* 2010 Aug; 19(4):323–9.
128. Oates TW, Dowell S, Robinson M, McMahan CA. Glycemic control and implant stabilization in type 2 diabetes mellitus. *J Dent Res.* 2009 Apr; 88(4):367–71.
129. Edelman SV. Importance of glucose control. *Med Clin North Am.* 1998 Jul; 82(4):665–87.
130. Ismail-Beigi F. Clinical Practice. Glycemic management of type 2 diabetes mellitus. *N Engl J Med.* 2012 Apr; 366(14):1319–27.
131. Oates TW, Huynh-Ba G, Vargas A, Alexander P, Feine J. A critical review of diabetes, glycemic control, and dental implant therapy. *Clin Oral Implants Res.* 2013 Feb; 24(2):117–27.
132. Retzepi M, Donos N. The effect of diabetes mellitus on osseous healing. *Clin Oral Implants Res.* 2010 Jul; 21(7):673–81.
133. Javed F, Romanos GE. Impact of diabetes mellitus and glycemic control on the osseointegration of dental implants: a systematic literature review. *J Periodontol.* 2009 Nov; 80(11):1719–30.
134. Courtney MW Jr., Snider TN, Cottrell DA. Dental implant placement in type II diabetics: a review of the literature. *J Mass Dent Soc.* 2010 Spring; 59(1):12–4.
135. Marchand F, Raskin A, Dionnes-Hornes A, Barry T, Dubois N, Valéro R, et al. Dental implants and diabetes: conditions for success. *Diabetes Metab.* 2012 Feb; 38(1):14–9.
136. Moore PA, Orchard T, Guggenheimer J, Weyant RJ. Diabetes and oral health promotion: a survey of disease prevention behaviors. *J Am Dent Assoc.* 2000 Sep; 131(9):1333–41.
137. Tomar SL, Lester A. Dental and other health care visits among U.S. adults with diabetes. *Diabetes Care.* 2000 Oct; 23(10):1505–10.
138. Macek MD, Taylor GW, Tomar SL. Dental care visits among dentate adults with diabetes, United States, 2003. *J Public Health Dent.* 2008 Spring; 68:102–10.
139. Macek MD, Tomar SL. Dental care visits among dentate adults with diabetes and periodontitis. *J Public Health Dent.* 2009 Fall; 69(4):284–9.
140. Moffet HH, Schillinger D, Weintraub JA, Adler N, Liu JY, Selby JV, et al. Social disparities in dental insurance and annual dental visits among medically insured patients with diabetes: the Diabetes Study of Northern California (DISTANCE) Survey. *Prev Chronic Dis.* 2010 May; 7(3):A57.
141. Thorstensson H, Falk H, Hugoson A, Kuylenstierna J. Dental care habits and knowledge of oral health in insulin-dependent diabetics. *Scand J Dent Res.* 1989 Jun; 97(3):207–15.
142. Allen EM, Ziada HM, O'Halloran D, Clerehugh V, Allen PF. Attitudes, awareness and oral health-related quality of life in patients with diabetes. *J Oral Rehabil.* 2008 Mar; 35:218–23.

143. Al Habashneh R, Khader Y, Hammad MM, Almuradi M. Knowledge and awareness about diabetes and periodontal health among Jordanians. *J Diabetes Complications.* 2010 Nov-Dec; 24(6):409–14.

144. Kneckt MC, Keinänen-Kiukaanniemi SM, Knuuttila ML, Syrjälä AM. Self-esteem as a characteristic of adherence to diabetes and dental self-care regimens. *J Clin Periodontol.* 2001 Feb; 28(2):175–80.

145. Mosen DM, Pihlstrom DJ, Snyder JJ, Shuster E. Assessing the association between receipt of dental care, diabetes control measures and health care utilization. *J Am Dent Assoc.* 2012 Jan; 143(1):20–30.

# Chapter 9

# Identification of dental patients with undiagnosed diabetes

*Evanthia Lalla, DDS, MS; Dana Wolf, DMD, MS; and Ira B. Lamster, DDS, MMSc*

Diabetes mellitus is estimated to affect 371 million people worldwide [1]. Approximately half of these individuals remain undiagnosed and a very large number of individuals are at-risk. In the United States, approximately 8.3% of the total population has diabetes and about a quarter of those affected are undiagnosed [2]. Type 2 diabetes is a preventable disease, and so are its complications, yet in most countries primary prevention is minimal. Early diagnosis is a particular problem for type 2 diabetes, in which there is a long asymptomatic period [3] and where diagnosis usually occurs when patients present to healthcare providers with signs, symptoms, or even complications of the disease [4]. Early identification of affected individuals may lead to earlier intervention and a subsequent decrease in the significant morbidity and mortality associated with diabetes.

In this chapter, we will first briefly review a number of the screening recommendations that exist in the medical community and then review in more detail screening models that have incorporated oral findings to identify individuals with diabetes mellitus. We will also discuss the potential for a more active role by dentists in diabetes screening and the barriers that exist to implementation of a more active role.

## Medical models for diabetes screening

In 2003, the World Health Organization and the International Diabetes Federation held a meeting on the topic of screening for type 2 diabetes. The aims of the meeting were to review the evidence for the usefulness of screening for early detection of type 2 diabetes and to make recommendations relevant to health care policy, action, and future research. At that time, the organizations found no direct evidence that earlier detection of type 2 diabetes has an impact on health outcomes. They did, however, find direct evidence that the incidence of diabetes can be reduced in high-risk individuals who may be identified via diabetes screening. Additionally, they acknowledged that screening may help raise disease awareness. The meeting report addressed a number of issues surrounding screening such as cost-effectiveness, sensitivity, and specificity of the screening test; the psychological and social effects of testing; and the ability of the health care system

*Diabetes Mellitus and Oral Health: An Interprofessional Approach*, First Edition. Edited by Ira B. Lamster.
© 2014 John Wiley & Sons, Inc. Published 2014 by John Wiley & Sons, Inc.

Table 9.1   Risk factors for type 2 diabetes mellitus.

**Non-modifiable**
- High risk race/ethnicity [African-American, Hispanic/Latino, Alaska Native, American Indian, Asian American, or Pacific Islander]
- Age greater than 40 years [or younger for high-risk race/ethnicity individuals]
- Family history of diabetes
- History of cardiovascular disease
- For females:
  History of gestational diabetes
  Delivery of infant greater than 9 lbs.
  Polycystic ovary syndrome

**Modifiable**
- Physical inactivity
- Overweight/obesity [body mass index equal to or greater than 25 kg/m² for most ethnic groups]
- Hypertension [equal to or greater than 140/90 mm Hg]
- Dyslipidemia [HDL cholesterol equal to or less than 35 mg/dl or triglycerides equal to or greater than 250 mg/dl]
- HbA1c 5.7–6.4%, impaired glucose tolerance [IGT], or impaired fasting glucose [IFG]

to intervene if the disease is identified. Rather than put forward specific screening recommendations, the report urged health authorities and professional organizations to formulate their own screening protocols for type 2 diabetes.

The American Diabetes Association (ADA) currently recommends screening to detect type 2 diabetes in asymptomatic individuals of any age who are overweight or obese and have one or more additional risk factors for diabetes (Table 9.1) [4]. The recommended test is either a hemoglobin A1c (HbA1c), a fasting plasma glucose (FPG), or a two-hour oral glucose tolerance test. In the absence of any risk factors for diabetes, the ADA recommends testing for diabetes starting at age 45 with repeat testing at three-year intervals if the results are normal. Because the incidence of type 2 diabetes has increased dramatically over the last ten years, especially in minority populations, the ADA also recommends testing overweight children and adolescents who have two or more additional risk factors for diabetes. They recommend that testing be initiated at age 10 or at onset of puberty, and repeated every three years if results are negative.

The U.S. Preventive Service Task Force recommends screening for type 2 diabetes in asymptomatic adults with sustained blood pressure greater than 135/80 mm Hg [5]. This recommendation is based on the fact that in individuals with diabetes and hypertension, lowering blood pressure below conventional targets reduces the incidence of cardiovascular events and associated mortality.

## Diabetes identification in dental care settings

Dental care facilities represent, for a number of reasons, alternative health care settings to detect unrecognized diabetes in a large segment of the population. First, as reviewed in detail in Chapter 6, multiple studies have demonstrated that diabetes adversely affects periodontal status [6], and that these effects appear to operate early in life [7, 8], suggesting that periodontitis may be one of the earliest complications of diabetes. There are also other oral manifestations of diabetes [9] (reviewed in Chapter 8), and patients with undiagnosed disease may be seen in the dental office with diabetes-related oral signs or symptoms. Second, according to the Centers for Disease Control and Prevention, nearly 70% of American adults have seen a dental provider in the preceding year, and health-care utilization patterns indicate that individuals tend to seek routine and preventive dental care more frequently than routine and preventive medical care [10, 11]. Lastly, dental patients often return for multiple non-emergent and recall/maintenance visits during which dental professionals can assess risk factors, advise on healthy lifestyle, perform or order blood screening tests, refer to a physician for diagnostic testing and treatment, and follow up on outcomes.

The concept of screening for diabetes in the dental office is not new [12–16], since the link between diabetes and periodontitis has been known for many decades. The first large-scale effort to systematically assess whether dental findings can contribute to the identification of people with undiagnosed diabetes was published in 2007 [17]. The study used National Health and Nutrition Examination Survey (NHANES) III data to develop a predictive equation that could determine the probability of undiagnosed diabetes using patient-reported information and periodontal clinical parameters routinely assessed in the dental office. The analyses performed revealed that individuals with family history of diabetes, self-reported hypertension and high cholesterol, and clinical evidence of periodontal disease bear a probability of 27–53% of having undiagnosed diabetes, with Mexican-American men exhibiting the highest probability and white women the lowest. These findings suggested that the dental office could provide an opportunity to identify individuals unaware of their diabetic status.

Three subsequent reports [18–20], all using NHANES data, approached the same concept in different ways and confirmed the potential for a role of dental professionals in diabetes identification. The first report (reviewed in more detail in Chapter 7) showed that periodontal disease at baseline is an independent predictor of incident diabetes [18]. Although conflicting data are available [21] and this topic warrants further investigation, the result of this study supports the use of periodontal parameters in the identification of diabetes risk. The second of these studies aimed to compare the proportion of subjects who would be recommended for screening according to ADA guidelines between dental patients with and without periodontitis. Additionally, the authors assessed whether at-risk individuals with periodontitis had visited a dental professional recently, and thus would have had a screening opportunity [19]. The findings indicated that more than 60% of those without periodontitis and more than 90% of those with periodontitis met ADA guidelines for diabetes screening. Of those at-risk with periodontitis, 50% had seen a dentist in the past year and 60% in the past two years. The third study [20] suggested that dental care providers should consider using a clinical guideline that includes the following parameters as predictors: waist circumference, age, self-reported oral health, self-reported weight and race/ethnicity, as well as any additional information on periodontal status and family history of diabetes. Although, arguably, some of these parameters are not easy to determine in a dental care setting, the proposed algorithm had good performance characteristics, corroborating the notion that the dental visit provides an important potential venue for this type of screening.

The first study that collected data *de novo* to assess the performance of targeted identification protocols for unrecognized prediabetes and diabetes in dental patients was published in 2011 [22]. Importantly, detection of prediabetes was part of the study design as well. Prediabetes often precedes type 2 diabetes and has emerged as a serious health concern because it independently places individuals at risk for serious micro- and macro-vascular complications [23]. In the study, 601 individuals who presented for care at a dental school clinic and had never been told they have prediabetes or diabetes were recruited. To target those at some level of risk for diabetes, the inclusion criteria encompassed being at least 40 years old if non-Hispanic white or at least 30 years old if Hispanic or non-white, and self-report of at least one diabetes risk factor (family history of diabetes, hypertension, high cholesterol, or overweight). This resulted in 535 subjects who then received a periodontal examination and a point-of-care fingerstick HbA1c test, which provided additional variables to be used in the prediction models.

Subjects were asked to return following an eight-hour fast for a venipuncture FPG test, the result of which was used as the study outcome to signify potential diabetes or prediabetes, per ADA guidelines at the time. In total, out of 506 subjects who returned for the FPG test, 182 were identified with an abnormal result: 21 (4.2%) potentially diabetic (FPG at least 126 mg/dL), and 161 (31.8%) prediabetic (FPG = 100–125 mg/dl). Performance characteristics of simple models to identify dysglycemia (FPG at least 100 mg/dl) using variables that are readily available in any dental care setting were evaluated and optimal cut-offs for each variable in a given model were identified. A model including only two dental variables (number of missing teeth and percent of teeth with deep periodontal pockets) had an estimated area under the receiver operating characteristic curve (AUC) of 0.65. The addition of the point-of-care HbA1c test improved the AUC to 0.79 ($p < 0.001$). The presence of at least 26% teeth with deep pockets or at least four missing teeth correctly identified 73% of true cases; the addition of a point-of-care HbA1c of at least 5.7% increased correct identification to 92%.

Because not all practitioners and/or patients will opt for a blood test in the dental setting, the finding that the use of just two dental variables provides high sensitivity is of significant merit. Indeed, both predictive models presented in this study have sensitivity similar to what has been reported for diabetes risk assessment approaches tested in medical settings [24], and because of their simplicity they have great potential for adoption. Interestingly, no diabetes prediction model has been universally accepted for use in medical settings, and it has been suggested that recalibration of algorithms might be necessary when models are applied to different populations [25]. A limitation of the study described above is that models were developed and assessed in a population that is predominantly Hispanic. Testing to assess external validity of these algorithms in diverse patient populations is needed.

More recently, additional studies exploring the notion of screening for undiagnosed diabetes in dental settings have been published. First, the early concept of using gingival blood for screening [12, 14–16, 26] was revisited in a highly vulnerable population in India [27], where almost half of the subjects tested had elevated blood glucose levels, suggestive of diabetes. Unfortunately, this report failed to provide critical information about the dental/periodontal status of the population and the specifics and performance characteristics of the screening approach used making the findings hard to interpret.

Subsequently, a pilot study [28] assessed the use of gingival crevicular blood for the measurement of HbA1c levels during a periodontal visit. The investigators were able to obtain an adequate gingival crevicular blood sample in 75 out of the 120 periodontitis patients included in their study; 18 subjects had no or insufficient bleeding on probing, and an additional 27 gingival crevicular blood samples had an unidentified component that interfered with the HbA1c assay. The authors reported good correlation in HbA1c results between the gingival crevicular blood and fingerstick blood samples. Similarly, a good correlation was shown in a small study that assessed glucose levels in gingival crevicular and fingerstick blood [29]. Obtaining enough gingival blood for a screening test is clearly not always feasible, even in periodontitis patients, but it presents an alternative for those clinicians and patients who feel uncomfortable with a fingerstick test.

Importantly, and as discussed in more detail in the section below, recent work has provided evidence that implementation of diabetes screening in dental practices is feasible and that both patients and dental providers believe that the dental visit is a good opportunity for early diabetes identification [30, 31]. A large study conducted in Sweden provided a glimpse into long-term outcomes following screening in a dental setting [32]. In this study, random blood glucose was measured using a fingerstick blood sample and a portable glucometer in 1,568 consecutive dental patients with no previous history of diabetes, and irrespective of risk profile or oral status. Subjects with a positive result for diabetes were referred to a primary health care center. The study outcome, diagnosis of diabetes, was obtained from medical patient records over the following three years. Of the 155 subjects who screened positive, 135 (90%) visited their primary health care center within the three-year follow-up period and 9 (6%) received a diabetes diagnosis. Of those who screened negative, 80% visited a primary healthcare center and 0.6% were found to have diabetes. The authors concluded that cooperation between dental professionals and primary care physicians for diabetes screening and follow-up appears to be a feasible method for early diabetes diagnosis.

Taken together, the evidence to date underscores that dental professionals have the opportunity to assume a role in identifying those with undiagnosed hyperglycemia among their patients (using parameters summarized in Table 9.2) and in directing them to receive appropriate medical evaluation and care. This approach may have important implications because both early/appropriate glycemic control in those with diabetes who remain unrecognized and a delay in the onset of diabetes among those with pre-diabetes are of great public health importance.

Table 9.2   Variables used for diabetes detection in dental settings and associated publications.

| Variable | Publication |
| --- | --- |
| Dental/periodontal parameters | Borell 2007 [17], Demmer 2008 [18], Lalla 2011 [22], Li 2011 [20] |
| Self-reported diabetes risk factors | Borell 2007 [17], Lalla 2011 [22], Li 2011 [20] |
| Gingival blood glucose | Stein 1969 [12], Tsutsui 1985 [14], Shetty 2011 [27], Parker 1993 [15], Beikler 2002 [16], Strauss 2009 [26], Gaikwad 2013 [29] |
| Gingival blood HbA1c | Strauss 2012 [28] |
| Finger-stick glucose | Barasch 2012 [30], Engström 2013 [32] |
| Finger-stick HbA1c | Lalla 2011 [22] |

## Acceptance by dentists and patients of diabetes testing in dental settings

Data from the retrospective and prospective studies discussed above suggest that the dental office can be a health care location where undiagnosed diabetes or pre-diabetes is identified. While the formal diagnosis is made by a medical provider, the willingness of dental providers to adopt a more active role in the detection and management of patients with diabetes requires a change in the traditional dental practice paradigm. The willingness of dentists to participate in the health care of their patients, and the attitude of dental patients about this new role, has been examined in a number of studies.

An early study by Greenberg and co-workers demonstrated that a substantial subset of patients presenting for dental care are at risk for serious health events, yet are unaware of that risk [33]. The study used the Framingham risk score, which was developed based on longitudinal data from the Framingham Heart Study, and was established to identify a person's risk of a cardiac event in the following 10 years [34]. Framingham risk scores were calculated for 100 patients presenting to an inner-city dental school clinic. For inclusion in the study, subjects had to be at least 40 years of age; without a history of hypertension, elevated cholesterol, diabetes mellitus, myocardial infarction or stroke; and without a visit to a physician in the previous year. Subjects received a questionnaire regarding established risk factors for cardiovascular disease, a chair-side assessment of hypertension, and finger-stick blood tests for total cholesterol, high-density lipoprotein, and HbA1c. Seventeen of the 100 participants demonstrated a Framingham risk score of 10% or greater. Fourteen individuals were at moderate risk (between 10% and 20%) and three were at high risk (greater than 20%) for a cardiac event. Nearly three-fourths of the participants demonstrated at least one important risk factor for coronary heart disease (i.e., elevated systolic blood pressure, current smoking, or elevated level of HbA1c).

A series of studies by Kunzel et al. examined dentists' attitudes regarding primary health care activities in the dental office [35–37]. Selected activities included screening for diabetes mellitus and smoking cessation activities because diabetes and smoking are important risk factors for periodontitis [38]. General dentists and periodontists were surveyed (response rate 80% and 73%, respectively). General dentists reported a lack of comfort with participating in diabetes management and smoking cessation activities due to a lack of knowledge about both activities. They also did not believe that such activities were central to their professional responsibilities and did not believe that their colleagues or their patients expected them to perform such activities. General dentists were more comfortable with assessing and advising patients, as opposed to a more active role in management. A comparison of the behavior of general dentists and periodontists revealed that specialists were more active in behaviors associated with risk identification and active management. However, both groups were more engaged in informational activities than they were in active management of these risk factors. For example, for their patients with diabetes, only 14% of generalists and 28% of periodontists reported that they often referred or monitored the level of blood glucose. One of the studies in this series aimed to identify factors that were associated with active participation of dentists in the management of patients with diabetes [37]. Confidence, professional responsibility, and relationships with other dental and medical professionals were influential predictors of active management for periodontists. Whereas periodontists where more influenced by colleagues, patient-related variables (discussions with patients, perception of patient expectations, and patients' socioeconomic level) were the significant predictors for general dentists.

Subsequently, Greenberg et al. examined the attitudes of dentists in regard to dental office screening for the risk of developing serious medical conditions [39]. A national sample of dentists was asked to respond to a series of questions in the following five categories:

1 The importance of dentist involvement in this activity
2 Which specific diseases would be assessed (i.e., hypertension, cardiovascular disease, diabetes)
3 The level of involvement in this new approach to practice (i.e., refer to a physician, perform chair-side tests, discuss results with the patient)
4 The type of data they would collect (i.e., physical measurements, collecting saliva for analysis, collecting blood for analysis)
5 The potential limitations (i.e., patient acceptance, liability, cost and time required)

All responses were provided on a five-point Likert scale, which ranged from 1 = very willing or very important to 5 = very unwilling or very unimportant. One thousand nine hundred and forty-five dentists responded to the survey (response rate = 26%). Nearly 90% of dentists believed it was somewhat important or very important for them to screen for specific medical conditions, and 77% believed it was somewhat important or very important to screen for diabetes. Only 56% of respondents were somewhat or very willing to take a fingerstick blood sample for a chair-side screening test.

Overall, the studies assessing the attitude of dentists toward diabetes screening and management in the dental office suggest a recognition that these activities are important but reluctance for more active involvement. Additionally, if there is to be increased participation of dentists in the screening for diabetes, patients would have to accept this change.

Greenberg et al. assessed patient attitudes toward screening for medical conditions in the dental setting [40]. Dental patients attending an inner-city dental school clinic and two private practices were asked to respond to a questionnaire about chair-side screening for medical conditions using the five-point Likert scale (1 = most favorable to 5 = least favorable). The mean scores for the questions about screening for medical disorders and monitoring for known medical disorders were 1.26 and 1.31 respectively, for the clinic patients and 1.83 and 1.60 for the private practice patients. This trend of more favorable scores given by the clinic patients was seen throughout, and likely relates to the greater access to care for medical services among patients using private practice dental offices.

In another study, Barasch et al. assessed acceptance of blood glucose testing in dental offices and found widespread acceptance of this procedure [30]. Data were gathered from the Dental Practice-Based Research Network, and therefore represent a wide geographic sampling (28 practices in the United States and Sweden). Most dentists and staff members surveyed (84%) felt that there would be important patient benefits from assessing blood glucose levels in the dental office. Eighty-eight percent of dental personnel agreed or strongly agreed that blood glucose testing promotes the perception that dentists are interested in patients' general health and increases patients' confidence in the practice (Figure 9.1).

When questions about the potential negative impact of testing were posed, the percentage of providers who agreed or strongly agreed was very low. Only 2% of dental personnel agreed or strongly agreed with the statement "blood glucose levels are not relevant to dental practice." The main concern of providers was the time required for such testing (22% agreed or strongly agreed that testing was time consuming). A majority of the patients agreed or strongly agreed that blood glucose testing was a good idea, easy, evidence of outstanding dental care, and provided them with useful information (Figure 9.2).

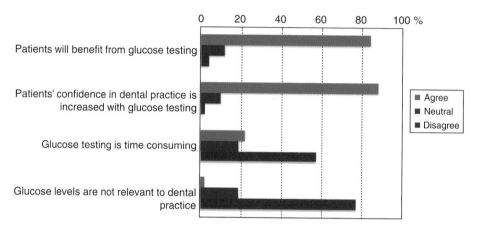

**Figure 9.1**   Attitudes of dental personnel toward blood glucose testing in the dental office. Barasch and co-workers [30] surveyed dentists and staff members from 28 practices who participated in a study of random blood glucose testing in dental patients at risk for diabetes using a fingerstick blood sample and a glucometer. Sixty-seven dentists and staff members participated in the survey. Four of the survey items and the percentage of respondents who agreed, were neutral, or disagreed with those statements are shown.

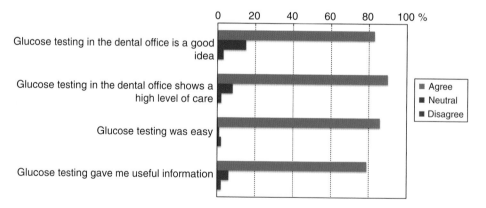

**Figure 9.2**   Attitudes of patients toward blood glucose testing in the dental office. Barasch and co-workers [30] surveyed patients from 28 dental practices who were identified as at risk for diabetes (n=498). Of those, 434 received a random blood glucose test using a fingerstick blood sample and a glucometer during a routine dental examination visit. Four of the survey items and the percentage of patients who agreed, were neutral, or disagreed with those statements are shown. The last two items were asked only of the 434 patients who underwent blood testing.

These data suggest that both patients and providers feel that greater involvement of dental professionals in the management of chronic diseases, and in particular diabetes, is beneficial. There are, however, other implementation issues that need to be addressed as an expanded role for the dentist in the identification and management of patients with diabetes is considered. These include state regulations regarding the scope of dental practice, regulatory issues concerning in-office laboratory testing, and reimbursement for these services.

Based on the evidence reviewed in the section above and in Chapter 5, protocols for dentists' involvement in diabetes identification and/or management of their patients will likely involve in-office testing for blood glucose or HbA1c. The use of in-office laboratory tests in the United States is regulated on a national level by the Clinical Laboratory Improvement Amendments (CLIA) [41]. Point-of-care tests for glucose and HbA1c are considered "CLIA-exempt" tests, and dental offices wanting to use point-of care testing would have to complete a simple application for a CLIA waiver.

Whether or not such testing is permissible as part of the scope of dental practice depends upon how the practice act is written in each state. Approximately half of the states have adopted some of the language contained in the scope of practice statement issued by the American Dental Association [42]. This statement is quite broad, and defines the practice of dentistry as "the evaluation, diagnosis, presentation and/or treatment (nonsurgical, surgical or related procedures) of diseases, disorders and/or conditions of the oral cavity, maxillofacial areas and/or the adjacent and associated structures and their impact on the human body…"

Finally, the issue of reimbursement has yet to be examined. If in fact, such testing falls within the scope of practice, and CLIA requirements for testing are met, then a patient can be billed for the service. In the previously discussed study by Greenberg et al. [40], dental patients responded that they were willing to pay a modest amount for blood testing. Whether third parties such as dental insurance companies will cover in-office tests for diabetes remains to be determined.

## Concluding remarks

More studies to dissect the best model(s) for diabetes and prediabetes detection among dental patients are warranted. Identification approaches need to be simple and capitalize on parameters routinely assessed as part of an individual's dental/periodontal examination so that they can be easily adopted in all types of dental care settings. Importantly, systems must also be in place so that identified patients are properly informed and advised about modifiable risk factors, and are directly referred for medical follow-up. Figure 9.3 proposes a decision-making tree that can be easily used in a dental setting. As the performance of such models of care is tested and validated in diverse populations in the future, assessment for undiagnosed dysglycemia may become part of the routine evaluation of each dental patient at risk.

Adopting the concepts described above into everyday practice is an important goal. It will allow dental professionals to achieve more predictable therapeutic outcomes, contribute to the fight to stop the diabetes epidemic, and play a significant role in promoting improved oral and overall health among their patients.

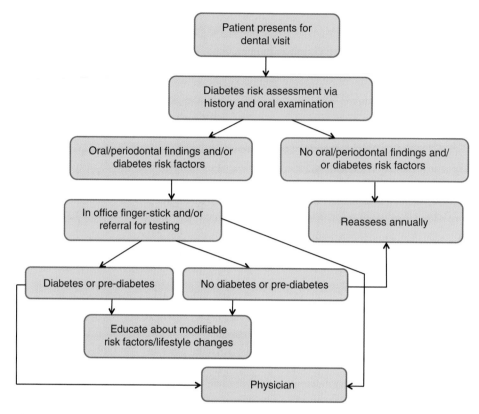

**Figure 9.3** A decision-making tree for diabetes and prediabetes detection in the dental setting. Dental professionals can contribute to the detection of dysglycemia among their patients by considering the simple activities outlined in this figure. Periodontitis or oral findings such as unexplained candidiasis or burning mouth syndrome should alert the dentist. Referral to a physician for formal diagnostic testing and treatment of those identified as potentially diabetic or prediabetic is of essence. Dental professionals should inquire about medical visit outcomes among those referred and reassess those who "screen negative" at future treatment or maintenance appointments.

## References

1. International Diabetes Federation Diabetes Atlas: International Diabetes Federation; 2012 [cited 2013 April 19]. 5th edition: Available from: http://www.diabetesatlas.org/content/diabetes-and-impaired-glucose-tolerance.
2. Centers for Disease Control and Prevention. *National diabetes fact sheet: national estimates and general information on diabetes and prediabetes in the United States*, 2010. Atlanta, GA: U.S. Department of Health and Human Services, Centers for Disease Control and Prevention; 2011.
3. World Healh Organization. Screening for Type 2 Diabetes 2003 [cited 2013 April 1]. Available from: http://www.who.int/diabetes/publications/en/screening_mnc03.pdf.
4. American Diabetes Association. Standards of Medical Care in Diabetes—2013. *Diabetes Care.* 2013 January 1, 2013; 36 (Suppl 1):S11–S66.

5. Screening for Type 2 Diabetes Mellitus in Adults: U.S. Preventive Services Task Force Recommendation Statement. *Ann Intern Med.* 2008; 148(11):846–54.
6. Lalla E, Papapanou PN. Diabetes mellitus and periodontitis: a tale of two common interrelated diseases. *Nat Rev Endocrinol.* 2011 12//print; 7(12):738–48.
7. Lalla E, Cheng B, Lal S, Tucker S, Greenberg E, Goland R, et al. Periodontal changes in children and adolescents with diabetes: a case-control study. *Diabetes Care.* 2006 Feb; 29(2):295–9.
8. Lalla E, Cheng B, Lal S, Kaplan S, Softness B, Greenberg E, et al. Diabetes mellitus promotes periodontal destruction in children. *J Clin Periodontol.* 2007 Apr; 34(4):294–8.
9. Lamster IB, Lalla E, Borgnakke WS, Taylor GW. The relationship between oral health and diabetes mellitus. *J Am Dent Assoc.* 2008 Oct; 139 (Suppl):S19–S24.
10. Centers for Disease Control and Prevention (CDC). *Behavioral Risk Factor Surveillance System Survey Data.* Atlanta, Georgia: U.S. Department of Health and Human Services, Centers for Disease Control and Prevention 2008. Available from: http://apps.nccd.cdc.gov/brfss/list.asp?cat=OH&yr=2008&qkey=6610&state=All.
11. Glick M, Greenberg BL. The potential role of dentists in identifying patients' risk of experiencing coronary heart disease events. *J Am Dent Assoc.* 2005 Nov; 136(11):1541–6.
12. Stein GM, Nebbia AA. A chairside method of diabetic screening with gingival blood. *Oral Surg, Oral Med, and Oral Pathol.* 1969 May; 27(5):607–12.
13. Chapnick L, Jolley HM, Newman S. Diabetic screening in the dental office. *Ont Dent.* 1974 Jul; 51(7):10–2.
14. Tsutsui P, Rich SK, Schonfeld SE. Reliability of intraoral blood for diabetes screening. *J Oral Med.* 1985 Apr-Jun; 40(2):62–6.
15. Parker RC, Rapley JW, Isley W, Spencer P, Killoy WJ. Gingival crevicular blood for assessment of blood glucose in diabetic patients. *J Periodontol.* 1993; 64(7):666–72.
16. Beikler T, Kuczek A, Petersilka G, Flemmig TF. In-dental-office screening for diabetes mellitus using gingival crevicular blood. *J Clin Periodontol.* 2002 Mar; 29(3):216–8.
17. Borrell LN, Kunzel C, Lamster I, Lalla E. Diabetes in the dental office: using NHANES III to estimate the probability of undiagnosed disease. *J Periodontal Res.* 2007; 42(6):559–65.
18. Demmer RT, Jacobs DR, Jr., Desvarieux M. Periodontal disease and incident type 2 diabetes: results from the First National Health and Nutrition Examination Survey and its epidemiologic follow-up study. *Diabetes Care.* 2008 Jul; 31(7):1373–9.
19. Strauss SM, Russell S, Wheeler A, Norman R, Borrell LN, Rindskopf D. The dental office visit as a potential opportunity for diabetes screening: an analysis using NHANES 2003–2004 data. *J Public Health Dent.* 2010; 70(2):156–62.
20. Li S, Williams PL, Douglass CW. Development of a clinical guideline to predict undiagnosed diabetes in dental patients. *J Am Dent Assoc.* 2011 January 2011; 142(1):28–37.
21. Ide R, Hoshuyama T, Wilson D, Takahashi K, Higashi T. Periodontal disease and incident diabetes: a seven-year study. *J Dent Res.* 2011 January 1, 2011; 90(1):41–6.
22. Lalla E, Kunzel C, Burkett S, Cheng B, Lamster IB. Identification of unrecognized diabetes and pre-diabetes in a dental setting. *J Dent Res.* 2011 July 1, 2011; 90(7):855–60.
23. Diabetes Prevention Program Research Group. The prevalence of retinopathy in impaired glucose tolerance and recent-onset diabetes in the Diabetes Prevention Program. *Diabet Med.* 2007 Feb; 24(2):137–44.
24. Lin JW, Chang YC, Li HY, Chien YF, Wu MY, Tsai RY, et al. Cross-sectional validation of diabetes risk scores for predicting diabetes, metabolic syndrome, and chronic kidney disease in Taiwanese. *Diabetes Care.* 2009 Dec; 32(12):2294–6.
25. Tabak AG, Herder C, Rathmann W, Brunner EJ, Kivimaki M. Prediabetes: a high-risk state for diabetes development. *Lancet.* 2012 Jun 16; 379(9833):2279–90.

26. Strauss SM, Wheeler AJ, Russell SL, Brodsky A, Davidson RM, Gluzman R, et al. The potential use of gingival crevicular blood for measuring glucose to screen for diabetes: an examination based on characteristics of the blood collection site. *J Periodontol*. 2009 Jun; 80(6):907–14.

27. Shetty S, Kohad R, Yeltiwar R, Shetty K. Gingival blood glucose estimation with reagent test strips: a method to detect diabetes in a periodontal population. *J Periodontol*. 2011 Nov; 82(11):1548–55.

28. Strauss SM, Tuthill J, Singh G, Rindskopf D, Maggiore JA, Schoor R, et al. A novel intraoral diabetes screening approach in periodontal patients: Results of a pilot study. *J Periodontol*. 2012 2012/06/01; 83(6):699–706.

29. Gaikwad S, Jadhav V, Gurav A, Shete AR, Dearda HM. Screening for diabetes mellitus using gingival crevicular blood with the help of a self-monitoring device. *J Periodontal Implant Sci*. 2013 Feb; 43(1):37–40.

30. Barasch A, Safford MM, Qvist V, Palmore R, Gesko D, Gilbert GH. Random blood glucose testing in dental practice: A community-based feasibility study from The Dental Practice-Based Research Network. *J Am Dent Assoc*. 2012 March 1, 2012; 143(3):262–9.

31. Rosedale MT, Strauss SM. Diabetes screening at the periodontal visit: patient and provider experiences with two screening approaches. *Int J Dent Hyg*. 2012; 10(4):250–8.

32. Engström S, Berne C, Gahnberg L, Svärdsudd K. Effectiveness of screening for diabetes mellitus in dental health care. *Diabet Med*. 2013; 30(2):239–45.

33. Greenberg BL, Glick M, Goodchild J, Duda PW, Conte NR, Conte M. Screening for cardiovascular risk factors in a dental setting. *J Am Dent Assoc*. 2007 Jun; 138(6):798–804.

34. Wilson PWF, D'Agostino RB, Levy D, Belanger AM, Silbershatz H, Kannel WB. Prediction of coronary heart disease using risk factor categories. *Circulation*. 1998 May 1, 1998;97(18):1837–47.

35. Kunzel C, Lalla E, Albert DA, Yin H, Lamster IB. On the primary care frontlines: The role of the general practitioner in smoking-cessation activities and diabetes management. *J Am Dent Assoc*. 2005 August 1, 2005;136(8):1144–53.

36. Kunzel C, Lalla E, Lamster I. Dentists' management of the diabetic patient: Contrasting generalists and specialists. *Am J Public Health*. 2007 April 1, 2007; 97(4):725–30.

37. Kunzel C, Lalla E, Lamster IB. Management of the patient who smokes and the diabetic patient in the dental office. *J Periodontol*. 2006 Mar; 77(3):331–40.

38. Papapanou PN. Periodontal diseases: epidemiology. *Ann Periodontol*. 1996;1(1):1–36.

39. Greenberg BL, Glick M, Frantsve-Hawley J, Kantor ML. Dentists' attitudes toward chairside screening for medical conditions. *J Am Dent Assoc*. 2010 Jan; 141(1):52–62.

40. Greenberg BL, Kantor ML, Jiang SS, Glick M. Patients' attitudes toward screening for medical conditions in a dental setting. *J Public Health Dent*. 2012;72(1):28–35.

41. Centers for Medicare and Medicaid Services. Clinical Laboratory Improvement Amendments (CLIA). Available from http://www.cms.gov/Regulations-and-Guidance/Legislation/CLIA/index.html

42. American Dental Association. Scope of Practice. Available from http://www.ada.org/2458.aspx.

# Section 3

# Case reports

*Ira B. Lamster, DDS, MMSc; Nurit Bittner, DDS, MS; and Daniel Lorber, MD*

## Introduction

The management of dental patients with diabetes mellitus depends upon communication between the dentist, physician, and other members of the health care team. Dental professionals must be familiar with the patient's medical history and how the patient's diabetes is managed, and determine if modifications to the usual clinical protocol are required. Physicians and other non-dental oral health care providers must have an understanding of the oral complications of diabetes, urge patients to see their dentist regularly, and refer patients for dental care when a problem is identified. Regular communication between the dentist and physician also emphasizes to patients the importance of oral self-care and the need for regular dental examinations.

Interprofessional practice often revolves around specific questions regarding patient management. The following are a number of general questions dentists routinely ask a patient's physician.

1 Does the patient with diabetes mellitus require prophylactic antibiotics for dental/periodontal procedures?
   The answer is "no" when there are no other underlying indications.
2 Should the patient's medications be altered in preparation for a dental procedure?
   Modifications may be needed, and this is decided on a patient-by-patient basis, based on a discussion between the physician and dentist.
3 Are there any other medical concerns that may influence oral health which the dentist should assess?
   Common comorbidities include decreased visual acuity, which may make self-examination of the mouth and performance of oral hygiene difficult. The presence of renal disease can affect drug metabolism, and for drugs metabolized by the kidney, adjustment of the dosage may be required.
4 What time of day should the dental procedure be performed?
   If possible, patients treated with insulin, or oral agents known to cause hypoglycemia (sulfonylureas or glinides), should be scheduled first thing in the morning. This minimizes the duration of fasting and the subsequent risk of hypoglycemia.

---

*Diabetes Mellitus and Oral Health: An Interprofessional Approach*, First Edition. Edited by Ira B. Lamster.
© 2014 John Wiley & Sons, Inc. Published 2014 by John Wiley & Sons, Inc.

5  How should meals and medications be managed?

Patients treated with sulfonylureas or glinides are at risk for hypoglycemia with fasting. These medications should not be taken until the patient is able to eat normal amounts of carbohydrate. Patients treated with anti-diabetes agents that are not associated with hypoglycemia (metformin, pioglitazone, DPP-4 inhibitors, SGLT-2 inhibitors, acarbose, GLP-1 agonists) alone tolerate prolonged fasting without an untoward event. Continued basal insulin treatment is necessary for people with type 1 diabetes and some with insulin-treated type 2 diabetes. Prolonged withholding of insulin for people with type 1 diabetes results in significant metabolic decompensation and diabetic ketoacidosis. Prandial (mealtime) insulin can be resumed with the first post-procedure meal. If a soft diet is recommended, suggest foods that contain amounts of carbohydrate similar to the patient's usual diet. In that case, the diabetes medications do not need to be altered. If the patient is limited to liquids, supplements such as Glucerna® provide a mixture of protein, fat, and carbohydrate similar to a mixed meal. In most cases, medications do not need to be adjusted.

6  Are there any precautions regarding post-operative medications?

If the patient has nephropathy, some concern must be given to drugs metabolized by the kidney, including the penicillin, cephalosporin, and aminoglycoside antibiotics. Caution is also required if steroids are to be used because these drugs can induce hyperglycemia.

The treating dentist must fully understand the nature of the patient's diabetes. Important information that should be obtained from the patient and confirmed with the patient's physician include:

1  What type of diabetes does the patient have?
2  When was the diagnosis first made?
3  How is the patient's disease managed (diet, exercise, oral medications, insulin)?
4  What is the level of metabolic control? This is often provided as percent glycosylated hemoglobin.
5  Does the patient have any clinical complications of diabetes?
6  Has the patient ever experienced hypoglycemia or hyperglycemia?

Following are six scenarios. The first three focus on medical management and the last three on the management of the patient's dental needs.

# Case 1

# A patient with type 1 diabetes mellitus is seen for dental care

*Ira B. Lamster, DDS, MMSc; Nurit Bittner, DDS, MS; and Daniel Lorber, MD*

---

**Case background**

A patient with well-controlled type 1 diabetes mellitus is seen for periodontal and prosthodontic care. The dentist is concerned about proper patient management during dental treatment, and in particular avoidance of hypoglycemia.

---

A 31-year-old woman with type 1 diabetes presents to her dentist for periodontal and prosthodontic care. A fixed partial denture is needed to replace tooth #4. Teeth #3 and #5 require crown lengthening procedures.

## Medical history

The patient was diagnosed with type 1 diabetes mellitus at the age of 15. Medical management of her diabetes is with a multiple-dose insulin regimen, consisting of insulin glargine 16 units hs (long-acting insulin, see Table 1) and insulin aspart (rapid-acting insulin, Table 1) before meals. The dose of insulin aspart is calculated based on the carbohydrate content of the planned meal and the blood glucose level as determined by a fingerstick test. Her most recent hemoglobin A1c (HbA1c) was 6.8%, indicating excellent metabolic control. She has no history of severe hypoglycemic events. She takes no other medications.

## Dental history and history of the current problem

Tooth #4 was extracted more than 10 years ago. The tooth was replaced with a fixed partial denture extending from #3 to #5. The patient visited her dentist intermittently, and received dental cleanings. She occasionally required amalgam and composite restorations, but noticed the fixed partial denture appeared loose approximately two months ago. Upon clinical evaluation, it was determined that the cement seal had been lost, and caries

---

*Diabetes Mellitus and Oral Health: An Interprofessional Approach*, First Edition. Edited by Ira B. Lamster.

**Table 1**   Insulin chart.*

| Insulin preparation | Onset of action | Peak | Duration of action |
|---|---|---|---|
| Lispro (Humalog®) | <15 minutes | 1–2 hours | 3–6 hours |
| Aspart (Novolog®) | <15 minutes | 1–2 hours | 3–6 hours |
| Glulisine (Apidra®) | <15 minutes | 1–2 hours | 3–6 hours |
| Regular (Novolin® R, Humulin® R) | 30–60 minutes | 2–4 hours | 6–10 hours |
| Humulin® R Regular U–500 | 30–60 minutes | 2–4 hours | Up to 24 hours |
| NPH (Novolin® N, Humulin® N, ReliOn®) | 2–4 hours | 4–8 hours | 10–18 hours |
| Glargine (Lantus®) | 1–2 hours | Usually no peak | Up to 24 hours |
| Determir (Levemir®) | 1–2 hours | Usually no peak** | Up to 24 hours** |
| **Premixed insulins**\*** | **Onset of action** | **Peak** | **Duration of action** |
| Novolin® 70/30, Humulin® 70/30 | 30–60 minutes | 2–10 hours | 10–18 hours |
| Humalog® 75/25, Novolog® 70/30, Humalog® 50/50 | 10–30 minutes | 1–6 hours | 10–24 hours |

*Information derived from a combination of manufacturer's prescribing information and clinical studies. Individual response to insulin preparations may vary.
**Peak and length of action may depend on size of dose and length of time since initiation of therapy.
***Premixed insulins are more variable in peak and duration of action. For instance, even though the literature states that the effects may last for up to 24 hours, many people find that they will need to take a dose every 10–12 hours.
Modified from www.dlife.com/diabetes/insulin/about_insulin/insulin–chart.

was present on the remaining tooth structure of the abutment teeth. In order to fabricate a new fixed restoration, periodontal surgery is necessary to expose sound tooth structure on the abutment teeth (crown lengthening procedure). The patient is scheduled for periodontal surgery in the morning and will not eat (NPO) after midnight in preparation for surgery. The dentist is concerned that she may become hypoglycemic before or during the procedure and contacts her endocrinologist for guidance.

**Comment**

A person with type 1 diabetes is absolutely dependent upon injected insulin for survival.

# Treatment

At this point, the dentist called the endocrinologist, and they reviewed the planned treatment. An important consideration is the food intake before the surgical procedure. The patient is concerned about the procedure, and has requested nitrous oxide/oxygen inhalation analgesia. Consequently, the patient is advised not to eat on the morning of the procedure, and the following guidelines are recommended: If the fasting blood glucose is consistently above 100 mg/dL, most endocrinologists would recommend that the patient take her usual insulin up to midnight before the morning of surgery. On the other hand, if the usual morning blood glucose levels are in the 70–80 range, the endocrinologist might recommend decreasing the nighttime dose by 20–25%. Inexperienced physicians and dentists may recommend that the patient hold the bedtime insulin if the patient is to be NPO in the morning. This is a not advisable. There usually is no indication to further reduce the dose, and doing so risks hyperglycemic decompensation or diabetic ketoacidosis.

In this case the patient reported that her usual morning glucose levels are in the 110–130 mg/dL range. She takes her usual hs insulin; on the day of surgery her morning capillary blood glucose was 140 mg/dL.

---

**Comment**

It is recommended that procedures requiring NPO status be scheduled first thing in the morning to minimize the risk of diabetes decompensation—either hypoglycemia or hyperglycemia.

---

Pre-operatively, if the patient awakens with hypoglycemia during the night or in the morning, the endocrinologist recommended 4 oz of apple juice to raise the blood glucose. Since low-fiber liquids are emptied from the stomach in 15–20 minutes, there is little risk of vomiting and aspiration during the procedure.

If the patient will have her morning meal, the following approach is suggested: If her usual glucose levels are acceptable after breakfast and before the next meal, she should take her usual dose of morning insulin. On the other hand, if she is either hypoglycemic or hyperglycemic, she should consult with her endocrinologist about whether and how to adjust her morning insulin.

The periodontal surgery is completed without incident. She resumes her usual insulin aspart with her first post-procedure meal.

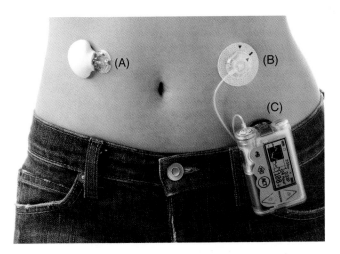

**Figure 1**   Continuous subcutaneous insulin infusion pump and associated equipment. (A) Continuous subcutaneous glucose sensor. (B) Infusion site. (C) MiniMed® insulin pump, with display of the continuous glucose monitor. www.diabetespharmacist.com/articles/insulin-pumps/

## Discussion

Most people with type 1 diabetes take a combination of long-acting insulins once or twice a day with rapid-acting analogs before each meal. Alternatively, increasing numbers of patients with type 1 diabetes are being treated with a continuous subcutaneous insulin infusion pump (CSII), using rapid-acting insulin alone. Intermediate, short-acting, and pre-mixed insulins are almost never used for type 1 diabetes, but are occasionally used for patients with type 2 diabetes.

If at some later point the patient's diabetes mellitus is treated with a CSII pump (Figure 1), and additional oral surgery or periodontal surgery is planned, a decision regarding NPO prior to the surgery must be made. The pump is programmed to deliver a constant subcutaneous infusion (basal insulin); at mealtimes, the patient programs in a bolus dose of insulin in which the dose of rapid-acting insulin is calculated based on the carbohydrate content of the planned meal and the current blood glucose level. In general, patients treated with the CSII are to continue their basal insulin infusion perioperatively, and take the usual calculated bolus with the next meal.

## Case 2

# A patient with type 2 diabetes mellitus requires oral surgery

*Ira B. Lamster, DDS, MMSc; Nurit Bittner, DDS, MS; and Daniel Lorber, MD*

---

**Case background**

A patient with well-controlled type 2 diabetes mellitus is seen for removal of two third molar teeth. The dentist consults with the patient's physician about alterations in the patients' routine that are required before and after the extractions.

---

A 63-year-old man with 15-year history of type 2 diabetes is scheduled for removal of two third molar teeth.

## Medical history

Based on discussions with the patient's physician, his metabolic control is good, with an HbA1c of 6.9%. Current medications for diabetes mellitus are metformin (1,000 mg in the morning, 500 mg in the evening) and pioglitazone (15 mg qd).

---

**Comment**

The dentist will ask several questions and should discuss the patient's medication schedule for the day of the oral surgery to diminish the risk of perioperative hypoglycemia.

---

Other medications include a statin (lovastatin 20 mg qd) and an ACE inhibitor (enalapril 5 mg qd) for mild hypertension.

## Dental history and history of the current problem

The patient demonstrates excellent oral hygiene, has minimal caries experience, and has mild gingivitis with a few areas of limited attachment loss. The two third molars on the left side (#16 and 17) have been affected by pericoronitis (interproximal to #15/16 and

---

*Diabetes Mellitus and Oral Health: An Interprofessional Approach*, First Edition. Edited by Ira B. Lamster.
© 2014 John Wiley & Sons, Inc. Published 2014 by John Wiley & Sons, Inc.

#17/18). The patient is often uncomfortable, abscesses occur intermittently, and there is concern for loss of bone on the distal surfaces of the second molar teeth. The two third molar teeth are not impacted but have a slight mesial inclination. Extraction is recommended.

## Treatment

A large number of oral medications are used to treat type 2 diabetes mellitus, and these are associated with different levels of risk of hypoglycemia (Table 1).

The most important question here is which oral agents is the patient using. There are two classes of currently used oral agents that are associated with an increased risk of hypoglycemia (if a patient takes them without eating). These are the sulfonylureas (examples include glyburide [generic only], glipizide [Glucotrol®], and glimepiride [Amaryl®]) and meglitinides (examples include nateglinide [Starlix®] and repaglinide [Prandin®]).

In general, procedures for patients treated with insulin or sulfonylureas are best scheduled in the early morning to minimize NPO duration and subsequent hypoglycemic risk.

On the morning of the procedure, the dentist will also ask:

1 When did you last take your diabetes medication?
2 When did you last check your blood sugar?
3 What was the level? What is the usual level?
4 Does the patient have a history of hypoglycemic episodes? Did this occur in the morning, or if meals are skipped, or if fasting?

The patient is taking a combination of metformin and pioglitazone (Actos®); neither drug is associated with an increased risk of hypoglycemia. His glucose control remains excellent with an HbA1c of 6.5%. He has no history of hypoglycemia, and in this case, there is a very low risk of hypoglycemia. Metformin should be taken with food to avoid gastrointestinal side effects, but no other adjustment in his diabetes regimen is necessary. The extractions are performed without any untoward reaction, and healing is uneventful.

The patient returns three years later with concern about the third molars on the right side. Now he is taking a combination of metformin and glyburide, a sulfonylurea. The dentist asks the same questions as above. The patient's morning capillary blood glucose level is generally about 100 mg/dL; he regularly eats three meals a day and does not report hypoglycemic symptoms. However, if oral surgery is required, this patient is now at increased risk for hypoglycemia if he is NPO for the procedure. Although sulfonylurea usage is declining significantly in the United States, many patients are still taking members of this class and are at increased risk of hypoglycemia. On the morning of the procedure, the patient should not take the morning dose of medication, but should take a dose with the first post-procedure meal. If the patient's morning blood glucose levels are tightly controlled (80–120 mg/dL), it may be advisable to stop the sulfonylurea on the day before surgery as well.

**Table 1**  Classes of hypoglycemic medications.

| Class | Mechanism | Advantages | Disadvantages | Cost | Generic | Brand |
|---|---|---|---|---|---|---|
| **DPP-4 inhibitors** | • Inhibits DPP-4<br>• Increases GLP-1, GIP | • No hypoglycemia<br>• Well tolerated | • Modest ↓HbA1c<br>• ? Pancreatitis<br>• Urticaria | High | Sitagliptin<br>Saxagliptin<br>linagliptin | Januvia®<br>Onglyza®<br>Tradjenta® |
| **GLP-1 receptor agonists** | • Activates GLP-1 R<br>• ↑ Insulin, ↓ glucagon<br>• ↓ gastric emptying<br>• ↑ satiety | • Weight loss<br>• No hypoglycemia<br>• ? β cell mass<br>• ? CV protection | • GI<br>• ? Pancreatitis<br>• Medullary ca<br>• Injectable | High | Exendin<br>Liraglutide<br>Exendin ER | Byetta®<br>Victoza®<br>Bydureon® |
| **Amylin mimetics** | • Activates amylin receptor<br>• ↓ glucagon<br>• ↓ gastric emptying<br>• ↑ satiety | • Weight loss<br>• ↓ PPG | • GI<br>• Modest ↓ HbA1c<br>• Injectable<br>• Hypo w/ insulin<br>• Dosing frequency | High | Pramlintide | Symlin® |
| **Bile acid sequestrants** | • Bind bile acids<br>• ↓ hepatic glucose production | • No hypoglycemia<br>• Nonsystemic<br>• ↓ post-prandial glucose<br>• ↓ CVD events | • GI<br>• Modest ↓ HbA1c<br>• Dosing frequency | High | Colesevelam | Welchol® |
| **Dopamine-2 agonists** | • Activates DA receptor<br>• Modulates hypothalamic control of metabolism<br>• ↑ insulin sensitivity | • No hypoglycemia<br>• ? ↓ CVD events | • Modest ↓ HbA1c<br>• Dizziness/syncope<br>• Nausea<br>• Fatigue | High | Bromocriptine | Cycloset® |
| **Biguanides** | • Activates AMP-kinase<br>• ↓ Hepatic glucose production | • Extensive experience<br>• No hypoglycemia<br>• Weight neutral<br>• ? ↓ CVD | • Gastrointestinal<br>• Lactic acidosis<br>• B₁₂ deficiency<br>• Contraindications | Low | Metformin | Glucophage® |

*(Continued)*

**Table 1** *(Continued)*

| Class | Mechanism | Advantages | Disadvantages | Cost | Generic | Brand |
|---|---|---|---|---|---|---|
| **SUs / Meglitinides** | • Closes KATP channels<br>• ↑ insulin secretion | • Extensive experience<br>• ↓ microvasc risk | • Hypoglycemia<br>• Weight gain<br>• Low durability<br>• ? ischemic preconditioning | Low | Su: lyburide, glipizide, glimepiride<br>Meg: Repaglinide, Nateglinide | Su: Glucotrol®, Amaryl®<br>Meg: Prandin®<br>Starlix® |
| **TZDs** | • PPAR-γ activator<br>• ↑ insulin sensitivity | • No hypoglycemia<br>• Durability<br>• ↓ TGs, ↑ HDL-C<br>• ? ↓ CVD (pio) | • Weight gain<br>• Edema/heart failure<br>• Bone fractures<br>• ? ↑ MI (rosi)<br>• ? bladder ca (pio) | High | Pioglitazone<br>Rosiglitazone | Actos®<br>Avandia® |
| **α-GIs** | • Inhibits α-glucosidase<br>• Slows carbohydrate absorption | • No hypoglycemia<br>• Nonsystemic<br>• ↓ post-prandial glucose<br>• ? ↓ CVD events | • Gastrointestinal<br>• Dosing frequency<br>• Modest ↓ HbA1c | Mod. | Acarbose<br>miglitol | Precose®<br>Glyset® |
| **SGLT2 inhibitors** | • Inhibits reabsorption in the kidney, causes glycosuria | • No hypoglycemia, weight loss, decreases blood pressure | • vaginitis/balanitis, volume depletion, fall risk in elderly | High | canagliflozin | Invokana |

Modified from *Diabetes Care* June 2012 vol. 35 no. 6 1364–1379.

## Discussion

It is essential that the treating dentist be fully aware of the patient's metabolic status over the course of the previous six to 12 months, as well as the patient's blood glucose level. Before beginning the procedure, the patient should be questioned about timing of medication ingestion, the last self-administered evaluation of the blood glucose level, and how she or he is feeling. Knowledge, planning, and preparation are the keys to avoiding hypoglycemia, and treating it effectively if it does occur.

# Case 3

# A patient with diabetes mellitus has a hypoglycemic episode in the dental office

*Ira B. Lamster, DDS, MMSc; Nurit Bittner, DDS, MS; and Daniel Lorber, MD*

---

**Case background**

A patient with type 2 diabetes mellitus experiences an acute physiologic reaction while receiving dental care. The dentist must immediately manage this suspected hypoglycemic episode.

---

A 56-year-old woman with type 2 diabetes is being seen for a lengthy appointment for prosthodontic rehabilitation of her maxillary and mandibular arches.

## Medical history

The patient is treated with a combination of levemir insulin (20 units hs) at bedtime and glimepiride (4 mg) in the morning. Her usual morning capillary blood glucose level is between 100 and 130 mg/dL. The only other medication she takes is levothyroxine (25 mcg qd).

## Dental history and history of the current problem

The patient provided a lengthy history of dental care from the time of early childhood to the present. New carious lesions occurred frequently as a child, requiring amalgam restorations in the posterior regions and composite restorations in the anterior regions. Recurrent caries and failure of existing restorations required larger restorations and single crowns. Tooth #8 was lost due to trauma and a four-unit fixed partial denture (#7–10) replaces #8. The esthetics are poor. Endodontic treatment was needed for a number of teeth, and tooth #19 was lost as a result of a failed endodontic treatment. A three-unit fixed partial denture now replaces #19.

---

*Diabetes Mellitus and Oral Health: An Interprofessional Approach*, First Edition. Edited by Ira B. Lamster.
© 2014 John Wiley & Sons, Inc. Published 2014 by John Wiley & Sons, Inc.

Many of the existing restorations demonstrate marginal deficiencies and recurrent caries. The patient is concerned with poor anterior esthetics. It was decided that a complete prosthodontic rehabilitation is required. Mild to moderate periodontitis is present. Periodontal surgery will be required to eliminate excessive probing depths before the final restorations are completed.

## Treatment

An early morning appointment is scheduled to begin the crown preparations.

The patient is not NPO for the procedure, eats breakfast, and takes her normal dose of insulin and oral medication. During the procedure, the patient suddenly becomes confused, diaphoretic, and tachycardic. How should this situation be managed?

## Discussion

The treating dentist suspects dysglycemia, but is unsure if the acute physiologic reaction is due to hypoglycemia or hyperglycemia (Figures 1 and 2). In either case, immediately discontinue the procedure. If possible, check the fingerstick glucose (the patient may have a meter with her and may have a family member who can assist; Figure 3). If the glucose level is less than 70 mg/dL or if a meter is not available, treat with 4 oz fruit juice or flat regular soda (one spoonful of sugar in a glass of soda will remove the carbonation).

---

**Comment**

If a dental patient monitors his or her blood glucose level regularly, he or she should be advised to have the glucose meter during dental appointments. Dentists should consider having a glucometer in the office to use in appropriate situations.

---

Observe the patient; repeat the fingerstick glucose 20 minutes later, and re-assess the patient once she returns to her normal state. Communicate with her physician to determine why hypoglycemia occurred.

In this case a glucose meter is available and the patient's capillary blood glucose is 54 mg/dL, indicative of significant hypoglycemia. She swallows 4 oz of juice and during the next 20 minutes, she becomes more lucid; the second blood glucose test indicates a level of 80 mg/dL. She is given several crackers; the dentist observes her for another 30 minutes and the blood glucose is 110 mg/dL. If at all possible, the prosthodontic situation should be stabilized (i.e., re-cement the provisional crowns). Her family member takes her home for a full meal. The patient re-schedules her procedure for one week later.

After discussion with her endocrinologist, she decreases her nighttime insulin dose by one-third for the next dental appointment and tests her blood sugar on awakening and immediately before the procedure. Both tests are in an acceptable range (110–140 mg/dL), she does not take her morning glimepiride, and the procedure is completed without incident.

| Hypoglycemia | |
|---|---|
| **CAUSES** | Too little food, too much insulin or diabetes medication, or excessive exercise. |
| **ONSET** | Sudden; may progress to insulin shock. |
| **BLOOD SUGAR** | Below 70 mg/dL. Normal range: 70–115 mg/dL. |
| **WHAT CAN YOU DO?** | Drink a cup of orange juice or eat several hard candies. Test blood sugar. Within 30 minutes after symptoms disappear, eat a snack (e.g., sandwich and a glass of milk). Contact physician if symptoms persist. |

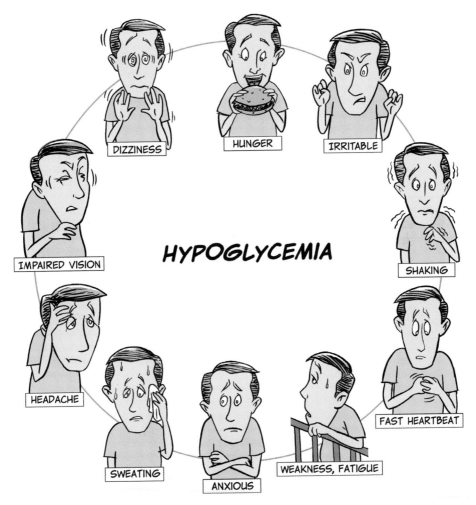

**Figure 1** Symptoms of hypoglycemia. Modified from http://www.lifeclinic.com/focus/diabetes/kids_symptoms.asp (accessed January 3, 2014).

| Hyperglycemia | |
|---|---|
| **CAUSES** | Too much food, too little insulin, illness or stress. |
| **ONSET** | Gradual, may progress to diabetic coma. |
| **BLOOD SUGAR** | Above 200 mg/dL. Normal range: 70–115 mg/dL. |
| **WHAT CAN YOU DO?** | Test blood sugar.<br>If over 250 mg/dL on repeat testing, an acute emergency exists and medical assistance should be sought. |

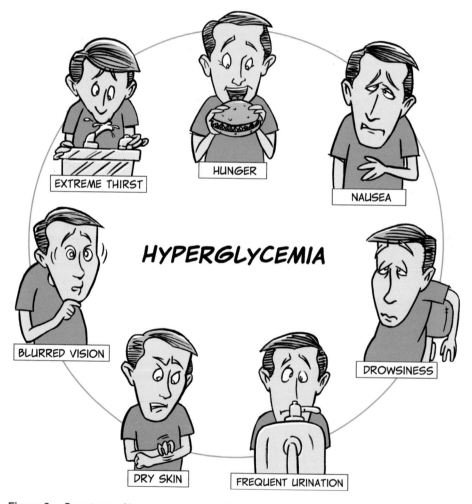

**Figure 2**    Symptoms of hyperglycemia. Modified from http://www.lifeclinic.com/focus/diabetes/kids_symptoms.asp (accessed January 3, 2014).

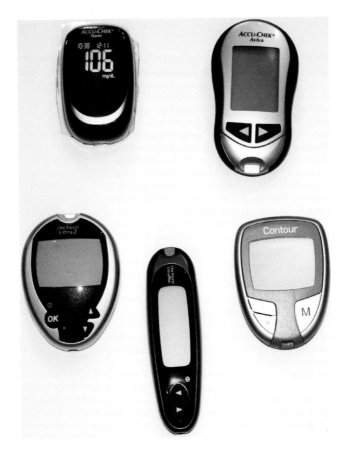

**Figure 3** There are more than 60 blood glucose meters on the U.S. market, and they vary in terms of cost, function, size, memory, and accuracy. The models shown are in common use at the time of this writing. Clockwise from upper left: Accu-check Nano®, Accu-check Aviva®, Bayer Contour®, One-touch Ultra Mini®, and One-touch Ultra®. Continuous glucose meters are also available, and provide a constant, real-time assessment of the blood glucose level. These devices are generally used as part of continuous subcutaneous insulin infusion, and an illustration is provided in Figure 1, in Case 1.

To review, the treatment of hypoglycemia should proceed as follows:

- If possible, confirm the diagnosis with blood glucose testing.
- If the blood glucose level is below 70 mg/dL or if you do not have access to a glucose monitor, initiate treatment by having the patient ingest sugar-containing drink or food. If the patient is able to swallow without aspiration, give 4–5 oz of juice or regular soda, glucose tablets, or hard candies.
- If the patient is obtunded, do not treat with oral carbohydrate because there is risk of aspiration. If hypoglycemia is confirmed, and if glucagon is available in the office emergency kit, consider giving the patient subcutaneous or intramuscular injection of this drug. The dose is 1 mg. The lyophilized drug and diluent are packaged

together in a "glucagon emergency kit." Glucagon needs to be reconstituted prior to injection.

• Wait 15 minutes and re-test the glucose. Re-test by having the patient ingest sugar every 15 minutes until the glucose is in the normal range (greater than 70 mg/dL).

---

**Comment**

The best way to treat hypoglycemia is to avoid it.

---

## Treatment of hyperglycemia

Hypoglycemia is far more likely the cause of an acute physiologic reaction in the dental office than is hyperglycemia. Again, knowing the patient's history, including the medications taken, is essential in managing an untoward reaction. If there is uncertainty as to whether the reaction is due to hyperglycemia, and the blood glucose cannot be assessed, treatment should proceed with the assumption that the patient's condition is due to hypoglycemia. If hyperglycemia is present the relatively small amount of added sugar will not add to the problems. Treatment of clinically significant hyperglycemia is best carried out under the supervision of the treating physician. Emergency services should be called (i.e., call 911).

# Case 4

## The patient with diabetes mellitus and xerostomia

*Ira B. Lamster, DDS, MMSc; Nurit Bittner, DDS, MS; and Daniel Lorber, MD*

---

**Case background**

A patient with diabetes presents with a complaint of xerostomia. Oral findings include recurrent caries and denture stomatitis. The xerostomia persists, making retention of the maxillary complete denture a problem.

---

A 67-year-old male presented with the chief complaint, "My top partial denture bothers me and the teeth on my top right hurt." The patient noticed some bleeding when brushing. He also mentioned that his mouth was feeling dry. The patient has not been to the dentist in the past three years.

## Medical history

The patient is 5′ 6″ tall and he weighs 185 pounds. He states that he has no allergies. The patient was diagnosed with type 2 diabetes mellitus eight years ago. At that time his HbA1c was 9.5%. He was given a course of treatment consisting of lifestyle changes (exercise and diet control) and oral medications (metformin 1,000 mg bid and glimepiride 2 mg qd). He has minimal follow-up with his primary care physician and does not see an endocrinologist.

With questioning, he notes paresthesia of his feet ("It feels like I am walking on clouds") and recently fractured his wrist with minimal trauma. The orthopedist noted bone loss on his examination and recommend a test for bone density, which has not yet been performed.

His last medical visit was three months ago, revealing an HbA1c of 9.1%. His primary care physician referred him to an endocrinologist; the appointment is pending.

The patient does not smoke cigarettes, and denies any history of alcohol abuse. He has not used recreational drugs for the past 20 years.

---

*Diabetes Mellitus and Oral Health: An Interprofessional Approach*, First Edition. Edited by Ira B. Lamster.
© 2014 John Wiley & Sons, Inc. Published 2014 by John Wiley & Sons, Inc.

# Dental history and history of the current problem

All of the patient's restorations, including the porcelain fused to metal splinted crowns on the maxillary premolars and the single crowns on the maxillary first molars, were delivered more than seven years ago, in conjunction with the maxillary and mandibular removable partial dentures.

The last dental visit was three years ago. At that time the patient's current maxillary removable partial denture was repaired as tooth #9 was added to the denture when the natural tooth fractured (Figure 1).

The muscles of mastication and facial expression were all within normal limits. The temporomandibular joint was also within normal limits. The skin around the lips appeared dry and flaky. Areas of the tongue, floor of the mouth, hard and soft palate, and buccal mucosa had an erythematous appearance. A screening for oral cancer was negative.

Moderate plaque and subgingival calculus deposits were observed; moderate to severe gingival inflammation was present. The mouth appeared dry, with minimal saliva. Probing depths ranged from 2 mm to 10 mm, with pronounced bleeding on probing. The maxillary right first molar and the mandibular left central incisor had grade three mobility. Furcation involvement was also noted on the maxillary right first molar. In some areas the papillae were absent, and more commonly hyperplasia and severe inflammation were noted (Figures 2 and 3). Recurrent caries were noted for many teeth. The patient claims to brush his teeth twice a day but he does not use dental floss.

All maxillary porcelain fused to metal crowns (#3, 4, 5, 12, 13, and 14) demonstrated recurrent caries. The root tip of tooth #9 was still present, with coronal decay. Teeth #21, 28, and 32 presented with defective amalgam restorations with recurrent caries. Tooth #27 presented with a defective porcelain fused to metal crown, and recurrent caries.

Pulp testing was completed for the maxillary right side because the patient complained of pain. It was determined that teeth #3 and 4 had irreversible pulpitis.

Although the patient was partially edentulous and an occlusal classification could not be made, with his current removable partial denture the patient showed an Angle's Class III occlusal scheme, which is related to the patient's maxillo-mandibular ridge relationship. No interferences were observed on excursive movements.

Full mouth series and panoramic radiographs were taken. The lamina dura was visible. Radiographic evaluation revealed minimum generalized horizontal bone loss. Teeth #9 and 13 had endodontic treatment, both demonstrating a periapical radiolucency.

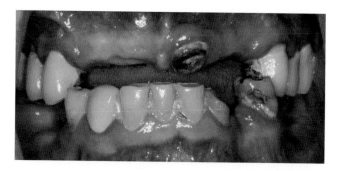

**Figure 1**   Maximum intercuspation, anterior view.

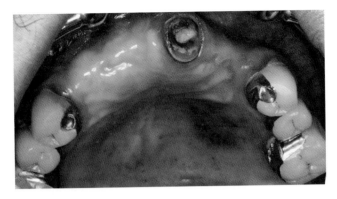

**Figure 2**  Maxillary occlusal view.

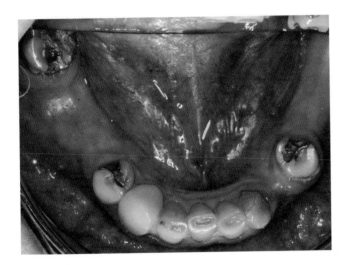

**Figure 3**  Mandibular occlusal view.

Teeth #3, 4, 5, 12, 13, 14, 21, 27, 28, and 31 presented with recurrent decay. The recurrent decay was more advanced on teeth #3, 4, 5, 12, 13, and 14, with both coronal and subgingival (root) involvement.

The following problem list was compiled after review of the history and clinical and radiographic data:

1 Generalized gingivitis.
2 Denture stomatitis.
3 Xerostomia.
4 Periapical lesion associated with teeth #9 and 13.
5 Irreversible pulpitis on teeth #3 and 4.
6 Recurrent caries/root caries on teeth #3, 4, 5, 12, 13, 14, 21, 27, 28, and 31.
7 Class III occlusion.

Based on the patient's medical history of poorly controlled type 2 diabetes mellitus and the current dental findings including xerostomia, papillary hyperplasia, and denture stomatitis, it was decided to evaluate the erythematous lesion on the patient's palate for *Candida albicans* infection.

Infection with *Candida* was confirmed via culture and microscopic evaluation of a tissue swab. The patient was treated with Nystatin suspension and was instructed to soak his current removable partial dentures in the Nystatin suspension overnight as well to eliminate fungus colonization of the denture. The xerostomia was believed to be a contributory factor to the fungal infection.

The patient's metabolic control remained poor on the current drug regimen. This was changed, and the patient was placed on a combination of long-acting insulin (detemir 40 units hs) with metformin (1,000 mg bid) and sitagliptin (100 mg qd) during the day.

## Treatment plan

The initial dental treatment plan consisted of reinforcement of the oral hygiene instructions, treatment for candidiasis, and palliative treatment for the xerostomia using rinses and lozenges and sipping water frequently. A full mouth scaling and root planning followed the initial patient education. Furthermore, the patient was urged to follow up with the endocrinologist because successful treatment of his dental problems depended upon achieving adequate metabolic control.

Due to the advanced recurrent and root caries affecting all remaining maxillary teeth, which was in close proximity to the pulp, the prognosis for all remaining maxillary teeth was poor and extraction was recommended (#3, 4, 5, 9, 12, 13, and 14).

Because the retention of the maxillary denture was a concern due to the patient's xerostomia, the possibility of a maxillary implant retained overdenture was discussed with the patient. Restoration with implants depended on the level of metabolic control, which has proven to be a challenge.

The restorative treatment plan for the mandibular arch consisted of a fixed partial denture on teeth #21– 23 and single porcelain fused to metal survey crowns on teeth #27, 28, and 31. A metal-based mandibular removable partial denture will be fabricated.

Upon completion of the prosthodontic treatment the patient will be placed on a frequent recall schedule (every three to four months). A restorative follow-up will be recommended as well to monitor recurrent caries and root caries on the mandibular restorations. Due to the patient's history and poor metabolic control, topical fluoride treatment will be part of the follow-up plan.

During the next few months, metabolic management of the diabetes was improved with an HbA1c of 6.9%. Considering the improved metabolic control, after discussion with the dentist, the endocrinologist felt that the comprehensive treatment plan could begin.

## Treatment

After the denture stomatitis was resolved (following treatment for *Candida* infection and improvement in metabolic control), and the initial phase of scaling and root planing, the restorative treatment began. The restorative treatment consisted first of fabrication of a maxillary immediate complete denture. All remaining maxillary teeth were extracted and the maxillary immediate complete denture was delivered with a tissue conditioner for the first week. The oral surgery was uneventful, but healing of the extraction sites was delayed. The tissue conditioner was replaced with a soft reline material that was changed periodically as deemed necessary by evaluation of the changes of the soft tissue, and to improve retention.

After healing of the maxillary extractions and after the immediate denture was completely adjusted and a final reline completed, the patient continued to complain of poor denture retention and difficulty in adapting to the complete denture due to mouth dryness and persistent mucosal irritation. An assessment of salivary function revealed increased flow compared to the initial assessment, but the amount of saliva was still below normal.

---

### Comment

Chronic hyperglycemia impairs healing and leukocyte function, thus increasing the risk of post-procedure complications. In this case there are no clear guidelines for use of post-operative antibiotics. Furthermore, although there are no absolute thresholds for diabetes control before dental implant surgery, the general recommendation of the American Diabetes Association is that the target HbA1c for patients should be as close to normal as possible without significant hypoglycemia. The level of control may be intensified for the otherwise healthy younger patient and less aggressive for the older patient with established diabetic sequelae or significant comorbidities.

---

Implant surgery was completed with six implants placed in the maxilla. The soft tissue was sutured to completely cover the implants. The maxillary denture was adjusted as necessary. During the four-month healing time after implant surgery, the patient was seen monthly for denture adjustments. He also maintained close follow-up with his physician to monitor his diabetes.

The restorative treatment for the mandibular arch was completed during the healing period for the maxillary implants. The treatment for the mandibular arch was removal of recurrent caries on teeth #21, 23, 27, 28, and 31. Endodontic treatment was performed on teeth #23 and 27 due to the extent of the carious lesions.

A porcelain fused to metal fixed partial denture was fabricated and inserted from tooth #21 to tooth #23. Porcelain fused to metal survey crowns were fabricated and inserted on teeth #27, 28, and 31. Lastly, a metal-based removable partial denture was fabricated and inserted for the mandibular arch with rest seats on teeth #21, 23, 27, 28, and 31. For the mandibular arch, it was important to reduce the time that the patient was in provisional restorations to avoid recurrent caries.

After second-stage surgery, the maxillary implant healing abutments were replaced with stud attachments (locator abutments) and a maxillary implant retained overdenture was fabricated and inserted, meeting the patient's esthetic and functional requirements with a bilateral balance occlusal scheme.

The patient was placed in a three-month periodontal recall program, which included full periodontal evaluation and scaling.

Due to the xerostomia and high caries rate at original presentation, a close recall program for caries risk was recommended. Also, mandibular trays were provided to the patient for topical fluoride delivery every night before bed.

The importance of maintaining the metabolic control of the patient's diabetes was emphasized to ensure a good long-term prognosis of the dental rehabilitation.

## Discussion

The importance of interdisciplinary treatment for the patient with diabetes mellitus is illustrated by this case. Based on the oral findings, dentists can help identify a person with poorly controlled diabetes mellitus. Conversely, as the patient's physician helped improve metabolic management, the dental treatment plan was modified to acknowledge this improvement.

Xerostomia is a recognized oral complication of diabetes mellitus [1–3]. Persistent xerostomia is related to other intraoral disorders, including increased root caries and candidiasis (Chapter 8).

This case illustrates how devastating xerostomia can be for the dentition. Caries control should be the emphasis of the preventive regimen, but reduction of xerostomia is an important determinant of the success of dental treatment.

Xerostomia is associated with dissatisfaction with removable dentures [4]. For restorative dentists the greatest obstacle is increasing the retention of the dentures for these patients. For some patients the only way to increase retention is the use of implants as part of an overdenture.

There are several approaches that should be considered when treating the patient with diabetes and xerostomia. The first is to improve metabolic control and see if the xerostomia improves. Local measures include application of fluoride varnishes to prevent additional carious lesions, rinsing with artificial saliva, and the use of sugar-free lozenges to increase salivary flow.

Another approach to reducing the symptoms of xerostomia for the edentulous patient with a complete denture is to incorporate a salivary reservoir into the removable appliance. Several salivary substitutes have been suggested for this use and a number of techniques have been proposed for fabrication of the reservoirs. These include a two-part denture design, addition of a soft liner, or fabrication of the prosthesis with a flexible acrylic (Valplast®; [5]).

The reservoir provides a small amount of saliva substitute, primarily during mastication. Good success has been reported when these techniques are used to improve denture retention for the xerostomic patient [6].

---

**Comment**

It is particularly important for physicians who care for patients with diabetes mellitus to ask them about their oral health, including intraoral symptoms and frequency of dental visits.

---

## References

1. Busato IM, Ignácio SA, Brancher JA, Moysés ST, Azevedo-Alanis LR. Impact of clinical status and salivary conditions on xerostomia and oral health-related quality of life of adolescents with type 1 diabetes mellitus. *Community Dent Oral Epidemiol* 2012 Feb; 40(1):62–9.
2. Moore PA, Guggenheimer J, Etzel KR, Weyant RJ, Orchard T. Type 1 diabetes mellitus, xerostomia, and salivary flow rates. *Oral Surg Oral Med Oral Pathol Oral Radiol Endod* 2001 Sep; 92(3):281-91.

3. Khovidhunkit SO, Suwantuntula T, Thaweboon S, Mitrirattanakul S, Chomkhakhai U, Khovidhunkit W. Xerostomia, hyposalivation, and oral microbiota in type 2 diabetic patients: a preliminary study. *J Med Assoc Thai* 2009 Sep; 92(9):1220–8.
4. Ikebe K, Morii K, Kashiwagi J, Nokubi T, Ettinger RL. Impact of dry mouth on oral symptoms and function in removable denture wearers in Japan. *Oral Surg Oral Med Oral Pathol Oral Radiol Endod* 2005 June; 99(6):704–10.
5. Sinclair GF, Frost PM, Walter JD. New design for an artificial saliva reservoir for the mandibular complete denture. *J Prosthet Dent* 1996 Mar; 75(3):276–80.
6. Frost PM, Gardner RM, Price AR, Sinclair GF. A preliminary assessment of intra-oral lubricating systems for dry mouth patients. *Gerodontology* 1997 July; 14(1):54–8.

# Case 5

# A patient diagnosed with diabetes mellitus after comprehensive prosthodontic rehabilitation

*Ira B. Lamster, DDS, MMSc; Nurit Bittner, DDS, MS; and Daniel Lorber, MD*

---

**Case background**

A patient who was restored with implants and fixed partial dentures three years ago now presents to the dental office with significant dental problems. Recently diagnosed with diabetes mellitus, the history suggests the metabolic syndrome was present before the development of diabetes mellitus.

---

A 62-year-old male presented with the chief complaint, "I want a check-up. I had a great deal of dental work three years ago, and now everything is coming apart."

He began to notice his teeth were shifting and his crowns were becoming loose about six months ago. The patient did not have any regular dental follow-up in the past three years. Three months ago he had an acute dental emergency, and a number of teeth were extracted.

## Medical history

The patient was diagnosed with type 2 diabetes mellitus six months ago. At that time his HbA1c was 9.8%. He was given a course of treatment consisting of lifestyle changes (exercise and diet control) and metformin. He was also diagnosed with high blood pressure, with an initial blood pressure of 160/100 mmHg. He is taking lisiniopril and hydrochlorthiazide for his blood pressure. He also takes atorvastatin (Lipitor® 10 mg daily) for elevated cholesterol, but is otherwise well. At this time his HbA1c is 7.6%, representing improved metabolic control.

The dentist reviewed the patient's history, and discussed the patient's status with the treating physician. It was suggested that prior to the diagnosis of diabetes, the metabolic syndrome likely was present at the time of the prosthodontic rehabilitation three years ago.

The patient has smoked eight cigarettes a day for the past 25 years (10 pack years). He denies recreational drug use. He drinks alcohol socially (one glass of wine/day).

---

## Dental history and history of the current problem

The mandibular anterior implant-supported fixed partial denture and the right maxillary first and second molar implant-supported crowns were completed six years ago. Ceramic crowns for the maxillary incisors were completed three years ago (Figures 1 and 2).

The last dental visit was three months ago. The patient did not have a regular dentist and went to a hospital dental clinic for emergency care. The maxillary lateral incisors and maxillary left first molar were extracted due to infection and advanced alveolar bone loss.

There were no significant findings on the extraoral examination. Muscles of mastication and facial expression were all within normal limits. The function of the temporomandibular joints was within normal limits. The intraoral examination of the soft tissues, including the tongue, floor of the mouth, hard and soft palate and buccal mucosa, did not reveal any abnormalities. The oral cancer screen was negative. The patient was partially edentulous,

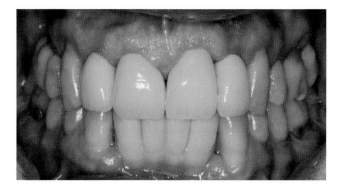

**Figure 1**    Maximum intercuspation, anterior view (after initial prosthodontic rehabilitation).

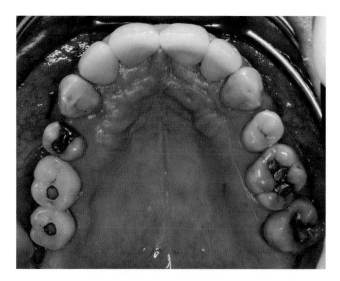

**Figure 2**    Maxillary occlusal view (after initial prosthodontic rehabilitation).

missing teeth #1, 2, 3, 5, 7, 10, 12, 14, 16, 17, 23, 24, 25, 26, and 32. Light plaque and calculus accumulations were present. The gingiva was fibrotic and demonstrated moderate inflammation. Two weeks after an initial scaling and root planning session, slight inflammation remained, generalized 3–4 mm probing depths, with some localized areas of 5 mm or greater, with bleeding on probing (Figures 3 and 4).

The maxillary central incisors presented with grade-two mobility. The maxillary left second premolar and the mandibular first molars demonstrated class 2 furcation involvement. No carious lesions were observed. The canine relationship was Class I Angle's classification. The occlusal scheme observed was anterior guidance in protrusion and canine guidance on lateral movements. There were no interferences observed on any of the excursive movements. The maxillary central incisors demonstrated fremitus.

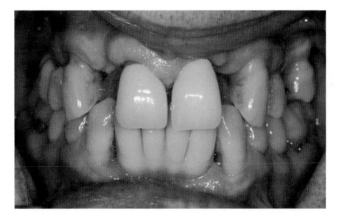

**Figure 3**  Maximum intercuspation, anterior view (current presentation).

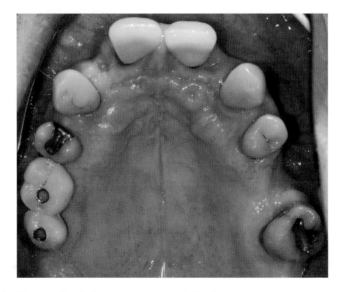

**Figure 4**  Maxillary occlusal view (current presentation).

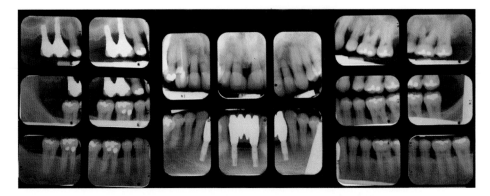

**Figure 5**   Full mouth series of radiographs (after initial prosthodontic rehabilitation).

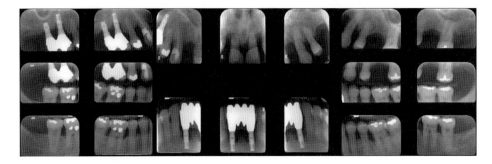

**Figure 6**   Full mouth series of radiographs (current presentation).

Full-mouth series of radiographs were taken. Radiographic evaluation revealed generalized horizontal bone loss. The implants placed in the mandibular lateral incisors and the maxillary right first and second molar sites demonstrated bone loss of more than 2 mm, with a trough-like appearance.

Radiographs were obtained from three years ago, taken after the completion of care. Radiographs were taken after the recent extractions and demonstrated progression of bone loss in the three-year period (Figures 5 and 6).

After evaluation of the medical and dental history and clinical and radiographic findings, the following problems list was identified:

1  Severe chronic periodontitis, second to diabetes mellitus.
2  Peri-implantitis associated with implants in sites #3, 4, 23, 26.
3  Partial edentulism.

## Treatment plan

The initial dental treatment plan consisted of full mouth scaling and root planing. Based on the gingival response, pocket reduction periodontal surgery may be necessary in the mandibular posterior sextants.

Extractions were suggested due to the poor periodontal prognosis of the maxillary central incisors. At this time, a maxillary removable partial denture was the best prosthodontic option. This denture will ensure that the remaining teeth are maintained as long as possible until acceptable metabolic control, and control of blood pressure, are demonstrated over a longer period of time. If good metabolic control is not maintained, this will be the final restoration. A removable denture will facilitate the transition to a complete denture if other teeth in the maxillary arch display continued bone loss and require extraction. An alternate treatment plan was proposed if the patient demonstrates good metabolic control over an extended period of time (six months). This would involve implant placement in the maxillary lateral incisors and maxillary left first molar sites. The final prosthesis will be a porcelain fused to metal implant-supported fixed partial denture for the maxillary incisors with the central incisors as pontics and a single implant crown on the maxillary left first molar.

Upon completion of the prosthodontic treatment the patient will be closely followed for periodontal maintenance, including scaling and root planning every three months.

## Treatment

After initial scaling and root planing, the maxillary central incisors were extracted, and a maxillary immediate interim removable partial denture was inserted.

After re-evaluation of the periodontal condition following scaling and root planning, it was decided that periodontal surgery for pocket reduction was necessary in the mandibular posterior areas. Periodontal surgery would ideally be performed if the patient demonstrates adequate metabolic control. At this time metabolic control is improved (HbA1c=7.9%). Periodontal surgery was performed as open debridement for root access. Pocket elimination surgery was not attempted, because it was felt that there was a risk of poor wound healing. It is also conceivable that the existing periodontal disease was contributing to the less than ideal metabolic control. The areas demonstrating peri-implantitis were treated with open surgical debridement and debridement of the implant surface with adjunctive use of antibiotics.

During the three-month healing time after the last periodontal surgery, the patient was seen by his physician to monitor the metabolic status. His last medical evaluation revealed that the patient continued smoking six cigarettes a day, his blood pressure was 135/90 mmHg, and his HbA1c was 8.1% on metformin alone. Following recommendation from his physician, due to the poor metabolic control heightened by the patient's high blood pressure, implant surgery was postponed. After discussion with the patient, his physician recommended addition of a GLP-1 agonist to his metabolic management. The GLP-1 agonists are injectable medications given twice daily (Byetta®), once daily (Victoza®), or once weekly (Bydureon®). GLP-1 agonists enhance insulin secretion, suppress glucagon, slow gastric emptying, and enhance satiety. The patient lost 8 lbs and his HbA1c decreased to 6.9%.

The interim maxillary partial denture that was delivered was fabricated with a metal base and rest seats on #4, 6, 11, 13, and 15.

## Discussion

As evidenced by a detailed history, it was suggested that this patient had "metabolic syndrome" at the time of initial presentation three years ago. The metabolic syndrome is a complex of insulin resistance, abdominal obesity, hypertension, dyslipidemia (high triglycerides and low HDL cholesterol), and elevated fasting glucose (greater than 100 mg/dL). The metabolic syndrome is associated with a significantly increased risk of atherosclerotic cardiovascular disease and type 2 diabetes mellitus (Table 1 [1]). Data from the NHANES 2003–2006 revealed that more than one-third of American adults have the metabolic syndrome [2]. A systematic review found a significant association between periodontal disease and the presence of the metabolic syndrome [3].

The Diabetes Prevention Program (DPP) investigated the effects of lifestyle change or metformin on incidence of type 2 diabetes in a high risk cohort. Approximately 53% of the participants in the Diabetes Prevention Program had metabolic syndrome. Lifestyle change in the DPP consisted of intensive coaching, with the aim of achieving and maintaining at least 7% weight reduction by diet and at least 150 minutes a week of moderate exercise [4].

Lifestyle change resulted in a 58% reduction in development of type 2 diabetes over a 2.8-year follow-up. Metformin was somewhat less effective, resulting in a 31% reduction in diabetes incidence. Lifestyle change reduced the prevalence of metabolic syndrome by one-third. Metformin, although decreasing the incidence of new diabetes mellitus, had no impact on the prevalence of metabolic syndrome.

This case illustrates the importance of complete patient evaluation prior to beginning dental care. It also illustrates the importance of close follow-up after prosthodontic care. In this case the re-established masticatory function was adversely affected by the medical status of the patient, specifically the onset of the diabetes mellitus, and the loss of support about teeth and implants.

Diabetes mellitus adversely affects the severity of periodontitis, and poor periodontal health may also adversely influence metabolic control [5]. Furthermore, the effect of poor metabolic control on dental implant outcomes is controversial [6], as there is evidence of delayed healing of implants when the HbA1c level is above 8% [7]. In addition, medical

**Table 1**    Criteria for the diagnosis of metabolic syndrome (National Cholesterol Education Program Adult Treatment Panel III).

| **Any three of the following:** |
| --- |
| Waist circumference > 102 cm (men); 88 cm (women) |
| Triglycerides ≥ 150 mg/dL |
| HDL cholesterol < 40 mg/dl (men); < 50 mg/dL (women) |
| BP ≥ 130/85 |
| Fasting glucose ≥ 100 mg/dL |

Grundy SM, Brewer HB Jr., Cleeman JI, Smith SC Jr., Lenfant C; American Heart Association: National Heart, Lung, and Blood Institute. Definition of metabolic syndrome: report of the National Heart, Lung, and Blood Institute/American Heart Association conference on scientific issues related to definition. *Circulation*, 2004 Jan 27; 109(3):433–8.

complications of diabetes mellitus occur more commonly when metabolic control is poor. If the HbA1c level is above 8–8.5% the diabetes is considered poorly controlled and a more conservative restorative approach may be advisable.

In patients with poorly controlled diabetes, the dental restorative treatment should focus on maintaining the remaining teeth for as long as possible because treatment with implants is invasive, time consuming, and expensive. Fixed partial dentures to replace the missing teeth is the treatment of choice for small edentulous areas. For large edentulous areas, removable partial dentures are indicated.

In this case, the decision was made to retain the implants that had previously been placed and restored, but to treat the peri-implantitis. A conservative approach was chosen. A systematic review [8] has shown this approach to be an effective means of reducing clinical signs of inflammation and halting the progression of bone loss about the implants.

However, when a removable complete or partial denture is necessary for poorly controlled diabetic patients, a closer follow-up schedule should be reinforced, which may include assessment of salivary flow, and if required, treatment of xerostomia with rinses and special chewing gums [9]. Also, to improve retention of the dentures, periodic relining of the prosthesis may be necessary; the patient should be made aware of the importance of a frequent recall schedule to monitor all possible complications.

These patients should also be periodically evaluated for carious lesions because an elevated prevalence of root caries in type 2 diabetic patients has been reported [10]. To prevent caries, a topical fluoride supplement protocol (fluoride rinse and fluoride varnish) should be considered [11].

---

**Comment**

Patients who develop poorly controlled diabetes mellitus are at increased risk for oral complications, and this can be a particular challenge when the patient has received a major prosthodontic rehabilitation.

---

# References

1. Grundy SM, Brewer HB Jr., Cleeman JI, Smith SC Jr., Lenfant C; American Heart Association: National Heart, Lung, and Blood Institute. Definition of metabolic syndrome: report of the National Heart, Lung, and Blood Institute/American Heart Association conference on scientific issues related to definition. *Circulation.* 2004 Jan 27; 109(3):433–8.
2. Ervin RB. Prevalence of metabolic syndrome among adults 20 years of age and over by sex, age, race and ethnicity, and body mass index. United States, 2003–2006. National health statistic reports, no. 13. Hyattsville, MD: National Center for Health Statistics, 2009.
3. Nibali L, Tatarakis N, Needleman I, Tu YK, D'Aiuto F, Rizzo M, Donos N. Association between metabolic syndrome and periodontitis: a systematic review and meta-analysis. *J Clin Endocrinol Metab.* 2013 Mar; 98(3):913–20.
4. Knowler WC, Barrett-Connor E, Fowler SE, Hamman RF, Lachin JM, Walker EA, et al. Diabetes Prevention Program Research Group. Reduction in the incidence of type 2 diabetes with lifestyle intervention or metformin. *N Engl J Med.* 2002 Feb 7; 346(6):393–403.
5. Preshaw PM, Alba AL, Herrera D, Jepsen S, Konstantinidis A, Makrilakis K, Taylor R. Periodontitis and diabetes: a two-way relationship. *Diabetologia* 2012 Jan; 55(1):21–31.

6.  Marchand F, Raskin A, Dionnes-Hornes A, Barry T, Dubois N, Valéro R, et al. Dental implants and diabetes: conditions for success. *Diabetes Metab.* 2012 Feb; 38(1):14–9.

7.  Oates TW, Dowell S, Robinson M, McMahan CA. Glycemic control and implant stabilization in type 2 diabetes mellitus. *J Dent Res.* 2009 Apr; 88(4):367–71.

8.  Renvert S, Polyzois I, Claffey N. Surgical therapy for the control of peri-implantitis. *Clin Oral Implants Res.* 2012 Oct; 23 (Suppl 6):84–94.

9.  Ettinger RL. Xerostomia—a complication of ageing. *Aust Dent J.* 1981 Dec; 26(6):365–71.

10. Hintao J, Teanpaisan R, Chongsuvivatwong V, Dahlen G, Rattarasarn C. Root surface and coronal caries in adults with type 2 diabetes mellitus. *Community Dent Oral Epidemiol.* 2007 Aug; 35(4):302–9.

11. Tan HP, Lo EC, Dyson JE, Luo Y, Corbet EF. A randomized trial on root caries prevention in elders. *J Dent Res.* 2010 Oct; 89(10):1086–90.

# Case 6

# Prosthodontic treatment for the newly diagnosed patient with type 2 diabetes mellitus

*Ira B. Lamster, DDS, MMSc; Nurit Bittner, DDS, MS; and Daniel Lorber, MD*

---

**Case background**

A patient is seen in the dental office for a consult. Based on the intraoral findings at the initial examination, diabetes mellitus is suspected and the patient is referred to a physician for evaluation.

---

A 31-year-old female presented with the chief complaint, "I need braces; my teeth have shifted."

The patient noticed her teeth shifting about two years ago. She was always interested in orthodontic treatment to address the mandibular crowding and the palatal position of tooth #7, but postponed treatment for financial issues. She is now ready to begin.

The patient noticed some bleeding when brushing, but did not complain of pain or any other symptoms associated with her mouth.

She claimed to brush her teeth twice a day, but admitted to flossing "rarely."

## Medical history

The patient is 5′1″ tall and she weighs 165 pounds. She has a history of asthma; however, the last episode was more than 19 years ago. She does not take any regular medications, and does not have any allergies. She does not see a physician regularly. She reported, "I'm fine except for my gums." Her father died at age 55 of a "massive heart attack." His height was 5′9″ and weight was 195 lbs with increased abdominal obesity. Her mother is 63 years old and has "mild" diabetes and arthritis. On questioning by the dentist, the patient reveals that she was told her "sugar level was borderline" several years ago. At that time, she went on a diet, lost 15 lbs, and was then told that her blood sugar was "OK." She has regained the weight that was lost. Based on the patient's height and weight, her body mass index (BMI) is 31.2, which is considered obese (to calculate and classify BMI, go to http://nhlbisupport.com/bmi/bminojs.htm).

---

*Diabetes Mellitus and Oral Health: An Interprofessional Approach*, First Edition. Edited by Ira B. Lamster.
© 2014 John Wiley & Sons, Inc. Published 2014 by John Wiley & Sons, Inc.

## Dental history and history of the current problem

The last dental visit was six months ago for a "cleaning" in another office. The patient has had only intermittent dental care throughout her lifetime. At the initial examination, there were no significant extraoral findings. Muscles of mastication and facial expression were all within normal limits. The temporomandibular joint was also within normal limits. The intraoral examination did not reveal any abnormalities of the tongue, floor of the mouth, hard and soft palate, and buccal mucosa. The oral cancer screening was negative. The buccal mucosa in the anterior region appeared erythematous. The patient is partially edentulous; she is missing all third molars and the mandibular second molars (Figure 1).

Moderate plaque and subgingival calculus deposits were observed; moderate to severe gingival inflammation was present. Probing depths ranged from 2 mm to 10 mm, with heavy bleeding on probing. In some areas the papillae were absent, and more commonly hyperplasia and severe inflammation were noted (Figures 2 and 3).

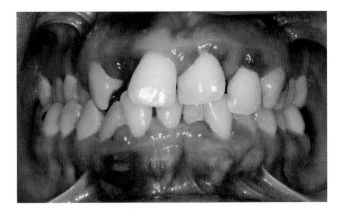

**Figure 1**    Maximum intercuspation, anterior view.

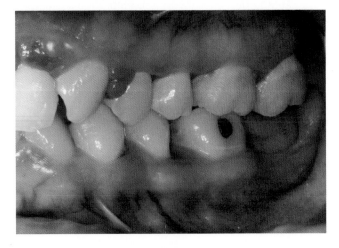

**Figure 2**    Maximum intercuspation, left lateral view.

The maxillary right second molar and the mandibular left central incisor had grade three mobility. Furcation involvement was also noted on the maxillary right second molar. No carious lesions were observed (Figures 4 and 5).

The patient has Class I Angle's classification on her first molars and canines, with right side posterior crossbite. Her maxillary right lateral incisor is palatally positioned, creating a localized anterior crossbite. The patient presents interferences in right working lateral movement on the non-working side with contacts between the premolars. She has group function contacts on laterotrussive movements. No fremitus was detected.

Full mouth series and panoramic radiographs were taken (Figures 6 and 7). Radiographic evaluation revealed generalized horizontal bone loss with localized vertical bone loss about the maxillary lateral incisors. The mandibular left central incisor demonstrated a periapical radiolucency.

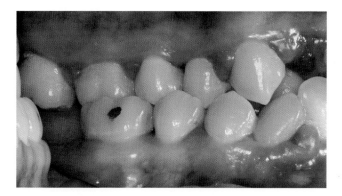

**Figure 3**  Maximum intercuspation, right lateral view.

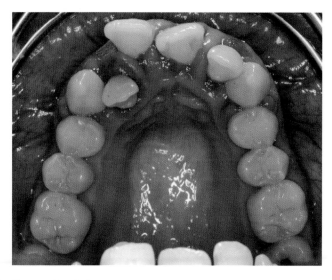

**Figure 4**  Maxillary occlusal view.

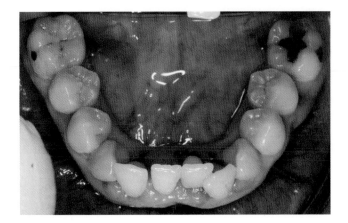

**Figure 5**   Mandibular occlusal view.

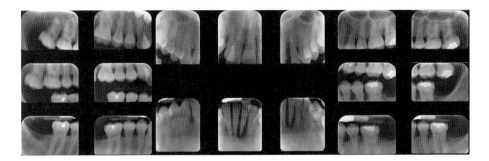

**Figure 6**   Full mouth series of radiographs.

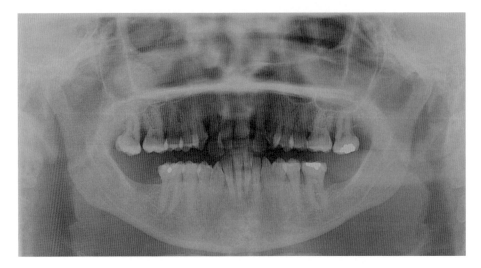

**Figure 7**   Panoramic radiograph.

The following problems list was compiled after review of the history and clinical and radiographic data:

1 Generalized moderate chronic periodontitis, with areas of severe inflammation.
2 Mucosal erythema.
3 Peri-apical lesion associated with the mandibular left central incisor.
4 Maloclusion with anterior and posterior crossbites.

Due to the nature of the gingival inflammation and erythematous mucosal lesions suggestive of *Candida albicans* infection, as well as her BMI, and since the patient's last medical examination was more than one year ago, it was recommended to the patient to have a full medical evaluation, including assessment of her risk for diabetes mellitus.

---

**Comment**

This patient has several risk factors for diabetes, including abdominal obesity, a parent with type 2 diabetes, and hypertension. A diabetes-focused history taken at the initial dental examination includes a history of hypertension, dyslipidemia, gestational diabetes, a baby over 9 lbs at birth, and first degree relative(s) with diabetes or heart disease. Another approach is asking the patient to complete a simple risk test from the American Diabetes Association (http:/www.diabetes.org/diabetes-basics/prevention/diabetes-risk-test/).

---

## Treatment plan

The patient realizes that she is at increased risk for diabetes. She then asks her dentist what she should do next. At this point, the dentist has several options:

1 Refer her to a primary physician for further evaluation.
2 Send her to a laboratory for an HbA1c determination and fasting blood glucose.
3 Perform a point-of-care blood glucose and/or HbA1c in the office.

The American Diabetes Association recommends testing to detect type 2 diabetes in adults of any age who are overweight and who have one or more additional risk factors. In those without these risk factors, testing should begin at age 45. To test for diabetes, laboratory determination of HbA1c, fasting plasma glucose, or a glucose tolerance test are appropriate (Table 1). The diagnosis of diabetes carries significant social, economic, and medical implications, and should not be made lightly. Thus, the American Diabetes Association recommends that any positive tests be repeated except in the presence of significant hyperglycemia. Although POC glucose or HbA1c are not sufficiently precise to make the diagnosis of diabetes, a clearly abnormal value on either test indicates the need for referral and complete evaluation.

After discussing the options with this patient, the dentist called the patient's physician who gave her a prescription for a fasting blood glucose and HbA1c determination. The HbA1c was 8.3% and the fasting blood glucose was 157 mg/dL, both indicative of a diagnosis of diabetes mellitus. She was referred back to the primary internist, who confirmed the diagnosis, began treatment with metformin, and referred her to a diabetes education program.

The patient returns for further dental care in four months. She has lost 17 lbs and her HbA1c is now 6.9%

The American Diabetes Association recommends that initial treatment for people with type 2 diabetes is lifestyle change with calorie restriction and increased physical activity, combined with metformin [1]. If monotherapy does not result in the desired level of glycemic control, additional medication is considered. The choice of a second medication depends upon consideration of efficacy and side effects (Table 2).

**Table 1**   Diagnostic criteria for diabetes mellitus in non-pregnant adults.

| |
|---|
| HbA1c ≥ 6.5%. The test should be performed in a laboratory using a method that is NGSP certified and standardized to the DCCT assay.*<br>OR<br>FPG ≥ 126 mg/dL (7.0 mmol/L). Fasting is defined as no caloric intake for at least 8h.*<br>OR<br>2-h plasma glucose ≥ 200 mg/dL (11.1 mmol/L) during an OGTT. The test should be performed as described by the WHO, using a gulcose load containing the equivalent of 75 g anhydrous  gulcose dissolved in water.*<br>OR<br>In a patient with classic symptoms of hyperglycemia or hyperglycemic crisis, a random plasma gulcose ≥ 200 mg/dL (11.1 mmol/L). |

*In the absence of unequivocal hyperglycemia, result should be confirmed by repeat testing.
American Diabetes Association. Standards of medical care in diabetes—2013. *Diab Care* 2013 Jan; 36 (Suppl 1): S11-S66.

**Table 2**   American Diabetes Association metabolic goals for adults with type 2 diabetes include:

| |
|---|
| • HbA1C <7%<br>• Pre-prandial glucose 70–130 mg/dL<br>• Peak postprandial glucose < 180 mg/dL<br><br>These goals should be individualized based on individual patient considerations, including:<br><br>• Duration of diabetes<br>  ○ Patients with long-standing diabetes may not benefit from aggressive glycemic control<br>• Age/life expectancy<br>  ○ Most microvascular complications of diabetes develop after 15–20 years of disease. Thus, elderly patients or those with shorter life expectancy might be appropriate for a less stringent level of glycemic control<br>• Comorbid conditions<br>  ○ Malignancy is more common in people with diabetes and its treatment often makes glycemic control more difficult<br>• Known CVD or advanced microvascular complications (retinopathy, nephropathy, neuropathy)<br>  ○ Although early intervention to improve glycemic control is likely to decrease the risk of later microvascular complications, there are no data to support the regression of existing advanced complications with tighter glycemic control<br>• Hypoglycemia unawareness<br>  ○ Patients with long-standing diabetes, particularly type 1, have decreased adrenergic signals of hypoglycemia and are at greater risk for severe hypoglycemia, including loss of consciousness or seizure |

American Diabetes Association. Standards of medical care in diabetes—2013. *Diab Care* 2013 Jan; 36 (Suppl 1): S11–S66.
*Note*: The American Association of Clinical Endocrinologists (AACE) has developed an alternative approach to initial treatment of type 2 diabetes (https://www.aace.com/files/glycemic-control-algorithm.pdf). The AACE recommends that the initial choice of medications be determined by the baseline HbA1c, with additional medications initiated for patients with higher HbA1c levels. For example, the AACE algorithm would suggest that this patient with an initial HbA1c of 9.1% be started on three oral agents or, if she is symptomatic, AACE would recommend initiating insulin directly.

Both epidemiologic studies and randomized control trials indicate that the long-term neurologic and microvascular complications of diabetes are directly related to glycemic control. The American Diabetes Association recommends that glycemic control should be as close to normal as possible, without hypoglycemia, and modified by other patient-specific factors [1].

The initial treatment plan consisted of full mouth scaling and root planing. Depending on the gingival response, a pocket reduction periodontal surgery may be necessary in some or all quadrants.

Due to the poor periodontal prognosis of tooth #2 and the mandibular and maxillary incisors, extraction was recommended. Implants were considered for teeth #2, 7, 10, 23, and 26. Implant placement was dependent on the level of metabolic control.

The restorative treatment plan presented to the patient consisted of immediate maxillary and mandibular interim removable partial dentures to be provided after the extractions.

After allowing time for implant integration, the implants would be restored with porcelain fused to metal fixed partial dentures from right lateral incisor to left lateral incisor on both the maxillary and mandibular arches, with pontics replacing the central incisors. Tooth #2 will be restored with a single implant and crown.

Upon completion of the prosthodontic treatment the patient will be placed on a close follow-up schedule for periodontal maintenance, including scaling and root planning every three to four months.

## Treatment

When surgical treatment began, the patient's HbA1c level was 6.7%. After an initial phase of scaling and root planing, all maxillary incisors (#7, 8, 9, and 10) were extracted. The granulomatous tissue was removed and was sent to the laboratory for histological examination. The extraction site was sutured before insertion of the maxillary interim removable partial denture (Figure 8). Tooth #2 extraction was completed at this time. The histological evaluation of the granulomatous tissue revealed normal tissues with a severe inflammatory infiltrate. The extraction sites healed uneventfully.

At the immediate follow-up, it was noted that the plaque and calculus accumulations were still abundant (Figure 9). At that point, the patient's diabetes management was considered as acceptable, with an HbA1c of 6.8%. Oral hygiene measures were again reinforced.

Extraction of the mandibular incisors was completed at the following appointment with delivery of the mandibular interim removable partial denture.

At the two-month follow-up after the extractions, it was decided that periodontal surgery for pocket reduction was necessary in all four quadrants. The patient's oral hygiene was significantly improved at this time. Periodontal surgery was completed without any complications and the patient continued to display excellent oral hygiene.

During the three-month healing time after the last periodontal surgery, the patient was seen monthly to monitor her periodontal condition. She also maintained close follow-up with her physician to control her diabetes.

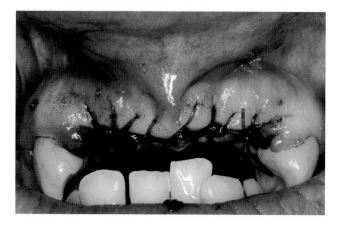

**Figure 8**   Immediately after removal of the maxillary incisors.

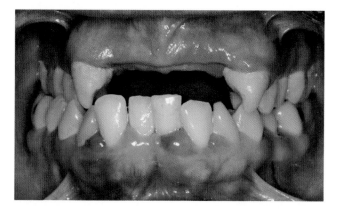

**Figure 9**   Maximum intercuspation, intraoral view, after healing of maxillary anterior extractions.

After communication with the physician and because the patient's HbA1c was 6.8% the previous three months, the physician and dentist agreed that the implant surgery could proceed. Implants were placed in the #2, 7, 10, 23, and 26 locations. After a four-month healing period, the implants were loaded with provisional screw-retained restorations to confirm osseointegration and implant stability as well to contour the soft tissues.

Six months after implant placement the implants were restored with porcelain fused to metal fixed partial dentures. A maxillary night guard was provided to the patient to protect the implant restorations against porcelain fracture.

The patient was placed in a three-month periodontal recall program, which included full periodontal evaluation and scaling. Even though the patient was not felt to be at high risk for caries, she will continue with a six-month recall program with the restorative dentist.

The dentist emphasized to the patient the importance of maintaining good metabolic control of her diabetes to ensure the best possible oral health and health outcomes.

## Discussion

This case demonstrated the important role that the dentist may have in identifying undiagnosed diabetes mellitus. Diabetes mellitus is associated with several intraoral conditions, including increased prevalence of periodontal disease, dental caries, reduced salivary flow, burning mouth syndrome, and *Candida* infection [2]. As illustrated here, it is possible for patients to be seen in the dental office for a chief complaint related directly to diabetes mellitus.

The presence of one or more of these oral conditions may be an indication to assess the risk for diabetes mellitus. In this case, a referral was given to the patient due to the severity of the periodontal disease, the deeply inflamed gingiva, and the appearance of the buccal mucosa, which was thought to be related to a *Candida* lesion. Other identified risk factors included her BMI and family history.

Evidence supports the relationship between diabetes and periodontal diseases as bidirectional; that is, diabetes is associated with increased occurrence and progression of periodontitis, and periodontal infection is associated with poorer glycemic control in people with diabetes [3].

The restorative treatment must also be customized to the patient's needs. Dental implants were a consideration, but a risk factor for implant complications was felt to be the presence of diabetes mellitus, and specifically the poor metabolic control at the initial assessment.

The literature is not clear regarding implant placement in patients with diabetes. Diabetes is not a contraindication for dental implants, as long as the blood glucose level is well controlled [4]. The success rate of implants in diabetic patients with better diabetes control has been reported to be as high as 94.3% [5]. Based on the data, the survival rate of dental implants in controlled diabetic patients is slightly lower than that documented for the general population, but is nonetheless still impressive. The increase in failure rate occurs during the first year following prosthetic loading [6]. The reason for this may be altered bone metabolism [7].

If the patient's diabetes is not well controlled, an alternative restorative approach is a maxillary removable partial denture without the use of dental implants. The dentist and physician must be in close communication regarding the patient's diabetes, representing an ideal example of proper inter-professional practice. The removable partial denture could be considered as an interim restoration. An implant-retained restoration would be fabricated if the patient demonstrates appropriate metabolic control.

Moreover, because the prognosis for teeth #23, 24, and 26 is more favorable than that for the mandibular right central incisor, another plan would include extraction of the mandibular right central incisor, and a resin bonded Maryland bridge would be fabricated to replace #25. The purpose of this approach is to try to maintain the remaining dentition as long as possible. Here, close post-operative monitoring is essential.

The re-establishment of a fully functional masticatory system and the improvement of the masticatory efficiency allow patients to maintain a more balanced diet and therefore proper nutrition. This should also be considered, especially in older patients with diabetes. Data suggest that patients with lower masticatory efficiency tend to be at higher risk for increased body fat, which in turn can be associated with a higher prevalence of type 2 diabetes mellitus [8]. This likely relates to the inability to chew fibrous foods and the need for a soft diet.

Dentists have an important role in establishing normal masticatory function for patients, and maintaining oral health in patients with diabetes mellitus. In addition, they can also play an important role in identifying patients with undiagnosed or poorly managed diabetes. A number of recent studies have suggested that the use of data collected at a dental examination can be used as part of an identification protocol for patients with suspected diabetes mellitus [9, 10]. These studies have suggested that the dental office can be a health care location that actively participates in the management of patients with diabetes mellitus.

# References

1. American Diabetes Association. Standards of medical care in diabetes—2013. *Diab Care* 2013 Jan; 36 (Suppl 1): S11–S66.
2. Lamster IBL, Lalla E, Borgnakke WS, Taylor GW. The relationship between oral health and diabetes mellitus. *J Am Dent Assoc* 2008 Oct; 139 (Suppl): S19–S24.
3. Lalla E, Papapanou PN. Diabetes mellitus and periodontitis: a tale of two common interrelated diseases. *Nat Rev Endocrinol* 2011 June 28; 7(12):738–48.
4. Oates TW, Huynh-Ba G, Vargas A, Alexander P, Feine J. A critical review of diabetes, glycemic control, and dental implant therapy. *Clin Oral Implants Res* 2013 Feb; 24(2):117–27.
5. Balshi TJ, Wolfinger GJ. Dental implants in the diabetic patient: a retrospective study. *Implant Dent* 1999; 8(4):355–9.
6. Fiorellini JP, Chen PK, Nevins M, Nevins ML. A retrospective study of dental implants in diabetic patients. *Int J Periodontics Restorative Dent* 2000 Aug; 20(4):366–73.
7. Retzepi M, Donos N. The effect of diabetes mellitus on osseous healing. *Clin Oral Implants Res* 2010 Jul; 21(7):673–81.
8. Sánchez-Ayala A, Campanha NH, Garcia RC. Relationship between body fat and masticatory function. *J Prosthodont* 2013 Feb; 22(2):120–5.
9. Li S, Williams PL, Douglass CW. Development of a clinical guideline to predict undiagnosed diabetes in dental patients. *J Am Dent Assoc* 2011 Jan; 142(1):28–37.
10. Lalla E, Kunzel C, Burkett S, Cheng B, Lamster IB. Identification of unrecognized diabetes and pre-diabetes in a dental setting. *J Dent Res* 2011 Jul; 90(7):855–60.

# Index